KT-520-178

Contents

Acknowledgements

Contributors to the UK edition

Tracey Edwards, DCR(R)
Senior Radiographer, Morriston Hospital, Abertawe Bro
Morgannwg University Health Board, Swansea, Wales

**Emyr I. Phillips, MSc, MBA, BN, PGCEd, RN, Cert A&E, PGCert
Infection Prevention & Control**
Lead Nurse: Emergency Care & Emergency Planning Morriston
Hospital, Abertawe Bro Morgannwg University Health Board,
Swansea, Wales

Frances Thornton, BA (Hons), MMAA, RMIP
Medical Animator, College of Human & Health Sciences, Swansea
University, Wales

Catherine Williams, Dip N, part 12 BSc (Hons), RNT MSc
Skills tutor College of Human and Health Sciences
Swansea University
Wales, UK

Reviewers of the UK edition

Denise Aspland, RGN, RSCN, DipHE Child Health
Practice Development Nurse Emergency Nursing, Emergency
Department

Amanda Y. Blaber, MSc, BSc, Dip A&E Nursing (ENB 199), RGN
Senior Lecturer, School of Nursing & Midwifery, University of
Brighton

Phil Downing, RN, BSc (Hons), MSc, ATHE
Lead Nurse Emergency Care, Gloucestershire Hospitals NHS
Foundation Trust

Rebecca Hoskins, BSc (Hons), MA, RGN, RN (Child)
Consultant Nurse & Senior Lecturer in Emergency Care,
Emergency Department, Bristol Royal Infirmary, University Bristol
Hospitals NHS Foundation Trust & Department of Nursing &
Midwifery, Health & Life Sciences, University of the West
of England

**Maria Kisiel, RN, BA (Hons) MSc Health Science (Education
Route)**
Head of Department, Adult & Critical Care, Birmingham
City University

Foreword to the UK edition

Emergency departments (EDs) in the UK face an increasing workload due to high level of attendees and increased levels of activities. To cope with this situation, the Department of Health in 2001 implemented a 'reforming emergency care modernisation programme'.

One key innovation that is vital in transforming care delivery in EDs is based around the principle that a decision-maker, who can make an assessment and decide on the appropriate next steps for investigation and treatment, sees a patient first. As such, it's crucial that emergency nurses ensure they have the knowledge and skills to provide the best possible care. *Emergency Nursing Made Incredibly Easy!* will help nurses hone these vital skills. This book covers the basics of triage, such as the evidence-based triage process, and holistic care issues, such as cultural and pain considerations. Subsequent chapters focus on physiological systems, covering shock, trauma and musculoskeletal, cardiac, respiratory, neurological, gastrointestinal, genitourinary, gynaecological and childbirth, maxillofacial and ophthalmic and general environmental emergencies.

Revision of anatomy and physiology of the specified systems is very important to your learning and understanding of the chapters in the book.

The clear language and illustrations will help readers anticipate and assess certain diagnoses, and prevent predictable complications. Recurring topics for each section include how to assess the patient, diagnostic tests that should be done, treatment options and common disorders for each body system. A *Quick quiz* at the end of each chapter tests the reader's knowledge on the information presented.

Humour plays a part to team survival in emergency care. Throughout the book are illustrations of cartoons demonstrating key issues which you'll find valuable. In addition, icons draw your attention to important issues:

Ages and stages – highlight age-related changes and how they affect your patient's health.

Stay on the ball – focuses on critical areas involving possible dangers, risks, complications or contraindications.

Education edge – offers patient-teaching tips.

    Although some EDs function differently and the role of the emergency nurse varies from novice to expert, this book can help emergency nurses learn more about their current practice. It can also help student nurses or nurses from other departments build enough confidence to consider joining this extremely worthwhile specialty. We are proud to introduce to you *Emergency Nursing Made Incredibly Easy* – a wonderful new tool in the challenging but rewarding world of emergency nursing.

    Enjoy!

Mark Edwards, RGN, BSc, tHE, Ddip in Emergency Nursing
Senior emergency nurse tutor/advance practice team coordinator
College of Human & Health Sciences
Swansea University
Wales

Dr Pauline Griffiths, RN, PhD, MSc, BN, PGCE, PG Dip in Health Care Law
Director of pre-qualifying undergraduate studies
College of Human & Health Sciences
Swansea University
Wales

Contributors and consultants to the US edition

Ann White, RN, MSN, CCNS, CEN
Clinical Nurse Specialist
Emergency Services
Department of Advanced Practice Nursing
Duke University Health System
Clinical Associate Faculty
Duke University College of Nursing
Durham, NC

Cynthia Francis Bechtel, RN, MS, CEN, EMT-1
Professor
MassBay Community College
Framingham, MA

Laura M. Criddle, RN, MS, CCNS, CCRN, CEN
Doctoral Student, Nursing
Oregon Health & Science University
Portland, OR

Laurie Donaghy, RN, CEN
Staff Nurse
Frankford Hospital
Philadelphia, PA

Nancy A. Emma, RN, BSN
Officer in Charge
U.S. Army EMS Programs Office
U.S. Army DCMT
Fort Sam Houston, TX

Lisa Kosits, RN, BC, MSN, CCRN, CEN
Clinical In-service Instructor
Montefiore Medical Center
Bronx, NY

Charles Kunkle, PHRN, BSN, CCRN, CEN, CNA
Nurse Manager, Emergency Department
St. Mary Medical Center
Langhorne, PA

Sharon L. Lee, FNP, MS, CCRN, CEN
Faculty
Bryan LGH College of Health Sciences
FNP
Gastroenterology Specialities
Lincoln, NE

Ruthie Robinson, RN, PhD(C), CEN, CCRN, FAEN
Director of the Magnet Program & Clinical Research
Christus Hospital
Beaumont, TX

Donna M. Roe, RN, MS, CEN
Clinical Education Manager
St. Joseph Hospital
Nashua, NH

Melissa S. Wafer, RN, MSN, CEN
Instructor
Southeastern Louisiana University
Baton Rouge, LA

Robin Walsh, RN, BSN
Clinical Nurse Supervisor
University of Massachusetts
Amherst, MA

① The nurse and emergency departments

Just the facts

In this chapter, you'll learn:

♦ Roles and responsibilities of an emergency nurse

♦ Credentials required for emergency nurses

♦ Ways to work with a multidisciplinary team (MDT)

♦ Ways to incorporate clinical tools and evidence-based practice into your care.

What is emergency nursing?

Emergency nursing is the immediate assessment and delivery of specialised care to a variety of ill or injured patients, such as in cases of cardiac arrest or polytrauma. Patients may be physically unstable, have complex needs and require intensive and vigilant nursing care. Others may have minor problems. No matter the reason for coming to the emergency department (ED), often called Accident and Emergency department (A&E), all patients feel that their problems are emergencies.

Some of the illnesses and injuries that patients present with in EDs include:

• Orthopaedic injuries, including fractures, strains and sprains

• Traumatic injuries from such events as road traffic collisions (RTCs) and falls

• Cardiovascular disorders, such as heart failure and acute coronary syndromes (unstable angina and myocardial infarction (MI)

• Respiratory disorders, such as acute respiratory failure, chronic obstructive pulmonary disease (COPD), pulmonary embolism and asthma

• Gastrointestinal (GI) and hepatic disorders, such as acute pancreatitis, GI bleeding, acute liver failure, acute cholecystitis and bowel obstructions

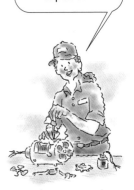

Emergency complaints come in all makes and models. This chapter will tune up your ED expertise!

- Renal disorders, such as acute and chronic renal failure, kidney stones and urinary tract infections
- Shock due to hypovolaemia, sepsis, cardiac dysfunction, acute spinal cord injury and anaphylaxis
- Mental health problems
- Paediatric ailments, such as gastroenteritis, bronchiolitis, febrile seizures and appendicitis
- Deliberate self-harm
- Minor injuries, including lacerations and abrasions
- Gynaecological and obstetric problems (although these emergencies may be directed straight to a specialist unit)
- Injuries resulting from violence and abuse, including knife injuries.

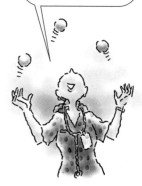

Juggling the variety of patient ailments in the ED can be tough, but we'll make sure you're prepared!

Meet the emergency nurse

An emergency nurse is responsible for making sure that all patients and members of their families receive close attention and the best care possible.

What do you do?

As an emergency nurse, you may progress in many roles in the emergency setting, such as staff nurse, nurse practitioner, nurse-educator, nurse-manager, consultant nurse. (See *Role call*.)

Where do you work?

As an emergency nurse, you may work in various settings, including:
- EDs
- Minor injury units
- Walk in centres
- Prehospital care environments
- General practitioner (GP) clinics
- Call centres.

What makes you a good ED nurse?

A nurse who specialises in emergencies accepts a wide range of responsibilities, including:
- Being an advocate
- Using sound clinical judgement
- Demonstrating caring practices
- Collaborating with an MDT
- Demonstrating a understanding of cultural diversity
- Providing patient and family teaching
- Health promoter.

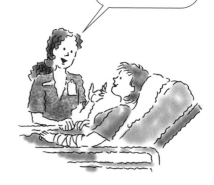

Patient advocacy is one of the most important aspects of emergency nursing.

Role call

By filling various nursing and management roles, an emergency nurse helps promote optimum health, prevent illness and aid coping with illness or death. Depending on the education and competencies achieved by various levels of nurses, here are some capacities in which an emergency nurse may function.

Health care support worker

In some EDs, health care support workers (HCSWs) are members of the health care team. Generally, an HCSW collaborates with a registered nurse (RN) to deliver patient care. The RN is responsible for and delegates specific tasks to the HCSW, whose duties may include caring directly for patients and collecting data. The HCSW may also take blood samples, assist with procedures and record vital signs.

Staff nurse

- Makes independent assessments
- Plans prioritises and implements patient care
- Provides direct nursing care
- Makes clinical observations and executes interventions
- Administers medications and treatments, such as pain control
- Promotes activities of daily living
- Depending on level of competence, may carry out extended skills, such as requesting X-rays.

Nurse practitioner

- Provides health care to patients and families; can function independently
- Obtains patient history and conducts physical examinations
- Requests laboratory and diagnostic tests and interprets results
- Makes a clinical diagnoses
- Prescribes and/or dispenses pharmacologic and nonpharmacologic treatments.
- Discharges patients or refers to specialist care
- Counsels and educates patients and families.

Nurse-educator

- Works clinically alongside all grades of staff: teaching, supervising and developing practice
- Contributes to the setting and monitoring standards of direct nursing care
- Provides advice and support to nurses and other professionals within the team
- Assesses and promotes of staff development by monitoring and teaching nursing and non-nursing staff
- In conjunction with other members of the MDT, sets standards and evaluates clinical outcomes in the management of the ED
- Develops evidence-based innovations and educational programmes, which lead to improved quality of care for patients.

Nurse-manager

- Acts as an administrative representative of the unit
- Is responsible for leading the provision of an emergency service for patients
- Ensures that effective and quality nursing care is provided in a timely sound environment
- Education
- Recruitment of staff.

Consultant nurse

- Is an expert in emergency nursing practice
- Is responsible for education and service development
- Has expert leadership and visionary qualities
- Works as a clinician providing senior clinical expertise
- Applies information in practice
- Conducts research studies and implements appropriate changes.

Multidisciplinary teamwork

Collaboration

Collaboration allows a health care team to use all available resources for the patient. Emergency nurses commonly collaborate with a MDT of health care professionals. The team approach helps caregivers to meet the diverse needs of individual patients by contributing their expertise.

As a nurse, you may often serve as the coordinator of such collaborative teams.

The whole goal

The goal of collaboration is to provide effective and comprehensive (holistic) care. Holistic care addresses the biological, psychological, social and spiritual dimensions of a person.

Team huddle

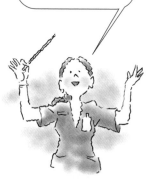

When we coordinate efforts, ED professionals make beautiful music together.

A MDT providing direct patient care may consist of many professionals, including:
- RNs
- Doctors
- Paramedics, emergency care practitioners and others. (See *Meet the team*.)

Working with RNs

Teamwork is essential in the stressful environment of the ED. The emergency nurse must work well with the other professionals within the department.

The buddy system

It's important to have a colleague to assure moral support, physical assistance with a patient and problem solving. No one person has all the answers, but together nurses have a better chance of solving problems.

Working with other MDTs

Patients in the ED are usually seen by an ED doctor or nurse practitioner who will probably have no prior knowledge of the patient. Consultations made to the patient's GP can help complete specific details of the patient, as can assessments from other specialists. Specialists commonly called to the ED to assess and treat patients include:
- Cardiologists
- General medical doctors
- General surgeons
- Neurologists

Meet the team

Although most EDs treat patients with their own staff, within their own department, some EDs have a collaborative relationship with other MDTs. Here are some examples.

Medical emergency team

- An appointed MDT that can respond to deteriorating patients or someone in a cardiopulmonary arrest caused by a medical problem
- Commonly includes a nurse, medical doctor, radiographer, anaesthetist and an operating department practitioner (ODP).

Emergency trauma team

- An appointed MDT that can respond to patients with major trauma and/or polytrauma
- May include a nurse, surgical doctor, neurosurgeon, orthopaedic doctor, radiographer, bed manager, anaesthetist, physiotherapist and an ODP.

Stroke team

- Assesses people coming to the ED with symptoms of an acute stroke
- Assesses patients for appropriateness of thrombolytic therapy and other needed treatments
- Commonly includes a nurse, a neurologist and a radiologist
- Can participate in hospital and community education related to stroke prevention, detecting early signs and symptoms, and treatments.

Social services

- Assist patients and families with such problems as difficulty paying for medications, follow-up physician visits and other health-related issues
- Assist patients with travel and housing if needed
- Develop social discharge plans.

Child protection services

- Designed to protect children from abusive situations
- Preserves the family unit, if possible, while ensuring the safety of children.

Pastoral caregiver

- Also known as a *chaplain*
- Meets the patient's and family's spiritual and religious needs
- Provides support and empathy to the patient and his/her family
- Delivers the patient's last rites if appropriate.

- Psychiatrist or psychiatric liaison nurses
- Orthopaedic doctors
- Gynaecologists
- Paediatricians
- Maxillofacial and oral surgeons.

Cultural diversity

Culture is defined as the way people live and how they behave in a social group. This behaviour is learned and passed on from generation to generation. Acknowledging and respecting patients' diverse cultural beliefs is a necessary part of high-quality care.

Keep an open mind

An emergency nurse is expected to demonstrate awareness and sensitivity towards a patient's religion, lifestyle, family makeup, socioeconomic status, age, gender and values. Be sure to assess cultural factors and concerns and integrate them into the care plan.

Education

As an educator, an emergency nurse is the facilitator of patient, family and staff education. Patient education involves teaching patients and their families about:

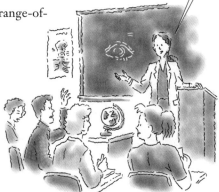

Patients, families, and staff members – everyone needs some education from an emergency nurse.

- The patient's illness
- The importance of managing comorbid disorders (such as diabetes, arthritis and hypertension)
- Diagnostic and laboratory testing
- Preoperative and postoperative expectations
- Instructions on specific patient care, such as wound care and range-of-movement exercises
- Medications that are prescribed
- Illness and injury prevention
- Home care instructions and follow-up appointments.

Staff as students

Emergency nurses also commonly serve as staff educators and role models. Examples of staff teaching topics you may need to address include:

- How to use new equipment
- How to interpret diagnostic test results
- How to administer a new medication.

Becoming an emergency nurse

Most nursing students are only briefly exposed to emergency nursing. Much of the preparation required to become an emergency nurse is achieved through good underpinning theoretical knowledge, exposure and experience.

Learning by doing

On-the-job education is central to gaining the extensive skills required of an emergency nurse. Your department may provide a competency-based orientation programme for new emergency nurses. In such a programme, you gain knowledge and experience while working in the ED and a preceptor (a staff nurse or clinical nurse specialist with specialised training in emergency nursing) provides guidance.

An orientation period allows the nurse time to acquire the knowledge and technical skills needed to work in the emergency environment. Such technical skills include working with cardiac monitoring systems, mechanical ventilators, haemodynamic monitoring devices and autotransfusers.

Gaining credentials

There are many Higher Education Intuitions (HEIs) across the UK that provide postgraduate qualifications for emergency nurses.

The primary goal of achieving such qualifications is to promote excellence in emergency nursing through leadership, education, research and advocacy.

Continual professional development (CPD) and competence, demonstrated by gaining your postgraduate qualification in emergency nursing, states you're a professional, with proficiency and skill in a highly specialised area of nursing. Be aware that obtaining a 'recognised' certificate from a course or study day doesn't mean that you are competent in a particular skill. Your competency of the knowledge and skill must be assessed by a current competent practitioner. You also have a professional requirement to maintain and update your skills.

Other emergency qualifications

There are also a number of courses that are generally accepted by EDs in the UK.

Some of these include:

- ATNC – Advanced trauma nursing course
- ALS – Advanced life support
- APLS – Advanced paediatric life support
- ATLS – Advanced trauma life support
- pILS – Paediatric immediate life support
- ILS – Immediate life support
- e-ATLS e-learning – Advanced trauma life support
- MIMMS – Major incident medical management and support.

Most certification for these courses requires competencies in certain skills and renewal after 4 years. Nurses can recertify by accessing the whole course again or by attending a 1-day recertification course.

Help wanted

Certification isn't mandatory to work as an emergency nurse, but it's certainly encouraged. Many units prefer to employ nurses with certification, because it means that they have demonstrated competence, expertise and commitment to emergency nursing.

Safety first

The goal of any nursing certification programme is to promote safe nursing care. Competency is evidence that a nurse has demonstrated clinical excellence and recognises the importance of patient safety. It validates the nurse's qualifications and specialised clinical knowledge.

What's in it for me?

For most nurses, the main reason for seeking competency is personal fulfilment, but there are other rewards as well. Some health employers reimburse nurses gaining further qualifications, and it will assist you in progressing to a more senior level.

Nursing responsibilities

As an emergency nurse, you're responsible for all parts of the nursing process: assessing, planning, implementing and evaluating care of all patients in your care. Remember that each of these steps gives you an opportunity to exercise your critical thinking skills.

Assessment

Emergency nursing requires that you constantly assess the patient for subtle changes in condition and monitor all equipment being used. Caring for emergency patients may involve the use of such highly specialised equipment as cardiac monitors and central venous pressure (CVP) and arterial line-monitoring devices. As part of the patient assessment, you should also assess the patient's physical, sociological and psychological statuses and interpret results of the investigations.

Planning

Planning requires you to consider the patient's psychological, sociological and physiological needs and set realistic patient goals. The result is an individualised care plan for your patient. To ensure safe passage through the emergency environment, you must also anticipate changes in the patient's condition. For example, for a patient admitted with a diagnosis of MI, you should monitor cardiac rhythm and anticipate rhythm changes. If an arrhythmia such as complete heart block develops, you may need to change the treatment plan and establish new goals.

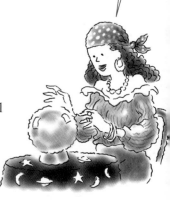

You don't need to be clairvoyant to prepare a patient care plan; just anticipate common problems.

What's the problem?

In planning, be sure to address present and potential problems, such as:
- Pain
- Altered conscious level
- Cardiac arrhythmias
- Altered haemodynamic status
- Impaired physical mobility
- Impaired skin integrity
- Fluid volume deficit.

Implementation

As a nurse, you must implement specific interventions to address existing and potential patient problems.

Examples of interventions include:
- Monitoring and treating cardiac arrhythmias
- Managing pain
- Monitoring responses to therapy.

Evaluation

It's necessary for you to continually evaluate a patient's response to interventions. Use such evaluations to change the care plan as needed to make sure that your patient continues to work towards achieving his outcome goals.

Clinical tools

The MDT uses various tools to promote safe and comprehensive holistic care. These tools include clinical pathways, practice guidelines and protocols.

Clinical pathways

Clinical pathways are care management plans for patients with a given diagnosis or condition.

Follow the path

Clinical pathways are typically generated and used by departments that deliver care for similar conditions to many patients. A multidisciplinary group of clinicians usually develop clinical pathways. The overall goals are to:
- Establish a standard approach to care for all providers in the department
- Establish roles for various members of the health care team
- Provide a framework for collecting data on patient outcomes
- Improve quality of care.

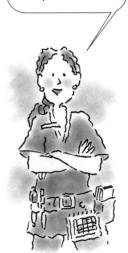

The tools of your trade? Clinical pathways, practice guidelines, and protocois.

Tried and true

Pathways are based on evidence from research and clinical practice. The committee gathers and uses information from peer-reviewed literature and experts outside the individual hospitals.

Outlines and timelines

Clinical pathways usually outline the duties of all professionals involved with patient care. They follow specific timelines for indicated actions. They also specify expected patient outcomes, which serve as checkpoints for the patient's progress and caregiver's performance.

Practice guidelines

Practice guidelines specify courses of action to be taken in response to a diagnosis or condition. Practice guidelines also aid decision-making by practitioners and patients. They're multidisciplinary in nature and can be used to coordinate care by multiple providers.

Let an expert be your guide

Expert health care providers usually write practice guidelines. They condense large amounts of information into easily usable formats, combining clinical expertise with the best available clinical evidence. Practice guidelines are used to:
- Streamline care
- Control variations in practice patterns
- Distribute health care resources more effectively.

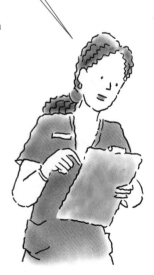

Always check where practice guidelines come from before you apply them to your patient.

The evidence is in

Practice guidelines are valuable sources of information. They indicate which tests and treatments are appropriate and provide a framework for building a standard of care (a statement describing an expected level of care or performance).

Consider the source

Like research-based information, clinical guidelines should be evaluated for the quality of their sources. It's a good idea to read the developer's policy statement about how evidence was selected and what values were applied in making recommendations for care.

Protocols

Protocols are established sets of procedures for a given circumstance. Their purpose is to outline actions that are most likely to produce optimal patient outcomes.

First things first

Protocols describe a sequence of actions a practitioner should take to establish a diagnosis or begin a treatment regimen. For example, a chest pain protocol outlines a bedside strategy for managing chest pain.

Protocols facilitate delivery of consistent, cost-effective care. They're also educational resources for clinicians who strive to keep abreast of current evidence-based practice. Protocols may be either highly directive or flexible, allowing practitioners to use clinical judgement.

Input from experts

Nursing or medical experts write protocols and standards of care, commonly with input from other health care providers, such as the faculty of emergency nursing. Protocols may be approved by legislative bodies, such as boards of nursing or medicine.

Evidence-based practice

As new procedures and medicines become available, nurses committed to excellence regularly update and adapt their practices. An approach known as *evidence-based practice* is an important tool for providing high-quality care.

Best for all concerned

The term *evidence-based practice* refers to clinical practices, treatments and interventions that result in the best possible outcomes for the patient and your department.

The best practice approach is generally a team effort that draws on various types of information. Common sources of information used to identify evidence-based practice are research data, personal experience and expert opinion.

Emergency research

The goal of emergency nursing research is to improve the delivery of care and thereby improve patient outcomes. Nursing care is commonly based on evidence that's derived from research. Evidence can be used to support current practices or to change practices.

The best way to get involved in research is to be a good consumer of nursing research. You can do so by reading nursing journals and being aware of the quality of research and reported results.

Share and share alike

Don't be afraid to share research findings with colleagues. Sharing promotes sound clinical care and all involved may learn about easier and more efficient ways to care for patients.

Evidence-based practice

Evidence-based practice isn't based on tradition, custom or intuition. It's derived from various concrete sources, such as:
- Formal nursing research
- Clinical knowledge
- Scientific knowledge.

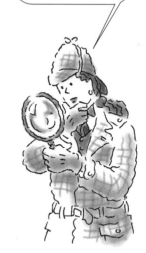

Hmmm ... the evidence points to an alternate treatment.

An evidence-based example

Research results may provide insight into the treatment of a patient who, for example, doesn't respond to a medication or treatment that seemed effective for other patients.

You may believe that a certain drug should be effective for pain relief, based on previous experience with that drug. The trouble with such an approach is that other factors can contribute to pain relief, such as the route of administration, the dosage, positioning of the patient and concurrent treatments.

First, last and always

Regardless of the value of evidence-based practice, you should always use professional clinical judgement when dealing with emergency patients and their families. Remember that each patient's condition ultimately dictates treatment.

Quick quiz

1. To work in an ED, you must:
   A. have a degree.
   B. have certification in emergency nursing.
   C. use the nursing process in delivering nursing care.
   D. possess an advanced nursing degree.

Answer: C. The professional nurse uses the nursing process (assessment, planning, implementation and evaluation) to care for emergency patients.

2. The purpose of the MDT is to:
   A. assist the nurse in performing patient care.
   B. replace the concept of primary care in the emergency setting.
   C. minimise lawsuits in the ED.
   D. provide holistic, comprehensive care to the patient.

Answer: D. The purpose of the MDT is to provide comprehensive care to the emergency patient.

3. Professional qualification/certification in emergency nursing allows you to:

    A.   function as an advanced practice nurse.

    B.   validate knowledge and skills in emergency nursing.

    C.   obtain an administrative position.

    D.   obtain a pay rise.

Answer: B. The purpose of professional certification is to validate knowledge and skill in a particular area. Certification is a demonstration of excellence and commitment to your chosen specialty area.

4. The easiest way to participate in research is to:

    A.   be a good consumer of research.

    B.   analyse related studies.

    C.   conduct a research study.

    D.   participate on your facility's internal review board.

Answer: A. Begin by reading valid research articles and judging whether they're applicable to your practice. Research findings aren't useful if they aren't incorporated into practice.

5. The purpose of evidence-based practice is to:

    A.   validate traditional nursing practices.

    B.   improve patient outcomes.

    C.   refute traditional nursing practices.

    D.   establish a body of knowledge unique to nursing.

Answer: B. Although evidence-based practices may validate or refute traditional practice, their purpose is to improve patient outcomes.

Scoring

☆☆☆   If you answered all five questions correctly, take a bow! You're basically a whiz when it comes to emergency nursing basics.

☆☆   If you answered three or four questions correctly, there's no room for criticism! Your critical thinking skills are basically intact.

☆   If you answered fewer than three questions correctly, the situation is emergent! Review the chapter, and you'll be on the right pathway.

Holistic care

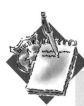

2

Just the facts

In this chapter, you'll learn:

♦ Family dynamics to consider when you provide care

♦ Issues that affect emergency patients, their families and carers

♦ Safety of the patient, the team and yourself

♦ Principles of legal and ethical decision making

♦ Concepts related to end-of-life decisions and how they're important to your care delivery

Advocacy

An advocate is a person who works on behalf of any other person. Advocacy is an important part of the nurse's role wherever care is given. The Emergency Department (ED) nurse's advocate role is of particular relevance due to the acute and often life threatening illnesses experienced by ED patients. Patients admitted to the ED often experience life-changing events, and this of course affects their families also. On the other hand, a patient may not have any family or friends who will speak up for his/her rights and best interests; in that case you will need to act as your patient's advocate. As an advocate, you should also address the concerns of family members and the community whenever possible.

As an advocate, you seek to:
• Protect patients' rights
• Assist the patient and his/her family and significant others in the decision-making process by providing information and support
• Negotiate with other members of the health care team on behalf of the patient and his family
• Keep the patient and his/her family and significant others informed about the care plan
• Advocate for family and key others involvement in decision making in the ED
• Respect and support the decisions of the patient

- Serve as a liaison between the patient and other members of the health care team
- Respect the patient's values and cultures
- Act in the patient's best interest
- Provide health promotion and safety advice, e.g. educating about poison storage, use of car restraints and safe sleeping tips for infants to prevent sudden infant death syndrome.

Stuck in the middle

Being a patient advocate can sometimes cause conflict between you and the patient's family or other concerned friends. For example, a patient may have an advance directive, requesting no resuscitation, but his family may not approve. It may also cause conflict between your professional duty and the patient's personal values. For example, the patient may be a Jehovah's Witness and refuse a blood transfusion even though this may have serious implications for the patient's health.

Considering vulnerable groups

You and the ED team have a particular responsibility to protect the safety and the rights of the vulnerable groups who access the ED. It is with such groups that the nurse's advocacy role takes on particular relevance. For instance, a patient with a profound learning impairment will need you to spend extra time with them to explain what you are doing and to lessen his fears. Patients subject to domestic violence may need to be protected from further harm or intimidation.

Clinical judgement

An emergency nurse needs to exercise clinical judgement in a fast-paced and stressful environment. To develop sound clinical judgement, you need critical thinking skills. Critical thinking is a complex mixture of knowledge, intuition, logic, common sense, experience and importantly a questioning and a curious approach to your nursing practice. Good nurses are always seeking to improve their knowledge, and an ED will provide you with constant opportunities to learn.

Critical thinking fosters understanding of issues and enables you to quickly find answers to difficult questions. Critical thinking enhances your ability to identify a patient's needs. It also enables you to use sound clinical decision-making to determine which nursing actions best meet a patient's needs and to be aware of the potential consequences of your actions.

Developing critical thinking skills

Critical thinking skills improve with increasing clinical experience supported by your theoretical learning. The best way for you to develop critical thinking skills is by asking questions and reflecting upon your learning needs.

Always asking questions

The first question you should find the answer to is 'What are the patient's symptoms or diagnosis?' If it's a diagnosis with which you aren't familiar, look it up and read about it. Find the answers to these questions:

- What are the signs and symptoms?
- What's the usual cause?
- What complications can occur?

In addition to the answers to diagnosis-related questions, also be sure to find out:

- What are the patient's physical examination findings?
- Which laboratory and diagnostic tests are necessary?
- Does the patient have risk factors? If so, are they significant? What interventions would minimise those risk factors?
- How can you best address the patient's cultural concerns?
- What are the possible complications? What type of monitoring is needed to watch for complications?
- What are the usual medications and treatments for the patient's condition? (If you aren't familiar with the medications or treatments, look them up in a reliable source or consult a colleague.)
- Is the patient in pain? Most patients attending the ED will be experiencing pain. Are you conducting appropriate pain assessments and providing the most effective pain relief interventions? (Pain management is discussed in greater detail in Chapter 3, *Initial assessment in emergency departments*.)
- What are the patient's nursing, medical and collaborative needs?

Critical thinking and the nursing process

Critical thinking skills are necessary when applying the nursing process. The making of evidenced patient-centred care decisions are based on holistic assessment, the formulation of statements of patient needs, planning care, implementation of evidence-based care, evaluation of outcomes and reassessment if required.

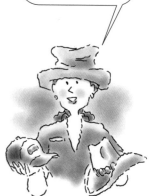

No matter what it looks like, be sure to put on your critical thinking cap for the next steps.

Caring practice

Caring practice is the use of a therapeutic and compassionate environment to focus on the patient's needs. Although care is based on standards and protocols, it must also be individualised to each patient. Caring practice also involves the following:

- Maintaining a safe environment
- Interacting with the patient and his family and friends in a compassionate and respectful manner throughout the ED stay
- Giving support to the family if a patient dies.

To act as the patient's and the family's advocate you need to understand the person from a holistic perspective.

What is holistic health care?

Holistic health care revolves around a notion of totality. The goal of holistic care is to meet not only the patient's physical needs, but also his/her social, spiritual and emotional needs.

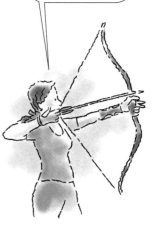

Holistic care aims to treat the entire patient from the inside out.

A new dimension

Holistic care addresses all dimensions of a person, including:
* Physical
* Emotional
* Social
* Spiritual.

Only by considering these dimensions can the health care team provide high-quality holistic care. You should strive to provide holistic care to all emergency patients, even if their physical needs seem more pressing than their other needs.

Holistic care issues

Delivering the best holistic care requires you to consider various issues, including:
* Issues related to the patient, his/her family and other concerned persons
* Cognitive impairment
* Ethical and legal considerations.

Patient and family issues

A *family* is a group of two or more persons who possibly live together in the same household, perform certain interrelated social tasks and share an emotional bond. Families can profoundly influence the individuals within them. The way that families are set up can be very different; so you must be alert to this and respectful of the rights and the sensitivities of individual groups.

Keep in mind that the stress from a medical emergency can really throw a family off-balance.

Family ties

A family is a dynamic system. During stress-free times, this system tends to maintain homoeostasis, meaning that it exists in a stable state of harmony and balance. However, when a crisis sends one family member into the ED, the rest may feel a tremendous strain and family homeostasis is disturbed. The major effects of such imbalances are:
* Increased stress levels
* Reorganisation of family roles.

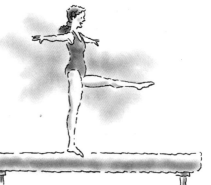

Slipping on emotional turmoil

The emergency patient's condition may change rapidly (within minutes or hours); the result of such physiological instability is emotional turmoil for the family. Family members may use whatever coping mechanisms they have, such as seeking support from friends, hospital chaplains or other faith leaders. The longer the patient remains in the ED, the psychological stress experienced by the patient and his/her family increases.

Circle out of round

When sudden critical illness or injury disrupts the family circle, a patient can no longer fulfill certain role responsibilities. Such roles are typically:
• Financial (if the patient is a major contributor to the family's monetary stability)
• Social (if the patient fills such roles as spouse, parent, mediator or disciplinarian).

Unprepared for the worst

Family members may also worry about the possible death of the patient. The suddenness of the illness or injury may overwhelm the family and put it into a crisis state. The ramifications of the patient's illness or injury may cause other family members to feel hopeless and helpless.

Nursing responsibilities

The patient's family needs guidance and support during his/her stay in the ED and beyond. An emergency nurse's responsibility to the family is to provide information about:
• Nursing care
• The patient's prognosis and expected treatments.

Lend a hand

Because you're exposed to members of the patient's family, you can help them during their time of crisis. For example, you can observe the family's anxiety level and, if necessary, refer them to another member of the multidisciplinary team, such as social services or faith leaders.

You can also help the family solve problems by encouraging them to:
• Verbalise the immediate problem
• Identify support systems
• Recall how they handled stress successfully in the past.

Such assistance helps the family focus on the present issue. It also allows them to solve problems and regain a sense of control over their lives.

Lend an ear, too

You can also help the family cope with their feelings during this stressful time. Two ways to do this are by encouraging expression of feelings (such as

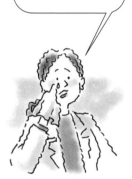

Encouraging families to express their feelings helps them relieve stress. 'sniff'

by crying or discussing the issue) and providing empathy. You can also help by realising that stress and grief can manifest in a variety of manners. The nurse must be sensitive to individual grief or stress reactions.

Because you asked

During a patient's stay in the ED, families will rely on the opinions of professionals and will commonly ask for advice. They need honest information that is given to them in terms that they can understand. In many cases, you will be the health care team member who provides this information or facilitates this information provision from another health professional.

Cultural considerations

Cultural influences can affect how a family copes with the hospitalisation of a loved one. A patient's cultural background can also affect many aspects of care, such as:

- Patient and family roles during illness
- Communication between health care providers and the patient and his family
- Feelings of the patient and his family regarding end-of-life issues
- Family views regarding health care practices and causes of ill health
- Pain management
- Nutrition
- Spiritual support.

Consider culture

To provide effective holistic care, you must honour the patient's cultural beliefs and values. Because culture can impact on care, you should perform a cultural assessment. Conducting a cultural assessment enables you to:

- Recognise a patient's cultural responses to illness and hospitalisation
- Determine how the patient and his family define health and illness
- Determine the family's beliefs about the cause of the illness.

Cognitive issues

A patient in an ED may feel overwhelmed by the technology around him. Although this equipment is essential for patient care, it can create an environment that's foreign to the patient that can result in disturbed cognition (thought-related function). In addition, the disease process can affect cognitive function in an emergency patient. For example, a patient with metabolic disturbances or hypoxia can experience confusion and changes in mental clarity.

Fair to compare

When assessing cognitive function, the first question you should ask is, 'What was your previous level of functioning?' If the patient can't answer this question, ask a family member.

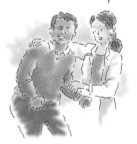

Culture affects many aspects of patient care, including pain management.

Si!

Assessing cultural considerations

A cultural assessment yields the information you need to administer high-quality nursing care to members of various cultural populations. The emergency nurse will collect such information as pertinent to the patient's current illness status, and this information will form part of the on-going assessment of the patient's needs. The goal of the cultural assessment is to gain awareness and understanding of cultural variations and their effects on the care you provide. For each patient, you and other members of the multidisciplinary team then use the findings of a cultural assessment to develop an individualised care plan. When performing a cultural assessment, be sure to ask questions that yield certain information about the patient and his family, including questions about:

- Cultural health beliefs
- Communication methods
- Cultural restrictions
- Social networks
- Nutritional status
- Religion
- Values and beliefs.

Some examples of the types of questions you should consider for each patient are depicted in the following sections.

Cultural health beliefs

- What does the patient believe caused his/her illness? A patient may believe for instance that his/her illness is the result of an imbalance in yin and yang, or it may be simply that he/she has no idea what caused the illness and has a poor understanding of the organs and systems of the body
- How does the patient express pain?
- What does the patient believe promotes health? Beliefs can range from eating certain foods to wearing amulets for good luck
- In what types of healing practices (such as herbal remedies and healing rituals) does the patient engage?

Communication differences

- What language does the patient speak?
- Does the patient require an interpreter?
- How does the patient want to be addressed?
- What are the styles of nonverbal communication (e.g. eye contact or touching)?

Cultural restrictions

- How are feelings about death, dying and grief expressed?
- How is modesty expressed?
- What are the cultural considerations regarding touching the patient?
- Does the patient have restrictions related to exposure of parts of the body?

Social networks

- What are the roles of each family member during health and illness?
- Who makes the decisions?

Nutrition

- What's the meaning of food and eating to the patient?
- What types of food does he/she eat?

Religion

- What's the role of religious beliefs and practices during illness?
- Does the patient or the family wish that special rites or blessings need to be performed?
- Are there any healing rituals or practices that must be followed?

It's a factor

Many factors impact on a patient's cognitive function while in the ED, including:
- Invasion of personal space
- Medications
- Pain
- Sensory input.

Invasion of personal space

Personal space is the unmarked boundary or territory around a person. Several factors – such as cultural background and social situation – influence a patient's interpretation of personal space. A patient's personal space is limited in many ways by the emergency environment – for example, due to the confines of bed rest, lack of privacy and use of invasive equipment.

You can try to increase your patient's sense of personal space – even within the emergency environment – by simply remembering to show common courtesy, such as:

- Asking permission to perform a procedure or look at a wound or dressing
- Pulling the curtain or closing the door
- Knocking before you enter the patient's cubicle.

Medications

Medications that can cause adverse central nervous system reactions and affect cognitive function include:

- Inotropics – such as digoxin that can cause agitation, hallucinations, malaise, dizziness, vertigo and paraesthesia
- Barbiturates – such as phenobarbitone that can cause drowsiness, lethargy, hangover symptoms, physical and psychological dependence, and paradoxical excitement (in older adults)
- Corticosteroids – such as prednisone that can cause euphoria, psychotic behaviour, insomnia, vertigo, headache, paraesthesia and seizures
- Benzodiazepines – such as lorazepam that can cause drowsiness, sedation, disorientation, amnesia, unsteadiness and agitation
- Opioid analgesics – such as morphine that can cause respiratory depression, vomiting, sedation, euphoria, dizziness, light-headedness and drowsiness.

Sensory input

Sensory stimulation in any environment may be perceived as pleasant or unpleasant and comfortable or painful. The emergency environment tends to stimulate all five senses:

 Auditory

 Visual

 Taste

 Olfactory (smell)

 Tactile.

> If you think finding personal space in the ED is hard, imagine what it's like for a patient!

Too much or too little

Patients in the ED don't have control over the environmental stimulation around them. They may experience sensory deprivation, sensory overload or both. *Sensory deprivation* can result from a reduction in the quantity and quality of normal and familiar sensory input, such as the normal sights and sounds encountered at home. *Sensory overload* results from an increase in the amount of unfamiliar sounds and sights in the emergency environment, such as beeping cardiac monitors, ringing telephones, paging systems and voices. The patient may become very anxious when hearing the resuscitation team in the next cubicle. When environmental stimuli exceed the patient's ability to cope with the stimulation, he/she may experience anxiety, confusion and panic as well as delusions.

Safety in EDs

Everyone, patients, visitors and staff, in the ED has the right to be safe and protected from harm. However, there are occasions when people in the department might be subjected to some form of abuse or violence. This can be very distressing for both the staff, the patient and the patient's relatives or companions and may lead to significant problems when assessing patients and providing appropriate care.

The nurse needs to be aware of contributory factors that may provoke or exacerbate situations which may cause anxiety, stress, emotions and fear. For example:
- A crisis resulting from an accident or illness, such as, self-image, social and financial
- How the health professional portrays their verbal and non verbal communication
- Alcohol or drugs
- Other people, including relatives
- Medical conditions, such as hypoxia or metabolic disturbances
- Pain
- Previous experience with health care
- History of violence
- Serious mental health problems
- Lack of communication
- Waiting times
- Poor facilities within the waiting area, e.g. drinks machine not working.

Although some incidents cannot be avoided, many violent or aggressive situations can be prevented. If the nurse is aware of circumstances similar to those noted above, then actions to reduce the potential for a violent or abusive reaction should be undertaken.

Be thoughtful

If a patient or relative report a problem to a member of staff, then obviously that problem is distressing that individual. If the problem is not dealt with effectively, then the situation becomes exacerbated, leading to the risk of violence or verbal abuse being directed towards staff. For example, if a person has been waiting for several hours to be seen and they report that the drink machine isn't working in the waiting room, action should be taken to rectify the problem or, if the problem cannot be rectified then this should be explained to the individual.

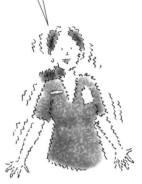

Overrrrstimulation of allll the senses can lllllead to ssssensory overload!

Communicate

Keeping people waiting will only increase their frustration. Updating the individuals will often reduce the anxiety and stress that can lead to aggressive behaviour. If the patient is told that the waiting time is increased because of unforeseen circumstances, such as a road traffic incident, the chances of them becoming aggressive or abusive should be reduced. Effective communication is essential.

However, as explained previously, some incidents cannot be avoided, and the nurse should recognise key warning signals:
- Abrupt conversational manner, including sarcasm
- Increased volume tone
- Showing tense/aggressive body language
- Rapid breathing
- Direct prolonged eye contact
- Increased breathing rate/nostrils flaring.

If any of these signs (or other indicators of increasing tension) are observed, then they should be dealt with appropriately. Junior nurses should seek help from more experienced personnel. It is essential that you stay calm and approach the situation in a supportive but confident manner. Lead the individual to a private but safe area with an open exit for you to escape from if necessary. Ensure there are no objects available that can be used as weapons. Make sure that you have at least an arm's length of space between you and the individual. Be empathetic and listen to the person's dilemma, encouraging them to discuss a potential solution to the problem with you and a colleague. Keep your voice in a conversational tone and try not to maintain constant eye contact: this will help to defuse the situation. The more you become confrontational, threatening or if you raise your voice, the more it will anger the person. Select your words carefully, and use language that is easily understood so that you don't aggravate the situation and try to solve the problem with achievable goals. However, it cannot always be possible to avoid situations of violent or aggressive behaviour but always try to use skills and interventions to avoid them occurring.

Practice pointers
- Give clear, short but assertive instructions
- Guide the person to a 'safer' location but not if to do so would put you at risk
- Use open questions and try and find the reason why they are angry
- Never threaten or become aggressive yourself
- Make sure you are at least an arm's length away from the aggressor at all times
- Be aware of your body posture and use of eye contact.

Many EDs have security guards who should be contacted immediately if there is an evident risk of violence or aggression. If violence should occur then the nurse should leave the person, activate their personal attack alarms and call the police. If you are attacked you should try and break away, leaving the situation to trained security personnel who may have to restrain the individual with a minimum of four members of staff. If possible, the situation should be left to be dealt with by the police. Restraint should be minimal while a decision is made for further care/treatment. A debriefing of the situation should be carried out within the department with incident forms/ statements completed. Any distressed staff requiring further help in dealing with the situation should be fully supported by the department, and the hospital and supportive 'debrief' and/or counselling should be available.

Legal and ethical issues

Nurses who work in EDs deal routinely with legal and ethical dilemmas. You'll recognise a situation as a dilemma in these circumstances:
• More than one solution exists; that is, there's no clear 'right' or 'wrong' way to handle a situation
• Competing values or beliefs about the best way to deal with an issue
• When the patient's wishes are at variance with medical advice.

Ethical dilemmas

Ethical dilemmas in EDs revolve commonly around quality-of-life issues for the patient, especially as they relate to end-of-life decisions – such as do-not-resuscitate orders and patients' requests for no heroic resuscitation measures.

When considering quality of life, make sure others don't impose their own value system on the patient. Each person has a set of personal values that are influenced by environment and culture. Nurses also have a set of professionally led values.

Professional standards

Nurses and midwives in the United Kingdom are professionally regulated by the Nursing and Midwifery Council (NMC). The NMC maintains the nursing and midwifery register and offers guidance on professional standards in practice and education. This professional guidance is found in *The Code. Standards of Conduct, Performance and Ethics for Nurses and Midwives*.

This guidance can be found in full at www.nmc-uk.org. The first statement in the Code requires that nurses and midwives 'Make the care of people your first concern, treating them as individuals and respecting their dignity'. Even in busy areas such as EDs nurses must at all times provide care that reflects this professional guidance.

Legal considerations

Clinical decision making in the ED is often done rapidly so the ED nurse should have a sound knowledge of the following basic legal concepts when faced with complex issues that have to be resolved promptly:
• Patients and their families have a legal right to expect that their information is kept confidential however patient information will be shared amongst the health care team appropriately

- The nurse will however have an overriding duty to society in cases of serious crime, such as murder and rape, to disclose evidence to the police that was gained whilst providing care
- No one can consent for an adult (an adult is anyone over 18 years of age)
- Adult patients have the legal (and ethical) right to personal autonomy and can refuse treatment should they wish. Only a legal ruling can overrule any such refusal except if the treatment is for a mental disorder and the patient is detained under the Mental Health Act (1983, amended 2007)
- Patients are entitled to enough information to allow them to make an informed choice
- Patients lacking mental capacity, for instance the unconscious patient, will be treated without consent in what would be their best interest
- Mental capacity is defined within The Mental Capacity Act (2005) to be demonstrated by the individual being able to:
    i.   Understand what the medical treatment is, its purpose and nature and why it is being proposed
    ii. Understand the benefits, risks and alternatives
    iii. Understand the consequences of not receiving the proposed treatment
    iv. Retain the information weigh it in balance in order to arrive at a decision
    v.   Communicate the decision
- If a patient has an appointed welfare attorney, or there is a court appointed deputy or guardian then this person, where practicable, must be consulted about treatment decisions
- All people aged 16 or over are presumed, in law, to have the capacity to consent to treatment
- Children under 16 years of age can make decisions regarding care if they have the ability to understand (Gillick Competence). Otherwise it is parents or those with parental responsibility who consent for children under 16
- If it is in the child or young person's (that is under 18 years of age) best interests the doctor may apply to a court to override the wishes of the child, parents or guardians.

A useful reader on the law as it relates to nurses is Griffith, R. and Tengnah, C. (2010). *Law and Professional Issues in Nursing*, 2nd edn. Exeter: Learning Matters.

End-of-life decisions

The threat of death is common in EDs. Perhaps at no other time is the holistic care of patients and their families as important as it is during this time. End-of-life decisions are almost always difficult for patients, families and health care professionals to make. Nurses are in a unique position to assist patients and their families through this process. Your primary role as a patient advocate is to promote the patient's wishes. In many instances, however, a patient's wishes aren't known. That's when ethical decision-making takes priority. Decisions aren't always easy to make, and the answers aren't usually clear-cut. At times, such ethical dilemmas may seem unsolvable, however in the ED a decision must be made and often with a short time span. Serving the patient's best interest is always the guiding principle.

A question of quality

It's sometimes difficult to determine what can be done to achieve good quality of life and what can simply be achieved, technologically speaking. Technological advances sometimes seem to exceed our ability to analyse the ethical dilemmas associated with them. Until fairly recently, death was considered a natural part of life, and most people died at home, surrounded by their families. Today, most people die in hospitals, and death is commonly regarded as a medical failure rather than a natural event. Sometimes it's hard for you to know whether you're assisting in extending the patient's life or delaying the patient's death. To reach a suitable decision the health care team will consult with the patient or if that is not possible with the family or key others. Remember that the decision to treat, or not to treat, must always be in patient's best interest.

Determining medical futility

Medical futility refers to treatment that's hopeless or interventions that aren't likely to benefit the patient even though they may appear to be effective. For example, a patient with a terminal illness who's expected to die experiences cardiac arrest. Cardiopulmonary resuscitation may be effective in restoring a heartbeat but may still be deemed futile because it doesn't change the patient's outcome.

Dealing with cardiac arrest

When cardiac arrest occurs, you must ensure that resuscitative efforts are initiated or that unwanted resuscitation doesn't take place. Any 'Do Not Attempt Resuscitation' (DNAR) orders must be clearly recorded by the doctor in the patient's notes. You need to check and be familiar with the DNAR hospital guidelines where you are working. Also check the ED's policy on relations or significant others witnessing resuscitation as increasingly this is seen as good practice. A patient in a hospital setting such as an ED will be treated using Advanced Life Support protocols. (This is discussed further in Chapter 6, *Cardiac emergencies*.) The senior clinician will make the final decision to stop the attempt, usually after consultation with the resuscitation team. Not every patient can be successfully resuscitated, however knowing that everything that could be done was done can be a real comfort to the patient's loved ones, and to the resuscitation team. There is lots of helpful and current information on the Resuscitation Council UK's web site found at: http://www.resus.org.uk

Who decides?

The wishes of a competent, informed patient should always be honoured. However, when a patient can't make decisions, the health care team – consisting of the patient's family, nursing staff, and doctors – may have to make end-of-life decisions for the patient.

Advance directives

Most people prefer to make their own decisions regarding end-of-life care. It's important that patients discuss their wishes with their loved ones; however, many don't. Instead, total strangers may be asked to make important health care decisions when patients can't do so. That's why it's important for people to make choices ahead of time and to make these choices known by developing advance directives.

Advance decisions to refuse treatment, that used to be known as living wills, allow patients to refuse all or some forms of medical treatment if they should lose their mental capacity. These advance decisions relate to refusal of treatment and cannot be used to request treatment. If the patient has a valid and applicable advanced decision, it carries the same legal weight as a refusal of treatment by a person with decision-making capacity. This means that the specified treatment noted by the advance decision cannot be given lawfully. If it were given the doctor or nurse might face civil liability or criminal prosecution. The Mental Capacity Act 2005 came into force in April 2007 and offers a legal basis for advance decisions. To be valid an advance decision must be made by a person 18 years old or over who has decision-making capacity at the time of making it. An advance decision to refuse treatment cannot:

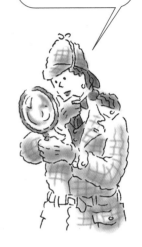

Although they aren't mandatory, advance directives can take a lot of the mystery out of end-of-life care decisions.

- Ask for anything unlawful such as active euthanasia
- Demand treatment
- Refuse food or drink by mouth
- Refuse basic care required for comfort and warmth
- Refuse basic nursing required for hygiene or pain relief.
    The health care team might not act on an advance decision if:
- the person has changed their circumstance so the advanced decision is no longer logically valid, for example the patient has changed their religious faith
- if medical developments to improve prognosis or to aid comfort were not taken into account
- it is not clear about what should happen (advanced decisions are difficult to write so as to consider all eventualities)
- if the person has been treated under the Mental Health Act (1983, amended 2007)
- if (in England and Wales) the patient has given someone lasting power of attorney to make that decision and so supersede the advance decision
- if the validity of the advance decision is being disputed or has been referred to the courts.
    To apply to the refusal of life saving treatment an advance decision must:
- be in writing
- be signed by the maker or signed on their behalf in their presence
- be witnessed in the maker's presence
- be verified by a statement that confirms that the advance decision to refuse treatment is to apply even if life is at risk.

Organ and tissue donation

Death used to be defined as the cessation of respiratory and cardiac function; however, developments in medical technology have made this definition obsolete. We now rely on brain death criteria to determine an individual's death. A person can be certified as dead even though the heart is still beating and beating maintained by artificial ventilation. The use of organ and tissue retrieved post-mortem has increased year by year.

When asked, most people say that they support organ and tissue donation. Organ and tissue transplantation is successful for many patients, giving them additional, high-quality years of life.

Organs including kidneys and hearts are obtained from patients in whom brain death has been confirmed; however, the heart must be kept beating, artificial ventilation provided and other support maintained to ensure adequate organ perfusion. Tissue donation, such as skin, bone and heart valves, can be retrieved up to 24 hours (and sometimes up to 48 hours) after death without the requirement to maintain a beating heart.

The nurse has an important contribution to the health care team when this process is underway. The need for sensitivity and compassion when dealing with the family in such cases cannot be overemphasised. Full information must be given and support provided for the family.

In 2009 in the UK, 3706 organs (an increase of 5% from 2008) were donated; however, in this same time frame 7877 people were still waiting. If patients have given prior permission to their organs being used after their death then their details are held on the NHS Organ Donor Register (ODR). The total number of people who have registered membership on the ODR on March 2010 was 17,077,105. A useful web site is: http://www.nhsbt.nhs.uk/index.html.

Your ED will have links with a transplant team who would be responsible for retrieving donated organs, and you are advised to read the local policy within the ED regarding organ donation. The law in this area is guided by the Human Tissue Act 2004, and this Act clarifies that organs may be removed from a donor if advanced permission has been given. If no such consent is available then consent from family members will be sought.

Quick Quiz

1. Which statement regarding a patient's culture and his hospitalisation experience is true?

    A. Culture affects a patient's experience during hospitalisation because the patient has to adapt to the hospital culture.

    B. Culture doesn't affect the patient's hospitalisation.

    C. Cultural factors can affect patient and family roles during illness.

    D. Culture rarely impacts decisions about health.

Answer: C. Cultural factors can have a major impact on patient and family roles during illness. Culture affects the patient's and family members' feelings about illness, pain and end-of-life issues, among other things.

2. Factors that can impact an emergency patient's cognitive function include:
- A. medications.
- B. health condition.
- C. sleep disturbances.
- D. all of the above.

Answer: D. All of these factors can impact the patient's cognitive function while in the ED.

3. An adult may not refuse treatment if:
- A. he/she has have religious objections to it.
- B. he/she just don't want the treatment.
- C. the treatment is for a mental disorder, and the patient is detained under the Mental Act (1983, amended 2007).
- D. he/she lacks mental capacity (Mental Capacity Act 2005)

Answer: C and D would be occasions when a patient would be given treatment without his/her consent. A and B are acceptable reasons to refuse treatment provided the patient has mental capacity.

Scoring

☆☆☆   If you answered all three questions correctly, jump for joy! You get the importance of holistic care issues.

☆☆   If you answered two questions correctly, we won't issue a complaint! You're ready to join the team.

☆   If you answered fewer than two questions correctly, don't worry; it isn't an ethical dilemma! Just review the chapter and try again.

Initial assessment in emergency departments

3

Just the facts

In this chapter, you'll learn:

♦ The assessment process

♦ Ways to control pain

♦ Special consideration to assessment

Emergency essentials

What comes to mind when you hear the word *emergency*? Do you think of a road traffic collision (RTC), a drowning or a patient with cardiac arrest coming through the doors of the emergency department (ED)? Or, do you visualise a postoperative patient experiencing respiratory distress or a patient falling while trying to walk to the bathroom? Emergencies occur everywhere. No matter what your area of expertise is, you'll encounter emergencies in your nursing career. This section will give an overview of assessing emergency situations and your role in responding to patients who need your help.

Triage

Triage is an assessment process which prioritises patient care according to the urgency of the patient's condition. It should be performed by an experienced competent emergency nurse. It is used to ensure that each patient receives care appropriate to his need in a timely manner and is a means of quickly identifying and treating those patients with more serious conditions. No patient should spend more than 4 hours from arrival in ED, to admission, transfer or discharge. In all EDs, patients who need life-saving treatment should be seen immediately. Other patients can wait up to 10 minutes to be seen and assessed by an experienced emergency nurse. The triage nurse must be able to rapidly assess the nature and urgency of problems for many patients and prioritise their care based on that assessment. Some people will present multiple problems, which the nurse must assess and categorise, making a decision based on the most serious complaint. Most EDs that use triage in the UK base their assessment on a five-tier principal system.

For example, if a cardiac arrest patient arrives in ED he will be assessed and prioritised as either an immediate, red or 1, depending on the specific tool used within different departments. Fundamentally, they all mean the same: this specific patient will wait 0 minutes before being seen by a doctor.

Number	Name	Colour	Maximum time (minutes)
1	Immediate	Red	0
2	Very urgent	Orange	10
3	Urgent	Yellow	60
4	Standard	Green	120
5	Nonurgent	Blue	240

The role of triage also includes the assessment from ambulance control informing the receiving department of a patient requiring immediate emergency care. Triage assessment of the patient should start before the patient arrives. By gathering essential information from ambulance control, the triage nurse can prioritise the patient and alert all the appropriate medical specialties to attend ED and carry out further assessment when the patient arrives.

How do you do it

It is a common practice that ED nurses get the training and experience in performing triage and are assessed in being competent before they carry out such an important element of patient assessment. As you perform triage, tell the patients you interview that you're the triage nurse and that you'll be performing an assessment. Be attentive to what's occurring beyond your current assessment, because it may be necessary to leave the patient if a patient with a more critical situation arrives in the ED.

Carefully document the patient's chief complaint and the vital signs if necessary, your triage assessment and the triage category to which you've assigned him. It's also important to document pertinent negatives. For example, if the patient is experiencing chest pain without cardiac symptoms, be sure to note 'patient complains of nonradiating left-sided chest pain, denies shortness of breath, sweating or nausea. Pain increases with movement and deep inspiration'. Quote the patient when appropriate.

Manchester triage

The Manchester triage approach was developed from 1994 onwards to formalise a standard of triage. The system relies on a list of presenting complaints, each with it's own flowchart. Within the flowchart are discriminators to determine the priority of the presenting complaint. A list of possible presenting complaints are:

Abdominal pain in adults	Falls
Abdominal pain in children	Fits
Abscesses and local infections	Foreign bodies
Allergy	Gastrointestinal bleeding
Apparently drunk	Headache
Assault	Head injury
Asthma	Irritable child
Back pain	Limb problems
Behaving strangely	Limping child
Bites and stings	Major trauma
Burns and scalds	Mental illness
Chest pain	Neck pain
Collapsed adult	Overdose and poisoning
Crying baby	Palpitations
Dental problems	Pregnancy
Diabetes	Per vaginum (vaginal bleeding)
Diarrhoea and vomiting	Rashes
Ear problems	Self-harm
Exposure to chemicals	Sexually acquired infection
Eye problems	Shortness of breath in adults
Facial problems	Shortness of breath in children
Sore throat	Unwell child
Testicular pain	Urinary problems
Torso injury	Worried parent
Unwell adult	Wounds

Atypical flowchart:

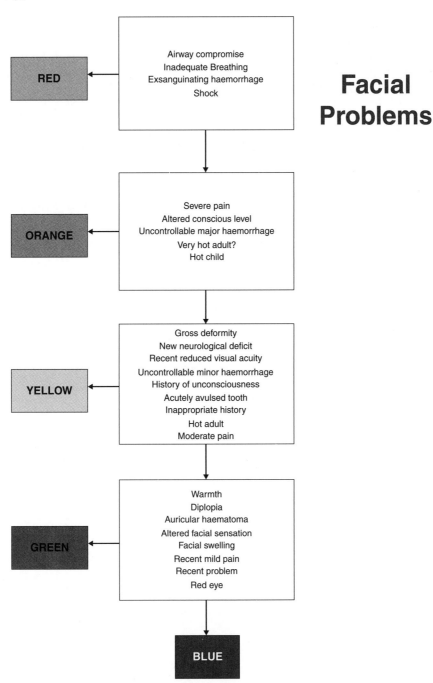

Facial Problems

RED
- Airway compromise
- Inadequate Breathing
- Exsanguinating haemorrhage
- Shock

ORANGE
- Severe pain
- Altered conscious level
- Uncontrollable major haemorrhage
- Very hot adult?
- Hot child

YELLOW
- Gross deformity
- New neurological deficit
- Recent reduced visual acuity
- Uncontrollable minor haemorrhage
- History of unconsciousness
- Acutely avulsed tooth
- Inappropriate history
- Hot adult
- Moderate pain

GREEN
- Warmth
- Diplopia
- Auricular haematoma
- Altered facial sensation
- Facial swelling
- Recent mild pain
- Recent problem
- Red eye

BLUE

SOAPE

The SOAPE model can be used to assess patients and assist the experienced triage nurse in prioritising patient care.

- **S** is for subjective: take a subjective history from the patient, relative or anyone that can provide information about the patient problem.
- **O** is for objective assessment: e.g. – examining a wound, palpating a potential fracture site, consideration for any suspicious injuries, judging if the injuries match the alleged mechanism of injury.
- **A** is for assessment: depending on the information you gain from the subjective and objective assessments as well as other information, e.g. vital signs, you can make a decision on what initial treatment can be implemented, e.g. any first aid measures or analgesia.
- **P** is for prioritise: the patient can then be given a priority or moved to a clinical area where further assessment can be carried out. Patients should be seen within their priority time.
- **E** is for evaluate: triage is dynamic, all initial treatment to patients should be evaluated and patients should be reviewed on a regular basis by the triage nurse until the patient is seen by an appropriate practitioner.

Stay in touch

Maintain communication with patients waiting to be summoned to a treatment room because a patient's status may change – improving or worsening – during an extended period in the waiting room. Ensure that advice and information is given to the patient of his triage category, expected waiting time and update him with any potential delays. Patients appreciate information on the reasons for waiting room delays.

Ambulance triage

When a patient arrives in the ED by ambulance, it's important to get as much information as you can from the prehospital care providers. For instance, if the patient was involved in an incident resulting in an injury, you'll want to know certain information.

Danger details

- How did the incident occur?
- What type of incident was it?
- If it was an RTC, did the vehicle sustain exterior or interior damage?
- What was the speed of the vehicle?
- Was the airbag activated?

Patient particulars

- Was the patient restrained?
- Did the patient have to be extricated from the vehicle?

- Was the patient ambulatory at the scene?
- If the patient sustained a burn injury, was he found in an enclosed space?
- If the burn resulted from a fire, was the fire accompanied by an explosion?

Injuries sustained

- What injuries have the prehospital care providers identified or suspected?
- What are the patient's chief complaints?

Vital vitals

- What vital signs have care providers obtained before arriving in the ED?
- What treatment has the patient received and how did he respond?

Systematic systems

All patients with traumatic injuries should be assessed rapidly with a systematic method used consistently for all patients. The Royal College of Surgeons has adopted the Advanced Trauma Nursing Course to teach nurses a systematic method of assessing trauma patients. The method uses primary and secondary surveys to rapidly identify life-threatening emergencies and prioritise care.

Primary survey

The primary survey is to assess and treat life-threatening injuries which follow a systematic review.

The primary survey begins with an assessment of airway, breathing and circulation – the ABCs learned in nurse education. Additional assessment parameters are recommended: neurologic status – designated as *disability (D)* – and exposure and environment – designated as *E*. (See *Primary assessment of the trauma patient*, page 36.) The ABCDE primary survey consists of – you guessed it – five steps.

It is important to know that each potential life-threatening problem should be treated before moving onto the next systematic assessment, e.g. the patient's airway and cervical (c) spine must be maintained before moving onto the assessment of breathing and adequate ventilation. If there is any change in the patient's condition, he or she should be reassessed from the beginning of the review, using ABCDE.

A is for airway with c-spine control

Before you assess a trauma patient's airway, immobilise the c-spine through initial stabilisation and by applying a triple immobilisation technique, including a cervical collar, head blocks and tape. Until proven otherwise, assume that the patient who has sustained a major trauma has a c-spine injury.

When continuing your assessment, note whether the patient can speak; if he can, he has a patent airway. Open the airway of an unresponsive patient with modified jaw thrust or a head tilt-chin-lift if there's no c-spine injury present or suspected. Check for obstructions to the airway, such as the tongue (the most common obstruction), blood, loose teeth/dentures or vomitus. Clear the airway obstructions immediately, using the jaw thrust to maintain c-spine immobilisation. You may need to use suction if blood or vomitus is present.

Primary assessment of the trauma patient

The chart below outlines the parameters for assessing the trauma patients along with their associated assessment steps and appropriate interventions.

Parameter	Assessment	Interventions
A = airway and c-spine control	• Airway patency	• Institute cervical spine immobilisation until X-rays or other imaging requests determine whether the patient has a cervical spine injury • Position the patient • To open the airway, make sure that the neck is midline and stabilised; next, perform the jaw-thrust manoeuvre.
B = breathing and ventilation	• Respirations (rate, depth, effort) • Breath sounds • Chest wall movement and chest injury • Position of trachea (midline or deviation)	• Administer 100% via a reservoir bag mask • Use airway adjuncts, such as a correctly sized nasopharyngeal airway (this is contraindicated in patients with severe head or facial injuries because of the possibility of insertion into brain tissue) or an oropharyngeal airway, endotracheal tube, cricothyrotomy, as indicated • Suction the patient as needed • Remove foreign bodies that may obstruct breathing • Treat life-threatening conditions, such as tension pneumothorax or pneumothorax.
C = circulation with haemorrhage control	• Pulse and blood pressure • Bleeding or haemorrhage • Capillary refill and colour of skin and mucous membranes • Cardiac rhythm	• Start cardiopulmonary resuscitation, medications and defibrillation or synchronised cardioversion • Control haemorrhaging with direct pressure or pneumatic devices • Establish I.V. access and fluid therapy (isotonic fluids and blood) • Treat life-threatening conditions, such as cardiac tamponade.
D = disability: neurologic status	• Neurologic assessment, including level of consciousness, pupils and motor and sensory function	• Institute cervical spine immobilisation until X-rays confirm the absence of cervical spine injury.
E = exposure and environment	• Environmental exposure (extreme cold or heat) and injuries	• Examine the patient to determine the extent of injuries • Institute appropriate therapy determined by environmental exposure (warming therapy for hypothermia or cooling therapy for hyperthermia).

Insert an appropriate airway adjunct, such as a nasopharyngeal or oropharyngeal airway if necessary; however, remember that an oropharyngeal airway can be used only on an unconscious patient. An oropharyngeal airway stimulates the gag reflex in a conscious or semiconscious patient. If a nasopharyngeal or oropharyngeal airway fails to provide a patent airway, the patient may require intubation.

B is for breathing with adequate ventilation

Assess the patient for spontaneous respirations, noting his rate, depth and symmetry. Obtain oxygen saturation with pulse oximetry. Is he using accessory muscles to breathe? Do you hear breath sounds bilaterally? Do you detect tracheal deviation or jugular vein distention? Does the patient have an open chest wound? All major trauma patients require high-flow oxygen. If the patient doesn't have spontaneous respirations or if his breathing is ineffective, ventilate him by using a bag-valve-mask device until intubation can be achieved.

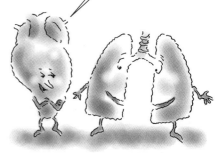

All right: just because the primary survey puts airway and breathing before circulation doesn't mean you can gloat.

C is for circulation with haemorrhage control

What's his skin colour? Does he exhibit pallor, flushing or some other discoloration? What's his skin temperature? Is it warm, cool or clammy to the touch? Is the patient sweating? Is there any obvious bleeding? Look and assess for internal bleeding to the chest, abdomen, pelvis or long bones. Check for the presence of peripheral pulses. Determine the patient's blood pressure. All major trauma patients need at least two large-bore I.V. lines because they may require large amounts of fluids and blood. A fluid warmer should be used if possible. If the patient exhibits external bleeding, apply direct pressure over the site. The patient may require surgery if internal bleeding is noted. If he has no pulse, initiate cardiopulmonary resuscitation immediately.

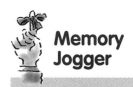

Memory Jogger

A Very **P**ractical **U**se (AVPU):

A = **A**lert, oriented patient
V = responds to **V**oice
P = responds to **P**ain
U = **U**nresponsive patient

D is for disability – neurological status

Perform a quick neurologic assessment by using the acronym AVPU. You may need to use the more in-depth Glasgow Coma Scale tool to assess the patient's baseline status. Obtain a blood sugar sample as a low reading may indicate reduced level of consciousness. Maintain c-spine immobilisation until X-rays or other imaging requests confirm that there's no cervical injury. If the patient isn't alert and oriented, conduct further assessments during the secondary survey.

E is for exposure and environment

Expose the patient to perform a thorough assessment. Remove all clothing to assess his injuries. Remember: if the patient has knife tears or bullet holes through his clothing, don't cut through these areas. The police will count on you to preserve evidence as necessary. Environmental control means keeping the patient warm. If you've removed the patient's clothes, cover him with warm blankets. You may need to use a warming device, especially with an infant or a small child. Use fluid warmers when administering large amounts of I.V. fluids. A cold patient has numerous problems with haemodynamics and healing.

Remember that the primary ABCDE survey is a rapid assessment intended to identify life-threatening emergencies that must be treated before assessment continues.

Secondary survey

After the primary survey is completed, perform and document a more detailed secondary survey, which includes a head-to-toe assessment. This part of the examination identifies all injuries sustained by the patient. At this time, a care plan is developed and diagnostic tests are ordered.

Attach a cardiac monitor and obtain a full set of vital signs initially, including respirations, pulse, blood pressure and temperature. If you suspect chest trauma, record blood pressures in both arms.

Pain control issues

Because pain is a major concern for many emergency patients, pain management is an important part of your care. Emergency patients are exposed to many types of procedures – such as an intravenous cannula, wound care or fracture manipulation that causes discomfort and pain. Pain is classified as acute or chronic.

Acute pain

Acute pain is caused by tissue damage due to injury or disease. It varies in intensity from mild to severe and lasts briefly. Acute pain is considered a protective mechanism because it warns of present or potential tissue damage or organ disease. It may result from a traumatic injury, surgical or diagnostic procedure or medical disorder.

Examples include:
- Pain experienced after a traumatic injury
- Pain experienced during invasive procedures
- Pain of acute myocardial infarction.

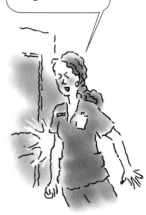

It isn't cute when it happens, but acute pain warns of potential tissue damage or organ disease.

Help is at hand

Acute pain can be managed effectively with interventions, such as positioning and splintage, also from analgesics, such as opioids, nonsteroidal anti-inflammatory drugs and Entonox gas. It generally subsides when the underlying problem is resolved.

Chronic pain

Chronic pain is ongoing pain that lasts 6 months or longer. It may be as intense as acute pain but isn't a warning of tissue damage. Some patients in the ED experience chronic as well as acute pain.

Examples of chronic pain include:
- Arthritis pain
- Chronic back pain
- Chronic pain from cancer.

Don't be fooled

The nervous system adapts to chronic pain. This adaptation means that many typical manifestations of pain – such as abnormal vital signs and facial grimacing – cease to exist. Therefore, chronic pain should be assessed as often as acute pain (generally, at least every 2 hours or more often, depending on the patient's condition). Assess chronic pain by questioning the patient.

Pain assessment

When it comes to pain assessment for emergency patients, it's especially important for the nurse to have good assessment skills. The most valid pain assessment comes from the patient's own reports.

A pain assessment includes questions about:
- *Location*. Ask the patient to tell you where the pain is; there may be more than one area of pain
- *Intensity*. Ask the patient to rate the pain using a pain scale
- *Quality*. Ask how the pain feels: sharp, dull, aching or burning
- *Onset, duration and frequency*. Ask when the pain started, how long it lasts and how often it occurs
- *Alleviating and aggravating factors*. Ask what makes the pain feel better and what makes it worse
- *Associated factors*. Ask whether other problems are associated with the pain, such as nausea and vomiting
- *Effects on lifestyle*. Ask whether appetite, sleep, relationships, emotions and work are affected.

Choose a tool

Many pain assessment tools are available. Whichever you choose, make sure it's used consistently so that everyone on the health care team is speaking the same language when addressing the patient's pain.

The three most common pain assessment tools used by clinicians are the visual analog scale, numeric rating scale and faces scale. (See *common pain-rating scales*, page 41.)

Silent suffering

Many patients can't verbally express feelings of pain. For example, a patient may be unable to speak because of intubation or have an altered level of consciousness ranging from confusion to unresponsiveness. In such cases, it's up to the nurse to ascertain the patient's pain level.

Body and mind

There are many physiologic and psychological responses to pain that a nurse should watch for during a pain assessment.

Some examples of the physiologic responses to pain are:
- Tachycardia
- Tachypnoea
- Dilated pupils
- Increased or decreased blood pressure
- Pallor
- Nausea and vomiting
- Loss of appetite
  Psychological responses to pain may manifest as:
- Fear
- Anxiety
- Confusion
- Depression
- Sleep deprivation.

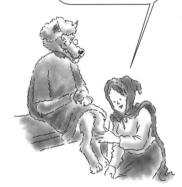

My, what a strange pallor you have, Grandmal. Are you sure you aren't in any pain?

Pain particulars

When communicating aspects of a patient's pain to other health care providers, make sure you:
- Describe the pain by location, intensity and duration
- Indicate possible causes of the pain if known
- Describe how the patient is responding to the pain or any treatment interventions.

Pain management

Achieving adequate pain control in the ED depends on effective pain assessment, effective re-evaluation of the intervention used to relieve the pain, the use of pharmacologic and nonpharmacologic treatments and essential documentation.

To provide the best holistic care possible, work with the doctor and other members of the health care team to develop an individualised pain management programme for each patient.

Common pain-rating scales

These common pain-rating scales are examples of the rating systems you can use to help a patient quantify pain levels.

Visual analog scale

To use the visual analog scale, ask the patient to place a line across the scale to indicate the current level of pain. The scale is a 10-cm line with 'No pain' at one end and 'Pain as bad as it can be' at the other end. The pain rating is determined by using a ruler to measure the distance, in millimeters, from 'No pain' to the patient's mark.

No pain | Pain as bad as it can be

Numeric rating scale

To use the numeric rating scale, ask the patient to choose a number from 0 (indicating no pain) to 10 (indicating the worst pain imaginable) to indicate his current pain level. The patient may circle the number on the scale or verbally state the number that best describes the pain.

No pain | 0   1   2   3   4   5   6   7   8   9   10 | Pain as bad as it can be

Faces scale

A paediatric or adult patient with language or cognitive difficulty may not be able to describe the current pain level using the visual analog scale or the numeric rating scale. In that case, use a face scale like the one below. Ask your patient to choose the face on a scale from 1 to 6 that best represents the severity of current pain.

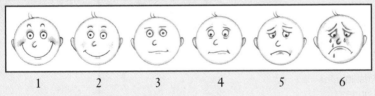

1   2   3   4   5   6

Pain management

All patients requiring pain relief need to be assessed with consideration to their physiological, emotional and psychological status. All individuals have different pain thresholds depending on influencing factors, such as:
- Nature of their injury/pain
- Environmental factors, e.g. losing their belongings in a house fire
- Their perception of pain.

Therefore, it is important to consider all methods of pain relief; some include:
- Reassurance for emotional and psychological help
- Universal analgesia (see pharmacologic pain management)
- Immobilisation of a limb (e.g. splints or plaster of Paris).

Nonpharmacologic pain management

Pain control isn't achieved solely with medications. Nonpharmacologic means are useful adjuncts in managing pain. Some common nonpharmacologic pain control methods are:

- Positioning the patient
- Splinting the affected limb
- Distraction – such as television viewing and reading
- Imagery – in which the patient visualises a soothing image while the nurse describes pleasant sensations (e.g. the patient may picture himself at the beach, while you describe the sounds of the waves and birds and the feel of the warm sun and a breeze on the patient's skin)
- Heat application (thermotherapy) – application of dry or moist heat to decrease pain (heat enhances blood flow, increases tissue metabolism and decreases vasomotor tone; it may also relieve pain because of muscle aches or spasms, itching or joint pain)
- Cold application (cryotherapy) – constricts blood vessels at the injury site, reducing blood flow to the site (Cold slows oedema development, prevents further tissue damage and minimises bruising; it may be more effective than heat in relieving such pain as muscle aches or spasms, itching, incision pain, headaches and joint pain)
- Relaxation therapy – a form of meditation used to focus attention on a single sound or image or on the rhythm of breathing.

Pharmacologic pain management

Local anaesthetic nerve block

This method of pain relief uses a local anaesthetic drug that reversibly blocks the transmission of nerve impulses. It can be used as an alternative or as well as systemic analgesics. Anatomical areas where this maybe effective are:

- Digital nerve block for fingers and wrist injuries
- Nerve blocks for forehead and ear injuries
- Dental anaesthesia
- Femoral nerve block for fractured shaft of femur
- Optical anaesthesia.

Inhalation analgesia

A common route of quick, short-acting pain medication administration in the ED is Entonox®. Entonox® is a mixture of 50% oxygen and 50% nitrous oxide. The patient needs to be alert, have the understanding, cognitive ability and coordination in order to self-administer this analgesia through a face mask or a mouthpiece and it can be an extremely effective method of pain relief in procedures such as:

- Reduction of dislocations or fractures
- Wound dressings
- Application of splints.

Other pharmacologic pain management

Other pharmacologic pain management common in EDs are:
- Nonopioids
- Opioids
- Adjuvant medications.

Nonopioids

Nonopioids are the first choice for managing mild pain. They decrease pain by inhibiting inflammation at the injury site. Examples of nonopioids are:

- Paracetamol
- Nonsteroidal anti-inflammatory drugs, such as ibuprofen
- Salicylates, such as aspirin.

Opioid option

A common route of pain medication administration in the ED is by I.V. bolus on an as-needed basis. It's the preferred route for opioid therapy. The benefit of this method is rapid pain control. On the downside, with I.V. bolus administration the patient can experience alternating periods of pain control and pain.

Opioids are narcotics that contain a derivative of the opium (poppy) plant and other synthetic drugs that imitate natural opioids. Opioids work by blocking the release of neurotransmitters involved in transmitting pain signals to the brain. There are three categories of opioids:

- Opioid agonists (opioid analgesics)
- Opioid antagonists (opioid reversal agents)
- Mixed agonist-antagonists.

Opioid agonists

Opioid agonists relieve pain by binding to pain receptors which, in effect, produce pain relief. Examples of opioid agonists are:

- Morphine
- Fentanyl
- Codeine.

Opioid antagonists

Opioid antagonists are used, if necessary, to reverse the effects of opioid overdose. They attach to opiate receptors without producing agonistic effects. They work by displacing the opioid at the receptor site and reversing the analgesic and respiratory depressant effects of the opioid. After the administration of an opioid antagonist you may observe withdrawal symptoms within minutes but the effect will subside in approximately 2 hours depending on the dose of the opioid antagonist and the amount and type of opioid administered.

An example of opioid antagonist is:

- Naloxone (Narcan).

(continued)

Mixed opioid agonist-antagonists

Mixed opioid agonist-antagonists, such as Temgesic (Buprenorphine), relieve pain by binding to opiate receptors to effect varying degrees of agonistic and antagonistic activity. They carry a lower risk of toxic effects and drug dependency than opioid agonists and opioid antagonists.

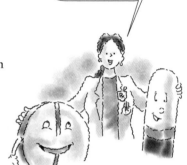

Adjuvant analgesics work alone or with a partner to help alleviate chronic pain.

Adjuvants are alright

Adjuvant analgesics are drugs that have other primary indications but are used as analgesics in some circumstances. Adjuvants may be given in combination with opioids or alone to treat patients with chronic pain. Drugs used as adjuvant analgesics include:
- Anticonvulsants, such as carbamazepine (Tegretol) and clonazepam
- Tricyclic antidepressants, such as amitriptyline
- Benzodiazepines, such as diazepam (Valium) and lorazepam
- Corticosteroids, such as dexamethasone.

Continue trauma management

Initiate cardiac monitoring.

Obtain continuous pulse oximetry readings. Be aware, however, that readings may be inaccurate if the patient is cold, has smoke inhalation/carbon monoxide poisoning or is in shock.

Consider the need to insert a urinary catheter to monitor accurate intake and output measurements. Many urinary catheters also record core body temperatures. Don't insert a urinary catheter if there's blood at the urinary meatus.

Consider the need to insert a nasogastric (NG) tube for stomach decompression. Injuries such as a facial fracture contraindicate the use of an NG tube; if a facial fracture is suspected, insert the tube orally instead. Depending on your department's policy and procedures, an anaesthetist may place an NG tube in an intubated patient under direct vision using a laryngoscope.

Obtain laboratory studies as ordered, such as type and crossmatching for blood; a full blood cell count and haemoglobin level; toxicology and alcohol screens, if indicated; a pregnancy test, if necessary and serum electrolyte levels.

Warning – patient at risk (PAR)

The triage nurse will make her assessment and assist in transferring the patient to the most appropriate environment within the department. However, if the patient is prioritised as a high priority such as category 1 or 2, strict monitoring and continual assessment should be continued.

Monitoring of the patient's condition, including his vital signs, will assist the nurse in the warning of a patient deteriorating. Some EDs have implemented early warning systems to assist in patients who are potentially at risk of deteriorating. This will include regular assessment of respiratory rate, neurological status, heart rate, systolic blood pressure and the patient's age. Points are allocated to individual observations and placed against a variation of acceptable ranges. The overall score is then used to alert the nurse of any deterioration. Although there are different adapted versions of patient at risk charts, in principle, they all do one thing – inform the nurse of how ill the patient is and whom to inform if the patient deteriorates.

An example for an adult:

	4	2	1	0	1	2	4
Heart rate/min	<40		41–50	51–100	101–110	111–129	>130
Systolic blood pressure (mm Hg)	<80 or unrecordable	81–90	91–99		>200		Unrecordable
Respiration rate/min	<9			10–14	15–20	21–29	>30
Oxygen SATs	<90	<93	<95				
Altered conscious level (AVPU)				Alert	Voice/confused	Pain	Unresponsive
Age				<71	>71		

If the patient scores >12, a cardiac arrest call should be made.
If the score is between 8 and 11, an urgent call (fast bleep) to the ED doctor should be made and review carried out urgently.
If the score is between 4 and 7, the ED doctor/senior nurse should be informed and a review of the patient should be made as soon as possible.

PAR >3 increase observations of vital signs to 4 hourly.
PAR >4 increase observations of vital signs to 1 hourly.
PAR >5 increase observations of vital signs to ½ hourly.

Reproduced with permission from: Abertawe Bro Morgannwg (ABM) University Health Board copyright 2010.

These early warning charts should NOT replace the nurses' experience and professional judgment of the patient's condition but used as an adjunct to the assessment and clinical decision-making process.

Family matters

Facilitate the presence of the patient's family. Many departments endorse the practice of allowing the patient's family to be present during resuscitation. It's important, however, to assess the family's needs before offering permission to be present. Family members may need emotional and spiritual support from you or from a member of the clergy. If a family member wishes to be present during resuscitation, assign a health care professional to explain procedures as they're performed.

A little tender loving care (TLC)

During a trauma situation, the urgency of the assessment and treatment processes may cause you to overlook the patient's fears. Remember to talk to the patient and explain the examination and interventions being administered. An encouraging word and tone can go a long way to comfort and calm a frightened patient. Comfort measures also include splintage, the administration of pain medication and sedation as needed.

Memory jogger

The acronym SAMPLE is a mnemonic that will help you remember the types of information you'll need to obtain for the patient's history.

Subjective: What does the patient say? How did the incident occur? Does he remember? What symptoms does he report?

Allergies: Does the patient have allergies and, if so, what's he allergic to? Is he wearing a medical identification bracelet?

Medications: Does the patient take medications on a regular basis and, if so, what medications? What medications has he taken in the past 24 hours?

Past medical history: Has the patient been treated for medical conditions and, if so, which ones? Has he had surgery and if so, what type of surgery?

Last meal eaten, **L**ast tetanus vaccination, **L**ast menstruation: When was the last time the patient had anything to eat or drink? When did he have his most recent tetanus? (If unknown, follow guidelines and maybe he will need to have one administered in the ED.) If the patient is a female of childbearing age, when was her last menstruation? Could she be pregnant?

Events leading to injury: How did the incident occur? Inquire about precipitating factors, if any. For instance, the patient being seen for injuries sustained in a RTC may have had the incident because he experienced a myocardial infarction while driving. Likewise, the patient who sustained a fall might have fallen because he tripped or became dizzy.

History counts

Obtain the patient's history, remembering to obtain as much information as possible to determine the presence of coexisting conditions, or alcohol or drug use that could affect his care or factors that might have precipitated the trauma.

Next, perform a head-to-toe assessment, starting at the patient's head and working your way down to his feet. Don't forget to check all posterior surfaces. You should be competent in logrolling the patient to assess for injuries to the back. Address life-threatening injuries immediately.

Transport

Patients who are hospitalised rarely stay in their ward for their entire visit; they're transported for diagnostic tests, procedures and surgery. The ED patient is no different. Transferring a patient can be a dangerous experience, e.g. it could cause malfunctioning of the equipment, tubes becoming dislodged and trapped, intravenous infusions running out, changes to bodily function and movement of life-saving equipment. Trauma patients can experience either an interhospital or an intrafacility transport journey.

Not so simple

Moving a patient from one place to another sounds simple. However, it isn't quite so easy when a patient is haemodynamically unstable, has airway or respiratory compromise, requires continuous cardiac monitoring, continuous infusion of I.V. fluids or medications or has an artificial airway or mechanical ventilation. In these instances, patients must be accompanied by an RN who's trained and prepared to handle any emergency situation that can happen.

Before any transport, the patient's condition must be reassessed to ensure his safety.

Interhospital transport

An *interhospital transport* is one that moves the patient from the ED to another health care facility. Interhospital transport happens on the ground with a paramedic ambulance or critical care transport, or by air (usually by helicopter).

ED on wheels (or wings)

Interhospital transport vehicles are like EDs on wheels. They can safely handle the transport of critically ill patients and are staffed with specially trained paramedics.

Movin' out

Trauma patients are moved from their original hospital to another for several reasons. The patient may be moved because he requires a higher level of medical care or special services not offered at the receiving hospital. Alternately, if the patient no longer requires specialised care he may be moved because of family or patient convenience.

Cha-ching

Interhospital transport doesn't come without a price. Air transport can be very costly in more ways than one; it's expensive, and helicopters can land only at approved heliport pads. This mode of travel usually requires the patient to be transported via an ambulance to the helicopter and then from the helicopter to the hospital. This loading and unloading can cause the patient unneeded stress. Its advantage is the ability to land at the scene of an incident and at hospitals equipped with heliport pads.

Intrafacility transport

An *intrafacility transport* involves transporting the patient from the ED to another area of the receiving hospital such as an inpatient unit, the X-ray or imaging department or the operating room.

Communication

Regardless of which type of transport the patient requires, communication is vital to the patient's survival in coming to your hospital, going to another hospital or just moving within your facility. Complete documentation of the patient's condition, procedures, laboratory test results, monitoring parameters and medications is paramount.

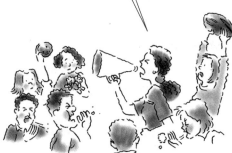

Communication is key during patient transport! Of course, it's a lot easier when someone is actually listening to you!

All in the know

Medication understanding should occur whenever a patient moves from one location to another.

When giving report about a patient, be sure to include:
- The patient's name, age, allergies, weight, medical history and daily medications
- When the current symptoms first occurred
- When the patient first arrived in the ED
- Critical laboratory values
- Diagnostic and interventional procedures that the patient received
- Intravenous sites and size of catheters as well as fluids infusing, rate of infusion and dose of any added medications
- Medications given to the patient and his response
- Endotracheal tube size (if the patient is intubated); depth of insertion and ventilator settings
- The patient's vital signs.

Family matters

Make sure that the patient's family is kept informed of plans to transport him. A traumatic event is stressful enough for the family, and being kept abreast of the patient's condition as well as plans for transporting him may help allay the patient's and his family's fears. The patient's condition ultimately dictates treatment.

Special consideration to assessment

The older adult

As with all patients attending EDs, the physical, psychological and social needs of the patient need to be thoroughly assessed. It is extremely important to gain as much history as possible from the patient, carers or ambulance personnel. Once the patient is referred by the paramedic the information can be easily lost. Listening to handover from paramedic crews regarding state of accommodation and relationships between family members during transit can have a significant effect on your care decisions for all vulnerable people, including the older person.

As people get older their general bodily function deteriorates, initiating the person to try to adapt to his or her ongoing lifestyle changes. However, some people are unaware of their deteriorating functions and may need assistance in recognising their need for support with their activities of daily living (ADL). Everyone ages at a different speed, but eventually the ageing process affects all body organs and systems.

Focused history

As with all consultations, they should be focused and carried out holistically. Although the older person may require some special consideration to his or her assessment:
- Be prepared to spend more time on your assessment
- Assess the individual's ability to carry out his or her ADL – does he or she require help?
- Be patient and explain things slowly and clearly
- You may want to include the family – they will know the individual better than you.

Physical examination: challenges

The ageing process presents the assessment of the older person with some degree of difficulty compared with someone younger:
- Patient often has coexisting illnesses
- Loss of pain sensation may obscure findings
- The older person will often wear several layers of clothing, which can be difficult to remove

- Must be handled gently to avoid additional injury
- Other underlining problems can be taken too lightly because of ambiguous presenting problems/complaints.

As we get older the ability to cope with ADL and physiological stress reduces. This can also have an effect on how we are cared for depending on how society or other individuals perceive the older person. When assessing the older adult you should consider some physiological changes that might affect his or her treatment or care management; some of these are:

- Reduced or loss of muscle strength
- Degeneration of bones and joints
- Eye problems, e.g. cataracts
- Reduced sensitivity, e.g. touch, pain and temperature
- Cerebral atrophy causing confusion.

Watch the pill

Be vigilant of the medication that the older person may be taking. Medication such as beta blockers, analgesia and diuretics will all have side effects that would have an effect on his body function, may affect his presenting complaint and subsequent further treatment.

Abuse

Unfortunately, EDs will treat an older person who has been subjected to some form of abuse. This may be difficult for the nurse to become aware of because abuse is sometimes blurred by the presenting injury or illness but it should always be a part of the assessment of any patient, especially the older patient. There are many forms of abuse, such as:

- Psychological – the patient may be quiet, letting the carer speak for the patient, they may show signs of anxiety, unexplained fidgeting, etc
- Physical – bruising, new or healing wounds, unusual fractures (fractures that don't match the mechanism of injury)
- Financial – carer keeping assets/money
- Sexual – unexplained vaginal discharge, sexually transmitted diseases, bruising around perineal area
- Neglect – loss of hearing aid/glasses, undernourished/dehydrated, unkempt/smelling.

The emergency nurse should be vigilant to this possibility, ensuring good communication with primary and community care; they must also be aware of local vulnerable adult protection policies and adhere to departmental guidelines.

Further advice on this topic may be obtained from:

http://www.dh.gov.uk/en/AdvanceSearchResult/index.htm?searchTerms=older+abuse

Is this vital

Body temperature

There's no real difference in the core body temperature of an older person. However, older people find it more difficult to regulate their body temperature and they tend to wear large amounts of layers of clothing in order to feel warm. They could potentially overheat due to the fact that they have a reduced ability to perspire. The older person is therefore at risk of hyper/hypothermia. Even moderate elevations or subnormal temperatures can be an indication for concern, especially when associated with confusion, loss of appetite or other behavioural changes.

It is difficult for the nurse to establish whether the older person has an infection because of his or her inability to reach a high temperature; therefore, it is essential for the nurse to take into account other vital signs and symptoms.

Respiratory rate

The respiratory rate does not change as we get older but the lung function decreases slightly and may cause some breathing problems from conditions, such as chronic obstructive pulmonary disease.

Heart rate

An older person's heart rate takes longer to increase when exercising and longer to slow back down after exercise. You need to be aware that if an older person has walked to the department, this should be taken into account.

Blood pressure

A gradual rise in systolic pressure over the years is normal and is often asymptomatic until severe complications are noted (i.e. stroke/heart attack).

Postural hypotension is experienced by some older people. They feel dizzy when they stand up too quickly. This is due to their blood pressure dropping suddenly leading to a disruption in the autonomic nervous system. As a result, systems like circulation and breathing can be significantly affected.

They may experience other primary cardiac problems that may contribute to falls or feeling generally unwell, such as:
- Hypertension
- Bradycardia
- Cardiac arrhythmias such as atrial fibrillation.

Psychological

A decline in overall well-being can occur from the effects of ageing:
- Increased health problems
- Death or dying of a spouse or friend
- Loss of support
- Reduced independence
- Increase in alcohol or drug abuse
- Depression
- Loss of self-worth
- Inability to work
- Increased financial burden.

Children and young adults

The key element of assessing this age group is to understand the physiological and psychological changes that occur with each stage of development. The stages of development can be broken down into seven groups:
- Newborn – birth to the first few hours
- Neonate – birth to 1 month
- Infancy – birth to 1 year
- Toddler – 1 to 3 years
- Preschool – 3 to 5 years
- School age – 5 to 12 years
- Adolescent (teenager) – 13 to 18 years.

A full assessment should be carried out as normal but if possible, you should also gain information from the parents/guardian as well as the child.

The assessment should be carried out observing the interaction between the child and parents/carers, and any sign of abuse should be acted upon with consultation of other colleagues and other health professionals.

If the parents or carers are not present then you should request that one of the emergency teams tries to contact them or maybe involve the police to help locate them. When there is no responsible adult available, the treatment can be carried out without consent but under 'the patient's best interest' or consent maybe obtained if the child or young person is regarded as 'competent'. A child aged 16 years and older is presumed by law to be competent to give consent himself or herself. (See Chapter 2.)

The assessment should be modified according to the age of the patient and consider the anatomical, cognitive and emotional differences of each group.

Anatomical significances include:
- Larger head size in proportion to the body
- Babies fontanelles can be used as an aid to assessing for dehydration/shock or rising intracranial pressure (ICP)
- Tongue is very large
- Small trachea is more anterior than an adult's airway (increased risk of a foreign body causing an airway obstruction)
- Nose breathers until 6 months (nasal secretions create obstruction)
- Neonates and infants are belly breathers because of immature respiratory muscles.

Toddlers

Keeping the child and the parents calm is a key factor for an accurate assessment and preventing the child from aggravating the current condition or injury. The nurses should be aware of their own facial expressions and body language, as the child will 'hone in' on this type of communication. Depending on how well or badly this is portrayed to the child will depend on the possibility of his or her cooperation towards the nurses and their assessment:
- Smile and talk gently in words that can be understood by the child
- Kneel down to the child's level so that he doesn't feel intimidated

- Demonstrate procedures on a toy or parent or yourself first
- Warm hands prior to touching
- Use distractors while you are assessing the child
- Save unpleasant/invasive procedures for last.

Preschool

This age group should have a basic understanding of communication and should be able to tell/point to what aspect of their body is hurting. Until you achieve a good rapport with the child, depending on home circumstances, he may cling to his or her parent/guardian for security, making assessment difficult. It is very important with this age group to be aware of your actions and of what you say, as they will tend to 'pick up' and 'focus' on mostly everything and anything you say or do.
- Do not lie
- Try and focus everything on the child as nothing else will matter apart from him or her
- Explain each step of your assessment
- They may require comfort from a/their toy.

School-aged child

Assessment can be quite 'tricky' with this age group as they are developing their independence and self-esteem. It is important not for them to feel different from other children and a sense of diplomacy should be adopted. Depending on their level of development the nurse should try to make decisions involving the child and verifying the information with a parent or a caregiver. This will sometimes allow the child to make minor choices and increase his or her sense of control.

Teenagers

This age group should be treated the same as adults with in respect of performing an assessment without their parents. This may not be without tribulations from the parents who may wish to being present, considering that their son or daughter is still their 'little child', but dignity and privacy must still prevail. Try to adopt an empathetic and considerate attitude and seriously listen to what the teenagers say, especially with any 'suicide' threats.

Abuse and neglect

This is an area of major concern which must not be taken lightly. All ED staff should attend safeguarding children updates and should be aware of the local, hospital and departmental policies.

The diagnosis of child abuse can be very complex and false allegations can cause unnecessary pain, suffering and aggression for all who are involved.

Situations like this should be dealt by experienced senior staff. The child could be subjected to any physical, psychological or sexual abuse and it is the nurse, who spends most of the time with the child whilst in ED, who is often in the best position to observe for such circumstances. If abuse or neglect is suspected, it is good practice to assess the siblings too. Some observations include:

- Relationship between the parents/carers and the child
- Different explanations of the mechanism of injury from the child and family/carers
- The mechanism of injury not correlating with the injury
- An injury that is inconsistent with the child development (a newborn falling out of a cot)
- Any fracture to a child younger than 1 year
- Unusual fractures
- Quiet child, letting the parent speak for the child (depending on age)
- Anxiety, unexplained fidgeting, etc
- Unexplained vaginal discharge, sexually transmitted diseases, bruising around perineal area
- Undernourished/dehydrated, unkempt/smelling
- Inappropriate delay in seeking treatment.

Nonaccidental injury should be considered in all patients, including children; if any suspicion of neglect is noted, the local children's services of safeguarding office or social services should be contacted. Be aware of your department's policies.

The care of the child is of paramount importance and he or she should be treated for his or her injuries in the most appropriate manner and location (admission to hospital if needed). If abuse is suspected, the child may also be admitted to the ward while further investigations are carried out and other appropriate professionals, such as the general practitioner (GP)/police/social services are contacted and included into further decisions for the welfare of the child.

For more information on safeguarding children use the following link: http://www.safeguardingchildren.org.uk/Safeguarding-Children/2008-report/Download-the-report#top

Is this vital?

An awareness of the different age group vital sign measurements is needed when assessing children. It is also necessary to have the correct equipment as well as the appropriate sizes of equipment. It may be useful to have the different ranges of measurements for each age group nearby or in a pocket form for easy access. Depending on the development of the child, normally a child aged 12 years and older may have similar recordings to that of an adult.

Temperature

Young children have an immature thermal control mechanism and infants/small children are unable to shiver. Therefore, the temperature of a child is really important as a fever can lead to febrile seizures and serious consequences.

Pulse

It can be quite difficult palpating for a pulse in children. You can obtain an infant pulse by auscultating the apical heartbeat or palpating the brachial or femoral pulses. In older children the radial pulse (same as adults) can be palpated. Guides to the normal ranges are:

- Infant: 120 to 160 bpm
- Toddler: 80 to 130 bpm
- School age: 70 to 110 bpm
- Adolescent: 60 to 100 bpm.

Respiratory rate

To record the respiratory rate you should observe the abdomen in infants and small children. The respiratory rate for the older child can be recorded the same as for adults. Guides to the normal ranges are:

- Infant: 25 to 40 rpm
- Toddler: 20 to 35 rpm
- School age: 15 to 25 rpm
- Adolescent: 10 to 20 rpm.

Blood pressure

Blood pressure can be difficult to obtain in small children because of uncooperativeness, fear and their small anatomy; however, an exact blood pressure reading is not always necessary with most children as the recording of the skin colour, temperature, capillary refill and condition of the child will provide you with a more reliable indicator of the child's circulatory status. Guides to the normal systolic ranges are:

- Infant: 60 to 90 mm Hg
- Toddler: 70 to 100 mm Hg
- School age: 90 to 100 mm Hg
- Adolescent: 95 to 130 mm Hg.

An estimated systolic pressure can be carried out using the following formula:

$$80 + (age \times 2)$$

For an 8-year-old boy:

$$80 + (8 \times 2) = 96 \text{ systolic}$$

Weight

An important factor when assessing children in emergency care is the assessment of the child's weight. Treatment, such as medication, especially analgesia and fluids depends on the weight of the child. It makes life easier if the child is accompanied by the parents or the carer who knows how much the child weighs or indeed if the child is aware himself or herself. However, it can be potentially difficult to achieve the weight of a child who is triply immobilised and cannot stand on a weighing scale. To overcome this, an estimated weight can be carried out using the following formula:

Add 4 to the child's age and then multiply by 2. For example, an 8-year-old boy will be recorded as:

$$(\text{age} + 4) \times 2 = 24\,\text{kg} = (8 + 4) \times 2 = 24\,\text{kg}$$

For further reading: Devitt, P & Thain J (2011) Children's & Young People's Nursing Made Incredibly Easy. UK: Lippincott Williams & Wilkins.

Behavioural/mental health emergencies

The ED is a very difficult environment to assess patients with mental illness because of the complexity of the department and the nature of treating so many patients with so many different problems. You should be aware that the majority of aggressive, violent and strangely behaving patients are not experiencing a psychiatric illness. The same assessment approach should be carried out for everyone including ABCDE, taking a good history (maybe asking the relatives, bystanders or ambulance personnel) and examining the patient.

Recommendations by the Royal College of Psychiatrists state that EDs should have adequate knowledge of mental health issues to achieve an acceptable level of assessment and treatment of patients with mental health presentations.

You should recognise that if you haven't got the specific training to assess mental health patients you should refer any potential patients with mental health issues to the appropriate member of staff.

Nearly all patients attending the ED will attend with some degree of emotional/psychological factor. Some people, with/without a psychiatric history become stressed and overwhelmed or feel that they are 'losing control'. A patient attending ED may already have an underlining medical or psychiatric problem, such as a brain tumour or a personality disorder and acute events can feel like a 'crisis'. Reactions can include:
- Panic attack
- Severe depression
- Anxiety attack
- Paranoia.

Confusion, aggression and disorientation may be caused by other underlying physical problems which need to be investigated and ruled out. For example:
- Infection (chest/urinary tract infection, etc)
- Hypoxia
- Hypoglycaemia
- Renal/liver failure
- Convulsions
- Drugs/alcohol (prescribed or recreational)
- Stroke

- Head trauma
- Hyperparathyroidism.

Once a general examination has been performed and any medical reasons for such behaviour have been ruled out, a psychiatric assessment of the patient should be carried out. The assessment should be carried out by a member of staff with appropriate training (preferably qualified in mental health nursing), who is aware of his or her ability to assess the situation safely and without being threatening. The patient should be free of alcohol to allow for a comprehensive assessment. There should be local policies and guidance in each ED on assessing and treating patients with mental health problems. The department should contact the local mental health team/crisis resolution team and conduct an effective mental health risk assessment. The main priority is to instigate a safe, clinically appropriate treatment plan and transfer from ED. If for some reason this cannot be carried out, the patient should be admitted to a ward/observation area until such assessment can be carried out appropriately.

A guide to a general psychiatric assessment may include:
- What do they look like (appearance)?
- Presenting complaint
- Is their speech coherent?
- History of illness and why the emergency today
- Psychiatric history including any admissions
- Current medication
- Any substance misuse
- Any family psychiatric history
- Social stressors and support mechanisms
- Any previous involvement with police/prison/courts, etc
- What is their mood (depressed, suicidal, aggressive, dangerous)?
- Thoughts (fear, phobias, positive/negative)
- Perceptual abnormality (hallucination, delusion, vagueness)
- Concentration levels
- Awareness of their illness
- Who has referred the patient (self, family, other professional)?
- Social involvement (single or married, housing, etc).

If the assessment requires further investigations, there are a number of options that the nurse can refer to:
- Mental health care team for admission
- Discuss with liaison mental health psychiatrist/nurse/crises resolution team
- GP
- Other voluntary services
- Mental health team for outpatient appointment
- Depending on the appropriate level of risk there can be no follow-up if requested by the patient.

Is this a crisis?

Crisis resolution teams are a service which provides an organisation to manage a mental health crisis within the primary care system as well as organising admissions. The team consists of psychiatrists, psychiatric nurses, social workers, support workers and administrators. Their function is to provide a 24-hour service in order to assess patients, including interventions such as taking medication, counselling and other social/financial advice and devise an appropriate plan of care for intensive home treatment. Crisis resolution teams can offer frequent visits within the community and follow up patients as often as required. The community mental health care team takes over the care once the initial crisis is over.

The triage nurse must ensure that the safety of the patient, the staff and himself is of paramount importance and a triage waiting time is allocated and reflected with this in mind.

For further reading: Evans D & Allen H. (2009) Mental Health Nursing Made Incredibly Easy. UK: Lippincott Williams & Wilkins.

Major incidents

If a major incident is declared, the EDs will normally be notified by ambulance control. However, the EDs may receive an influx of high-priority patients who are brought to the department via other methods of transport other than the ambulance service. This rarely happens, but in situations like this it is the hospital's responsibility to declare a major incident and activate the hospital major incident plan, if they cannot cope with the increase of the number of patients or sometimes the number of high-priority patients. The hospital will then be declared the 'receiving hospital'. Under the Civil Contingency Act 2004, all identified receiving hospitals have a legal requirement to carry out a mock incident annually so that all the staff within the hospital are aware of their duties in such an event occurring. Even though the receiving hospital will be assessing and treating patients from a major incident, they still should be assessing and prioritising other patients that attend the department who have not been involved in the major incident.

Some episodes when major incidents are declared:
- Multiple injuries from RTC
- Sporting events
- Terrorism attack
- Fire/explosion
- Food poisoning
- Chemical inhalation
- Chemicals affecting eyesight
- Natural disasters.

All identified EDs will have their own individual hospital major incident plan. In principal, the ED will be set up to receive priority 1 patients; another part of the hospital will be set up for priority 2 patients and so on. Most priority 4 and 5 patients will more than likely be advised to seek other medical attention, such as their GP.

Even though it may not be the ultimate responsibility of the triage nurse, the department and hospital must maintain an efficient functioning and effective system which includes dealing with security, press, relatives and the general public.

Quick quiz

1. The purpose of triage assessment is to:
    A. Reduce patient complaints.
    B. Find out their personal details.
    C. Prioritise patient care according to their condition.
    D. Attain whether they need to be seen in ED.

Answer: C. An assessment is a process to determine the priority of treatment based on the severity of a patient condition.

2. The priority assessment in a primary survey consists of:
    A. Breathing, airway, circulation, disability, exposure and environment.
    B. Airway, disability, breathing, circulation and exposure.
    C. Airway breathing circulation, environment and disability.
    D. Airway, breathing, circulation, disability, exposure and environment.

Answer: D. The priority is to assess a patient in this systematic order as this allows the nurse to prioritise potential life-threatening problems.

3. Pain assessment in an unconscious patient:
    A. Isn't necessary because unconscious patients don't experience pain.
    B. Requires astute assessment skills by the nurse.
    C. Can be achieved through the use of visual analog scales.
    D. Is treated differently from pain in a conscious patient.

Answer: B. Nurses should be especially vigilant in assessing for nonverbal signs of pain in an unconscious patient.

4. When assessing the older person consideration should be paid to:
    A. An early discharge.
    B. Physiological changes affecting his or her problem/complaint.
    C. Being assessed by an older person triage nurse.
    D. All the above.

Answer: B. As we get older the human body is affected by the ageing process which might mask the patient's presenting complaint.

5. When assessing patients with mental illness:
    A. There is no need to carry out ABCDE.
    B. They always present with aggressiveness.
    C. They should be free of the effect of alcohol and drugs.
    D. No knowledge of mental illness assessment is required.

Answer: C. Alcohol and drug consumption by the patient will impede a comprehensive assessment.

Scoring

☆☆☆   If you answered all five questions correctly, take a bow! You're basically a whiz when it comes to emergency nursing basics.

☆☆   If you answered three or four questions correctly, there's no room for criticism! Your critical thinking skills are basically intact.

☆   If you answered fewer than three questions correctly, the situation is emergent! Review the chapter and you'll be on the right pathway.

(4) Shock

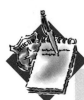

Just the facts

In this chapter, you'll learn:

♦ What shock is

♦ Emergency assessment of the patient experiencing shock

♦ Diagnostic tests and procedures for shock

♦ Shock disorders in the emergency department and their treatments

Understanding shock

Shock is a clinical presentation resulting from a generalised reduction in tissue perfusion and can affect the control of every system in the body. This reduction of blood supply (especially to the brain and the kidneys), unless rectified, can lead to cell death, multiple organ dysfunction and ultimately the patient's death. The emergency department (ED) nurse must understand the pathological processes of shock, be able to detect warning signs of deterioration and be ready to treat promptly.

Anatomy and Physiology Made Incredibly Easy (2004), *Pathophysiology Made Incredibly Easy (2009)* and *Critical Care Nursing Made Incredibly Easy (2010)* published by Lippincott Williams & Wilkins in the same series as this book will provide you with underpinning knowledge when seeking to understand the physiology of shock.

Truly shocking effects

Shock involves a disruption in the components responsible for maintaining normal circulation and cell perfusion. These components include cardiac output (CO), adequate circulating volume and correctly responsive systematic vascular resistance (SVR). Revise the important cardiology equations:

Cardiac output (CO) = Stroke volume (SV) × Heart rate (HR)
Blood pressure (BP) = Cardiac output (CO) × Systemic vascular resistance (SVR).

Useful terms

Stroke volume is the amount of blood pumped by the left ventricle in one contraction.

SVR is the resistance the left ventricle must overcome to pump blood through the arterial blood vessels of the systemic circulation. The arterioles and small arteries account for about 50% of the SVR.

Preload is the force that stretches the myofibrils of the cardiac myocardium. This force depends on the effectiveness of the myocardium and the volume of blood that stretches the myocardium.

Afterload is the pressure that the heart must pump to create the forward flow of blood.

Low BP, and subsequent tissue hypoperfusion, can be caused by low CO (for instance, reduced volume of blood returning to the heart or failure of the heart to pump effectively) or a decrease in the ability of the SVR to respond effectively to the need to control peripheral blood flow so as to maintain BP.

Shock is typically categorised by the underlying mechanism affected. Types of shock include:

• Hypovolaemic – caused by exogenous (or external) fluid loss, usually blood loss and endogenous (or internal) fluid loss such as in burns
• Cardiogenic – pump failure
• Distributive (which includes anaphylactic, neurogenic and septic shock) – caused by widespread dilation of the SVR system so that blood pools in these expanded vascular regions.

Physiology of shock

The clinical presentation will vary depending on the cause of the shock. A decrease in adequate perfusion is detected by baroreceptors (pressure receptors) and chemoreceptors (detecting blood acid-base balance). Reduction in brain perfusion (the brain is very sensitive to blood flow) causes a sympathetic nervous system response and the release of catecholamines (adrenaline and noradrenaline) from the adrenal glands. Much of the clinical presentation of the shocked patient is related directly to this response.

Early responses that raise BP

Neutrally mediated mechanisms and the release of catecholamines lead to an increase in HR and in its contractile force plus an increase in SVR. This may maintain or increase BP. If the brain detects poor perfusion despite this response, catecholamine release will be maintained.

Later responses that counteract volume deficiency

Volume deficiency and lower BP activates the renin-angiotensin-aldosterone mechanism. This causes the patient to experience thirst and lowers the renal excretion of salt and thus of water. Antidiuretic hormone is released from the pituitary gland and this reduces renal water loss also. Thirst and a low BP are late presentations and interventions should be in place before this.

Refractory or irreversible shock

If these homeostatic compensatory mechanisms are inadequate and the patient's body cannot adapt without interventions, such as an intravenous (I.V.) infusion, and if interventions are not provided promptly, or are inadequate, then self-reinforcing mechanisms can develop that worsen the condition so that a refractory, or irreversible, stage of shock is reached.

Assessment

When faced with an emergency involving shock, or the potential for shock, the patient must be assessed quickly yet thoroughly, always being alert for subtle changes that might indicate a potential deterioration in the patient's condition. Patients at risk, or showing signs, of shock require immediate attention because of possible wide-ranging negative effects on one or more body systems; prompt attention to the patient's vital functions is essential. Perform a primary survey ABCDE (**A**irway, **B**reathing, **C**irculation, **D**isability and **E**xposure) and only then a more focused history taking and assessment. You may need to intervene at any time. Your ED may have a 'track and trigger' or other early warning systems that detect signs and symptoms that indicate deterioration in the patient's condition. You must be aware of your local 'track and trigger' system and how to use it effectively.

If you can't interview the patient because of his condition, gather history information from his medical records and from family or friends. Important information will be given to you by the paramedic team that transported the patient to the ED.

Primary survey/assessment

The assessment of patients in the ED has been discussed in-depth in Chapter 3, *Initial assessment in emergency departments*. There it was noted that a primary survey consists of assessing the patient's airway (ensuring cervical spine immobilisation), breathing, circulation, alertness and orientation using the Alert, Voice, Pain, Unresponsive (AVPU) scale or the more in-depth Glasgow Coma Sale (GCS), and checking exposure, examination and environment by checking the patient 'head to toe' including his back.

Need oxygen-arterial blood oxygen saturations

All critically ill patients will require high-flow oxygen. The nurse must be aware that all oxygen use must be guided by the British Thoracic Society guidelines available at: http://www.brit-thoracic.org.uk. Remember in particular that oxygen is a treatment for hypoxaemia and has not been shown to have any effect on the experience of breathlessness. Oxygen is given to maintain oxygen saturations between prescribed target ranges – for adult patients this is 95% to 98% or 88% to 92% for adult patients at risk of hypercapnic (a raised arterial blood CO_2 level) respiratory failure. Pulse oximetry (the 'fifth vital sign') is therefore required, with the oxygen saturation and the delivery system details recorded on the patient's chart. This measurement is discussed in greater detail in Chapter 7, *Respiratory emergencies*.

Common features found in shock

- Postural hypotension, later systolic BP less than 90 mm Hg
- Tachycardia
- Respiratory rate above 20
- Reduced oxygen saturations
- Cool, clammy skin (may look mottled)
- Dry mouth, feeling of thirst
- Decreasing level of consciousness (LOC).

Focused history and physical examination

When the initial assessment is complete, you can start on a more focused assessment of each body system. (The body system chapters in this book will give you specific in-depth assessment information.)

Diagnostic tests

Numerous diagnostic tests may be performed, depending on the patient's underlying condition and overall status. Blood studies and radiologic and imaging studies are commonly performed.

Blood studies

Although specific blood studies may vary among facilities, common studies ordered for patients with shock include:
- Full blood count (FBC) and blood sugar
- Urea and electrolytes (U & Es)

- Coagulation studies, such as prothrombin time and partial thromboplastin time
- Blood type and cross match is done in anticipation of the need for a blood and blood products transfusion in trauma situations
- Serum amylase, lipase and lactate
- Liver function tests
- Blood cultures
- Arterial blood gases (ABGs).

Practice pointers
- Tell the patient that the test requires a blood sample and gain consent where feasible
- Check the patient's medication history for medications that might influence test results.

Radiologic and imaging studies

Specific radiologic and imaging studies completed for these patients depend on the underlying mechanism causing the shock and the body areas or organs affected. These include X-rays of the chest, pelvis, cervical spine, thoracic and lumbar spine and extremities. A focused assessment with sonography for trauma, a limited ultrasound examination directed solely at identifying the presence of free intraperitoneal or pericardial fluid, may be undertaken. In the context of traumatic injury, free fluid is usually due to haemorrhage and contributes to the assessment of the circulation. If safe to do so, computed tomography may be used to evaluate head injury or abdominal trauma.

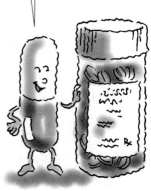

Some medications may influences blood test results, so be sure to check your patient's medication history.

Practice pointers
- Prepare the patient for the X-ray or scan to be performed, including the reason for the study and gain consent (where possible)
- Inform the patient's family of the investigation and what it entails
- Ensure that the appropriate checklist has been completed
- Verify that the order includes pertinent history, such as trauma, and identifies sites of injury, tenderness or pain
- Make sure that all jewellery is removed from the patient and handled in accordance with hospital policy.

Hypovolaemic shock

Hypovolaemic shock most commonly results from acute blood loss. Without sufficient blood or fluid replacement, it may cause irreversible damage to organs and systems.

What causes it?
Massive volume loss may result from:
- Gastrointestinal (GI) bleeding, internal or external haemorrhage or any condition that reduces circulating intravascular volume or other body fluids

- Intestinal obstruction
- Peritonitis
- Acute pancreatitis
- Ascites
- Dehydration from, e.g. excessive perspiration, severe diarrhoea, protracted vomiting, diabetes insipidus or inadequate fluid intake. (See *Estimating adult fluid loss*.)

How it happens

Potentially life-threatening, hypovolaemic shock stems from reduced intravascular blood volume, which leads to decreased CO and inadequate tissue perfusion. The subsequent tissue anoxia prompts a shift in cellular metabolism from aerobic to anaerobic pathways. This shift results in an accumulation of lactic acid, which produces metabolic acidosis.

Estimating adult fluid loss

Intravascular volume loss of less than 15%

A fluid loss of less than 750 ml results in:
- Slight tachycardia
- Normal supine BP
- Normal pulse pressure
- Normal respirations
- Urine output of 0.5 ml/kg/hour or more
- Capillary refill time (CRT) normal (less than 2 seconds)
- Skin colour normal
- Patient feeling slightly anxious.

Intravascular volume loss of 15% to 30%

A fluid loss of 750 to 1,500 ml results in:
- Tachycardia – more than 100 beats per minute (bpm)
- Pulse pressure narrowed – thready pulse
- BP normal systolic and elevated diastolic
- CRT normal (less than 2 seconds)
- Respirations 20 to 30 breaths per minute

- Urine output of 20 to 30 ml/hour
- Thirst
- Skin pale, cool and moist
- Anxious, restlessness, confusion or irritability.

Intravascular volume loss of 30% to 40%

A fluid loss of 1,500 to 2,000 ml results in:
- Marked tachycardia – more than 120 bpm
- Marked hypotension
- Feeling of thirst
- CRT – normal
- Pulse pressure barely palpable
- Weak peripheral pulses
- Weak rapid respirations 30 to 40 breaths per minute
- Urine output less than 5 to 15 ml/hour
- Skin extremely pale and sweaty. Will be cool to the touch
- Anxiety, confusion, maybe unconscious.

Intravascular volume loss of more than 40%

A fluid loss of more than 2,000 ml results in:
- Decreased cognition and perception. Maybe unconsciousness
- Rapid, shallow respirations. Rate more than 35 breaths per minute and hard to detect
- Possible anuria
- CRT not detectable
- Rapid, thready peripheral pulses. Pulse may only be detectable at the carotid arteries may detect pulse only at the carotid arteries
- Pale, cold, clammy skin
- Mean arterial pressure (MAP) less than 60 mm Hg and a narrowing pulse pressure
- Decreased central venous pressure (CVP), right atrial pressure and CO
- High risk for respiratory arrest followed by cardiac arrest.

Shock sequence

When compensatory mechanisms fail, hypovolaemic shock occurs in this sequence:
- Intravascular fluid volume decreases
- Venous return diminishes, which reduces preload and so decreases stroke volume
- CO is reduced, tissue perfusion is impaired and so oxygen and nutrient delivery to the cells decreases
- Arterial BP is reduced. (This monitoring requires a catheter to be inserted into the radial or femoral artery to measure BP and obtain samples of arterial blood)
- Multisystem organ failure occurs.

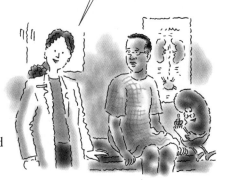

If urine specific gravity exceeds 1.020 while urine sodium levels fall to less than 50 mEq/L, your patient may have hypovolaemic shock.

What tests tell you

No single diagnostic test confirms hypovolaemic shock, but these tests results help support the diagnosis:
- Low haematocrit (Hct)
- Decreased haemoglobin (Hb) level
- Decreased red blood cell (RBC) and platelet counts
- Elevated serum potassium, sodium, creatinine and urea levels
- Increased urine specific gravity (greater than 1.020) and urine osmolality
- Decreased pH and PaO_2 and increased $PaCO_2$
- X-rays and scans
- Aspiration of gastric contents through a nasogastric tube and tests for occult blood
- Coagulation studies for coagulopathy from disseminated intravascular coagulation (DIC).

Other tests

- Chest X-ray (CXR) can detect blood in the thorax
- Ultrasound scan (scan maybe done in the resuscitation area, if the department has the equipment)
- Focused assessment with sonography for trauma scan.

How it's treated

Emergency treatment relies on prompt, adequate fluid and blood replacement to restore intravascular volume and to raise BP and maintain it above 80 mm Hg. Rapid infusion of normal saline or Hartmann's solution and, possibly, albumin or other plasma expanders may expand volume adequately until whole blood can be matched. If hypovolaemic shock is caused by massive bleeding, Hartmann's solution rather than normal saline is preferred for fluid replacement, because it minimises the risk of electrolyte imbalances. (See *When BP drops*, page 68.)

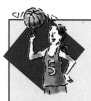

Stay on the ball

When BP drops

A drop below 80 mm Hg in systolic BP usually signals inadequate CO from reduced intravascular volume. Such a drop usually results in inadequate coronary artery blood flow, cardiac ischaemia, arrhythmias and other complications of low CO. If the patient's systolic BP drops below 80 mm Hg and the pulse is thready, call the doctor immediately. Check oxygen saturations and consider increasing the oxygen flow rate.

Treatment also includes oxygen administration, and may also control of bleeding, administration of dopamine or another inotropic drug and surgery if appropriate. (See *Hypovolaemic shock and children*.)

What to do
- Give information and reassurance to the patient and family or friends
- Assess ABCDEs, including cardiac monitoring
- If the patient experiences cardiac or respiratory arrest, start resuscitation protocols
- Administer oxygen and maintain oximetry
- Monitor the patient's oxygen saturation and ABG values for evidence of hypoxaemia and anticipate the need for endotracheal (ET) intubation and mechanical ventilation if the patient's respiratory status deteriorates
- Assess the patient for the extent of fluid loss and begin fluid replacement as ordered
- Measures to reduce external blood loss (direct pressure or pressure dressing and elevation)
- Obtain type and crossmatch for blood component therapy

Ages and stages

Hypovolaemic shock and children

- Suspect hypovolaemia in the infant or the child who has a capillary refill longer than 2 seconds and accompanying history and signs of hypovolaemic shock, such as tachycardia, altered level of consciousness, pale skin, lack of tears and depressed fontanelles.
- Keep in mind that fluid replacement for an infant and a child is generally a crystalloid at a volume of 20 ml/kg of body weight in a fluid bolus for the ill child (and 10 ml/kg for the child with trauma). If the response is poor, after 40 ml/kg has been given to the sick child, resuscitative measures, including intubation would be considered.

- Place the patient in a supported semi-recumbent position to maximise chest expansion and enhance oxygenation (not if spinal trauma or certain other skeletal injuries are suspected)
- Reassure the patient and keep him as calm as possible to minimise oxygen demands
- Monitor the patient's vital signs, neurologic status and cardiac rhythm continuously for changes such as cardiac arrhythmias and myocardial ischaemia
- Surgery also depends on the patient's underlying condition. For example, surgery may be indicated to repair a laceration of a wound or organ, repair a fracture, insert pins or a fixation device to stabilise bone or incise and drain an abscess. Exploratory surgery may be necessary to identify the source of haemorrhage in a patient experiencing hypovolaemic shock.

Capillary cues

- Observe the patient's skin colour and check capillary refill
- Notify the doctor if capillary refill takes longer than 2 seconds
- Monitor haemodynamic parameters – including CVP, CO and cardiac input – as often as every 15 minutes to evaluate the patient's status and response to treatment
- Monitor the patient's fluid intake and output closely
- An indwelling urinary catheter may be ordered and hourly urine output recorded.

Watch for blood

- If bleeding from the GI tract is the suspected cause, check all stools, vomit and gastric drainage for frank or occult blood
- If urine output falls below 0.5 ml/kg/hour in an adult, expect to increase the I.V. fluid infusion rate, but watch for signs of fluid overload such as elevated CVP
- Notify the doctor if urine output doesn't increase
- Administer blood component therapy as ordered; monitor serial Hb values and Hct to evaluate the effects of treatment
- Administer dobutamine and/or noradrenaline I.V. as ordered to increase cardiac contractility and renal perfusion
- Watch for signs of impending coagulopathy, such as petechiae, bruising and bleeding or oozing from gums or venipuncture sites, and report them immediately. (See *Understanding DIC*, page 88)
- Provide emotional support and reassurance as appropriate in the wake of massive fluid losses
- Prepare the patient for surgery as appropriate.

Perfusion pointers

- Monitor LOC for changes indicating decreased cerebral perfusion

- Evaluate peripheral tissue perfusion, including skin colour, temperature, pulses and capillary refill
- Reassure and give explanations to the patient and his family.

Blood transfusion therapy

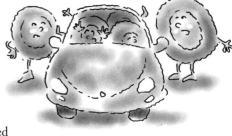

I know that "packed" RBCs are highly valued for transfusions, but this seems a little extreme.

Blood transfusions treat decreased Hb level and Hct. A whole blood transfusion replenishes the circulatory system's volume and oxygen-carrying capacity by increasing the mass of circulating RBCs. It's usually used in cases of haemorrhage.

Packed RBCs, a blood component from which 80% of the plasma has been removed, are transfused to restore the circulatory system's oxygen-carrying capacity. Packed RBCs are used when the patient has a normal blood volume to avoid possible fluid and circulatory overload. (See *Guide to whole blood and cellular products*, pages 72–75.)

Whole blood and packed RBCs contain cellular debris, requiring in-line filtration during administration. Washed packed RBCs, commonly used for patients previously sensitised to transfusions, are rinsed with a special solution that removes white blood cells and platelets, thus decreasing the chance of a transfusion reaction.

Refusal of transfusion

In some cases, a patient may refuse a blood transfusion; e.g. a Jehovah's Witness may refuse one because of his religious beliefs. A competent adult has the legal right to refuse treatment even if this could lead to his death. You may be able to use other treatment options if the patient refuses the blood transfusion, such as providing erythropoietin, iron and folic acid supplements before and after surgery. Using available alternative treatments supports the patient's right of self-determination and honours his wishes. A court order requiring the patient to undergo transfusion therapy can be obtained if the patient has diminished mental competency (see Chapter 2) or if the patient is a child.

It may be hard to stomach, but the patient's right of self-determination means he can choose to refuse a blood transfusion.

Practice pointers: right blood, right patient, right time, right place

- Verify the doctor's prescription or check electronic order
- Obtain baseline vital signs and ensure that an I.V. line is placed if one isn't already started. Use a large bore catheter. For adult trauma patients usually it will be a 14 G but will be smaller for groups such as older adults and children, so clinical judgement is required
- Identify the patient and check the blood bag identification number, ABO blood group, Rh compatibility and blood product expiration date. This step should be confirmed by another registered nurse or a doctor. Follow your hospital's policy for blood administration and the guidance from the United Kingdom Blood Services: http://www.transfusionguidelines.org.uk

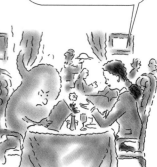

- Obtain the patient's vital signs after the first 15 minutes and then every 30 minutes (or according to your hospital's policy) for the remainder of transfusion therapy
- Record the date and time of the transfusion (time started and completed); the type and amount of transfusion product; the type and gauge of the catheter used for infusion; the patient's vital signs before, during and after transfusion; a verification check of all identification data (including the names of individuals verifying the information) and the patient's response
- Check that follow-up laboratory tests have been ordered to determine the effectiveness of therapy
- For rapid blood replacement, use a pressure bag or rapid transfusion device if necessary. Be aware that excessive pressure may develop, leading to broken blood vessels and extravasation with haematoma and haemolysis of the infusing RBCs. Large-gauge catheters and central lines are preferred for rapid and pressured transfusions
- If administering platelets or fresh frozen plasma, administer each unit immediately after obtaining it. Although some microaggregate filters can be used for up to 10 units of blood, always replace the filter and tubing if more than 1 hour elapses between transfusions. When administering multiple units of blood under pressure, use a blood warmer to avoid hypothermia
- Measures to be in place to ensure that the patient remains warm
- Document the patient's transfusion reaction and the treatment required (if any)
- Notify the doctor if the patient refuses the blood transfusion.

Cardiogenic shock

Sometimes called *pump failure*, cardiogenic shock is a condition of diminished CO due to a reduction in cardiac contractibility and SV that severely impairs tissue perfusion. Cardiogenic shock occurs as a serious complication in nearly 15% of patients who are hospitalised with acute myocardial infarction (MI). (See Chapter 6, *Cardiac emergencies*.)

It typically affects patients whose area of infarction involves 40% or more of left ventricular muscle mass; in such patients, mortality may exceed 85%. Most patients with cardiogenic shock die within 24 hours of onset. The prognosis for those who survive is poor.

What causes it?
Cardiogenic shock can result from any condition that causes significant left ventricular dysfunction with reduced CO, such as MI (the most common cause), myocardial ischaemia, papillary muscle dysfunction and end-stage cardiomyopathy.

Other causes include myocarditis and depression of myocardial contractility after cardiac arrest and prolonged cardiac surgery. Mechanical abnormalities of the ventricle, such as acute mitral or aortic insufficiency or an acutely acquired ventricular septal defect or ventricular aneurysm, may also result in cardiogenic shock.

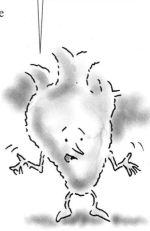

I feel so guilty – cardiogenic shock kills most patients within 24 hours of onset, and the prognosis for survivors is poor.

(*Text continues on page 74.*)

Guide to whole blood and cellular products

This chart lists blood components along with indications for their use and nursing considerations.

Blood component	Indications
Whole blood	
Complete (pure) blood	• To treat symptomatic chronic anaemia • To prevent morbidity from anaemia in patients at greatest risk for tissue hypoxia • To control active bleeding with signs and symptoms of hypovolaemia • To aid preoperatively; haemoglobin less than 9 g/dl with possibility of major blood loss • To treat sickle cell disease
Packed red blood cells (RBCs)	
Same RBC mass as whole blood with 80% of the plasma removed	• To treat symptomatic chronic anaemia • To prevent morbidity from anaemia in patients at greatest risk for tissue hypoxia • To control active bleeding with signs and symptoms of hypovolaemia • To aid preoperatively; haemoglobin less than 9 g/dl with possibility of major blood loss • To treat sickle cell disease
Leukocyte-poor RBCs	
Same as packed RBCs except 70% of the leukocytes are removed	• To treat symptomatic anaemia • To prevent morbidity from anaemia in patients at greatest risk for tissue hypoxia • To control active bleeding with signs and symptoms of hypovolaemia • To aid preoperatively; haemoglobin less than 9 g/dl with possibility of major blood loss • To treat sickle cell disease • To prevent febrile reactions from leukocyte antibodies • To treat immunosuppressed patients • To restore RBCs to patients who have had two or more nonhaemolytic febrile reactions
White blood cells (WBCs, leukocytes)	
Whole blood with all the RBCs and 80% of the plasma removed	• To treat sepsis that's unresponsive to antibiotics (especially if the patient has positive blood cultures or a persistent fever exceeding 101° F [38.3° C]) and life-threatening granulocytopenia (granulocyte count less than 500/μL)

Nursing considerations

- Compatibility is ABO identical
- Group A receives A; group B receives B; group AB receives AB; group O receives O. Rh type must match
- Use blood administration tubing You can infuse rapidly in emergencies, but adjust the rate to the patient's condition and the transfusion order, and don't infuse one unit over more than 4 hours
- Whole blood is seldom administered other than in emergency situations because its components can be extracted and administered separately
- Warm blood if giving a large quantity
- Use only with normal saline in the blood administration line
- Monitor the patient's volume status for fluid overload

- Compatibility: Group A receives A or O; group B receives B or O; group AB receives AB, A, B or O; group O receives O. Rh type must match
- Use blood administration tubing to infuse over more than 4 hours
- Packed RBCs shouldn't be used for anaemic conditions correctable by nutrition or drug therapy
- Use only with normal saline

- Compatibility: Group A receives A or O; group B receives B or O; group AB receives AB, A, B or O; group O receives O. Rh type must match
- Use blood administration tubing. May require a microaggregate filter (40-micron filter) for hard-spun, leukocyte-poor RBCs
- Cells expire 24 hours after washing
- Leukocyte-poor RBCs shouldn't be used for anaemic conditions correctable by nutrition or drug therapy

- Compatibility: Group A receives A or O; group B receives B or O; group AB receives AB, A, B or O; group O receives O. Rh type must match. WBCs are preferably human leukocyte antigen (HLA)–compatible, although compatibility isn't necessary unless the patient is HLA-sensitised from previous transfusions
- Use blood administration tubing. One unit daily is given for 4 to 6 days or until infection clears
- WBC infusion may induce fever and chills. To prevent this reaction, the patient is premedicated with antihistamines or steroids. If fever occurs, give an antipyretic, but don't stop the transfusion. Reduce the flow rate for the patient's comfort
- Because reactions are common, administer slowly over 2 to 4 hours. Check the patient's vital signs and assess him every 15 minutes throughout the transfusion
- Give the transfusion with antibiotics to treat infection

(continued)

Guide to whole blood and cellular products *(Continued)*	
Blood component	**Indications**
Platelets	
Platelet sediment from RBCs or plasma	• To treat bleeding due to critically decreased circulating platelet counts or functionally abnormal platelets • To prevent bleeding due to thrombocytopenia • To treat a patient with a platelet count less than 50,000/μL before surgery or a major invasive procedure

How it happens

Regardless of the cause, left ventricular dysfunction initiates a series of compensatory mechanisms that increases HR, strengthens myocardial contractions, promotes sodium and water retention and causes selective vasoconstriction. These mechanisms attempt to increase CO and maintain vital organ function.

Stable, but brief

However, these mechanisms also increase myocardial workload and oxygen consumption, thus reducing the heart's ability to pump blood, especially if the patient has myocardial ischaemia. As CO falls, aortic and carotid baroreceptors activate sympathetic nervous responses. These compensatory responses further increase HR, left ventricular filling pressure and peripheral resistance to flow in order to enhance venous return to the heart. These actions initially stabilise the patient but later cause deterioration with rising oxygen demands on the compromised myocardium.

Cardiac output cycle

These events constitute a vicious cycle of low CO, sympathetic compensation, myocardial ischaemia and even lower CO. Consequently, blood backs up, resulting in pulmonary oedema. Eventually, CO falls and Multi Organ Failure (MOF) develops as the compensatory mechanisms fail to maintain perfusion.

What to look for

• Sustained hypotension A systolic reading of less than 90 mm Hg for more than 30 minutes
• Tissue hypoperfusion and oliguria of less than 0.5 ml/kg/hour.
  Typically, the patient's history includes a disorder (such as MI or cardiomyopathy) that severely decreases left ventricular function. A patient with underlying cardiac disease may complain of anginal pain because of decreased myocardial perfusion and oxygenation. Inspection typically reveals

Nursing considerations

- Compatibility: ABO should be identical. Rh-negative recipients should receive Rh-negative platelets
- Use a blood filter or leukocyte-reduction filter. Don't use a microaggregate filter
- Platelet transfusions aren't usually indicated for thrombocytopenic autoimmune thrombocytopenia or thrombocytopenia purpura unless the patient has a life-threatening haemorrhage
- Patients with a history of platelet reaction require premedication with antipyretics and antihistamines
- Use single donor platelets if the patient has a need for repeated transfusions

pale skin that feels cold and clammy, decreased perception and rapid, shallow respirations. Palpation of peripheral pulses may detect a rapid, thready pulse.

Auscultation of BP usually discloses a Mean Arterial Pressure (MAP) of less than 60 mm Hg and a narrowing pulse pressure (the difference between systolic and diastolic BP). In a patient with chronic hypotension, the MAP may fall below 50 mm Hg before the patient exhibits signs of shock. Auscultation of the heart detects gallop rhythms, faint heart sounds and possibly (if shock results from rupture of the ventricular septum or papillary muscles) a holosystolic (pansystolic) murmur. You can listen to heart sounds at this link: http://www.med.ucla.edu/wilkes/intro.html.

Although many of these clinical features also occur in heart failure and other shock syndromes, they're usually more profound in cardiogenic shock. Patients with pericardial tamponade may have distant heart sounds.

Compensation clues

The patient's signs and symptoms may also provide clues to the stage of shock. For example, in the compensatory stage of shock, signs and symptoms may include:
- Tachycardia and bounding pulse due to sympathetic stimulation
- Restlessness and irritability related to cerebral hypoxia
- Tachypnoea to compensate for hypoxia
- Reduced urine output secondary to vasoconstriction
- Cool, pale skin associated with vasoconstriction.

That's progress for ya

In the progressive stage of shock, signs and symptoms may include:
- Hypotension as compensatory mechanisms begin to fail
- Narrowed pulse pressure associated with reduced stroke volume
- Weak, rapid, thready pulse caused by decreased CO
- Shallow respirations as the patient weakens
- Reduced urine output as poor renal perfusion continues
- Cold, clammy skin caused by vasoconstriction
- Cyanosis related to hypoxia.

> Cold, clammy skin is expected for me right now, but for a cardiogenic shock patient receiving therapy, it means the condition is progressing.

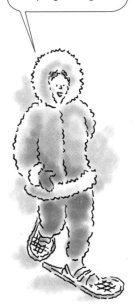

No going back

In the irreversible stage, clinical findings may include:
• Unconsciousness and absent reflexes caused by reduced cerebral perfusion, acid-base imbalance or electrolyte abnormalities
• Rapidly falling BP as decompensation occurs
• Weak pulse caused by reduced CO
• Slow, shallow or Cheyne-Stokes respirations secondary to respiratory centre depression
• Anuria related to renal failure.

What tests tell you

• Arterial pressure monitoring shows systolic arterial pressure less than 80 mm Hg caused by impaired ventricular ejection
• ABGs analysis may show metabolic and respiratory acidosis and hypoxia
• Electrocardiography (ECG) demonstrates possible evidence of acute MI, ischaemia or ventricular aneurysm
• ECG determines left ventricular function and reveals valvular abnormalities
• Serum enzyme measurements display elevated levels of troponins, creatine kinase, lactate dehydrogenase, aspartate aminotransferase and alanine aminotransferase, which indicate MI or ischaemia and suggest heart failure or shock. Creatine kinase-MB and lactate dehydrogenase isoenzyme levels may confirm acute MI
• Cardiac catheterisation and echocardiography may reveal other conditions that can lead to pump dysfunction and failure, such as pericardial tamponade, papillary muscle infarct or rupture, ventricular septal rupture, pulmonary emboli, venous pooling and hypovolaemia
• Brain natriuretic peptide low levels help exclude cardiogenic shock.

How it's treated – ABCDE

The goal of treatment is to enhance cardiovascular status by increasing CO, improving myocardial perfusion and decreasing cardiac workload with combinations of cardiovascular drugs and mechanically assistive techniques. These goals are accomplished by optimising preload, decreasing afterload, increasing contractility and optimising HR:
• Provide oxygen and respiratory support. Consider use of intubation and ventilator intervention
• Use opiate such as diamorphine if the patient's condition can sustain it
• ECG monitoring (including a 12-lead ECG)
• Treat any cardiac arrhythmia
• CXR can show pulmonary oedema, increase in heart size (cardiomegaly), aortic dissection, left ventricular failure and tension pneumothorax
• Blood tests will include U & Es, liver function tests, FBC and cardiac enzymes to include troponin
• Treat any electrolyte imbalance
• Echocardiography can detect pericardial tamponade and aortic dissection

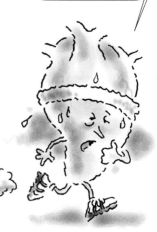

Cardiogenic shock treatment aims to decrease cardiac workload, among other things. Boy. I'd appreciate some of that right about now!

- Recommended I.V. drugs may include dopamine (a vasopressor that increases CO, BP and renal blood flow), dobutamine (inotropic agent that increases myocardial contractility and so increases CO) and noradrenaline (when a more potent vasoconstrictor is necessary).

And just for good measure

Additional treatment measures for cardiogenic shock may include:
- Thrombolytic therapy or coronary artery revascularisation to restore coronary artery blood flow if cardiogenic shock is due to acute MI
- Emergency surgery may be required to repair papillary muscle rupture or ventricular septal defect if either is the cause of cardiogenic shock
- Possible use of an intra-aortic balloon counterpulsation.

What to do

- If concurrent hypovolaemia is present I.V. fluids will be prescribed. Colloid challenges (100 to 200 ml) maybe requested
- Administer oxygen by face mask or artificial airway to ensure adequate tissue oxygenation. Adjust the oxygen flow rate to a higher or lower level as blood gas measurements indicate. Many patients will need 100% oxygen and some will require 5 to 15 cm H_2O of positive end-expiratory or continuous positive airway pressure ventilation
- Monitor and record the patient's BP, pulse, respiratory rate and peripheral pulses every 1 to 5 minutes until the patient stabilises.

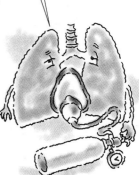

Administering oxygen by face mask ensures adequate tissue oxygenation.

Fascinating rhythm

- Monitor the patient's cardiac rhythm continuously. Systolic BP less than 80 mm Hg usually results in inadequate coronary artery blood flow, cardiac ischaemia, arrhythmias and further complications of low CO
- If BP drops below 80 mm Hg, notify the doctor immediately. A progressive drop in BP accompanied by a thready pulse generally signals inadequate CO from reduced intravascular volume
- Determine how much fluid to give by checking BP and urine output
- Keep in mind that, if the patient is hypovolaemic, as in a right ventricular infarction, preload may need to be increased, which is typically accomplished with I.V. fluids. However, I.V. fluids must be given cautiously and increased gradually while haemodynamic parameters are closely monitored.

I'm going in

- Insert an indwelling urinary catheter if necessary to measure hourly urine output. If output is less than 0.5 ml/kg/hour (in adults), increase the fluid infusion rate but watch for signs of fluid overload such as an increase in CVP. Notify the doctor if urine output doesn't improve
- Administer a diuretic, such as frusemide or bumetanide, as ordered to decrease preload and improve SV and CO

- Consider small dose of diamorphine to relieve anxiety, to cause vasodilation and to lower the metabolic rate
- Monitor ABG values, FBC and electrolyte levels. Administer electrolyte replacement therapy as prescribed and indicated by laboratory test results
- If metabolic acidosis isn't resolved then expect to administer sodium bicarbonate given as a small volume of hypertonic solution, such as 50 ml of 8.4% solution intravenously
- During therapy, assess skin colour and temperature and note changes. Cold, clammy skin may be a sign of continuing peripheral vascular constriction, indicating progressive shock
- Prepare the patient for possible emergency cardiac catheterisation, percutaneous transluminal coronary angioplasty or coronary artery bypass graft in an attempt to reperfuse areas with reversible possibility.

Distributive shock

This is a group of conditions that the clinical presentation is due to sudden blood vessel dilation and impairment of suitable adjustment to SVR systems leading to hypotension and generalised tissue hypoxia.

- Anaphylactic shock
- Neurogenic shock
- Septic shock.

Anaphylactic shock

A broad definition of anaphylaxis was proposed by the European Academy of Allergy and Clinical Immunology Nomenclature Committee and adapted by the UK Resuscitation Council. The current definition is that anaphylaxis is a severe, life-threatening, generalised or systemic hypersensitivity reaction, characterised by rapidly developing life-threatening airway, breathing and/or circulation problems, usually associated with skin and mucosal changes.

What causes it?

Anaphylaxis usually results from ingestion of, or other systemic exposure to, sensitising drugs or other substances. Such substances may include:

- Bee and wasp stings
- Food stuffs, such as legumes (beans, lentils and peanuts), nuts, berries, seafood and egg albumin and egg-based vaccines
- Penicillin or other antibiotics (which induce anaphylaxis in 1 to 4 of every 10,000 patients treated, most likely after parenteral administration or prolonged therapy and in patients with an inherited tendency to food or drug allergy)
- Anaesthetic drugs, such as suxamethonium
- Drugs, such as salicylates and other nonsteroidal anti-inflammatory drugs
- Diagnostic chemicals and radiographic contrast media
- Others may include latex and hair dye.

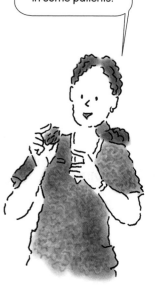

For some, it's a healthy snack; for others, it brings on an attack. In other words, nuts contain food proteins that cause anaphylaxis in some patients.

All about speed

With prompt recognition and treatment, the prognosis for anaphylaxis is good. However, a severe reaction may precipitate vascular collapse, leading to systemic shock and, sometimes, death. The reaction typically occurs within minutes but can occur up to 1 hour after exposure to an antigen.

How it happens

Anaphylaxis requires previous sensitisation or exposure to the specific antigen, resulting in immunoglobulin (Ig) E production by plasma cells in the lymph nodes and enhancement by helper T cells. IgE antibodies then bind to basophils and membrane receptors on mast cells in connective tissue.

Here it comes again!

Upon exposure, IgM and IgG recognise the antigen and bind to it. Activated IgE on the basophils promotes the release of histamine, serotonin and leukotrienes. An intensified response occurs as venule-weakening lesions form. Fluid then leaks into the cells, resulting in respiratory distress. Further deterioration occurs as the body's compensatory mechanisms fail to respond. (See *Understanding anaphylaxis*, pages 81–82.)

Recognising an anaphylactic reaction

- An anaphylactic reaction produces sudden physical distress within seconds or minutes after exposure to an allergen. The patient feels anxious and commonly has a feeling of impending doom
- Life-threatening **A**irway, **B**reathing and/or **C**irculation problems
- **Di**sability – confusion, agitation, lack of consciousness
- **E**xposure – skin and/or mucosal changes. (See *Anaphylaxis algorithm*, page 80.)

Assessment

The patient may present with airway swelling, wheezing, dyspnoea and complaints of chest tightness suggesting bronchial obstruction. These signs and symptoms are early indications of impending, potentially fatal respiratory failure. The patient may present signs of hypotension, physical signs of shock (pale clammy), tachycardia, dizziness, drowsiness, headache, restlessness and seizures and reduced level of consciousness (LOC). The leakage of large amounts of fluid from the patient's circulation and vasodilatation with the resultant low BP may precipitate vascular collapse and if untreated can lead to cardiac arrest. The patient is also at risk of cardiac arrhythmias.

On inspection, the patient's skin may display well-circumscribed, discrete cutaneous wheals with erythematous, raised, indented borders and blanched centres. They may coalesce to form urticarial rash. Other effects may follow rapidly. The patient may report GI and genitourinary effects,

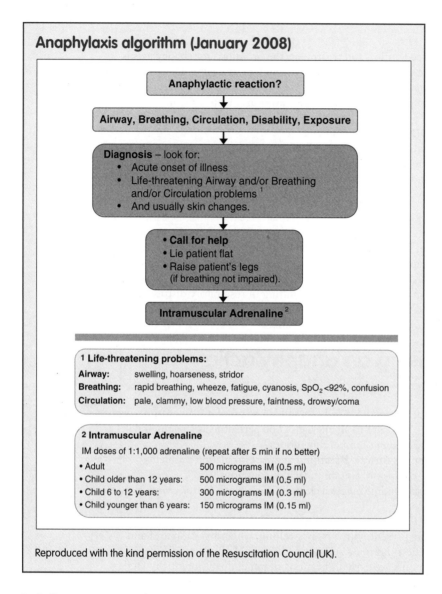

Anaphylaxis algorithm (January 2008)

Anaphylactic reaction?

↓

Airway, Breathing, Circulation, Disability, Exposure

↓

Diagnosis – look for:
- Acute onset of illness
- Life-threatening Airway and/or Breathing and/or Circulation problems [1]
- And usually skin changes.

↓

- **Call for help**
- Lie patient flat
- Raise patient's legs (if breathing not impaired).

↓

Intramuscular Adrenaline [2]

[1] **Life-threatening problems:**

Airway:	swelling, hoarseness, stridor
Breathing:	rapid breathing, wheeze, fatigue, cyanosis, $SpO_2 < 92\%$, confusion
Circulation:	pale, clammy, low blood pressure, faintness, drowsy/coma

[2] **Intramuscular Adrenaline**

IM doses of 1:1,000 adrenaline (repeat after 5 min if no better)

• Adult	500 micrograms IM (0.5 ml)
• Child older than 12 years:	500 micrograms IM (0.5 ml)
• Child 6 to 12 years:	300 micrograms IM (0.3 ml)
• Child younger than 6 years:	150 micrograms IM (0.15 ml)

Reproduced with the kind permission of the Resuscitation Council (UK).

including severe stomach cramps, nausea, diarrhoea and urinary urgency and incontinence.

What tests tell you

No single diagnostic test can identify anaphylaxis. It can be diagnosed by the rapid onset of severe respiratory or cardiovascular symptoms after ingestion or injection of a drug, vaccine, diagnostic agent, food or food additive or after an insect sting. If these symptoms occur without a known allergic stimulus, other possible causes of shock (such as acute MI, status asthmaticus or heart failure) must be ruled out.

(Text continues on page 83.)

Understanding anaphylaxis

An anaphylactic reaction occurs after previous sensitisation or exposure to a specific antigen. The sequence of events in anaphylaxis is described here.

Response to the antigen

IgM and IgG recognise the antigen as a foreign substance and attach to it. Destruction of the antigen by the complement cascade begins but remains unfinished because of insufficient amounts of the protein catalyst or the antigen inhibits certain complement enzymes. The patient has no signs or symptoms at this stage.

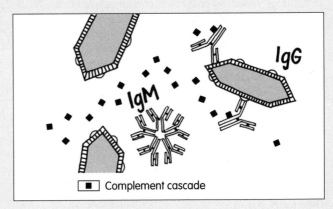

■ Complement cascade

Released chemical mediators

The antigen's continued presence activates IgE on basophils. The activated IgE promotes the release of mediators, including histamine, serotonin and leukotriene. The sudden release of histamine causes vasodilation and increases capillary permeability. The patient begins to have signs and symptoms, including sudden nasal congestion; itchy, watery eyes; flushing; sweating; weakness and anxiety.

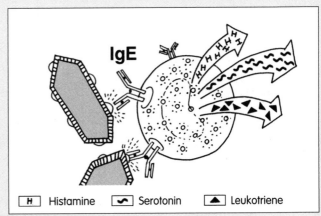

H Histamine   Serotonin   ▲ Leukotriene

Intensified response

The activated IgE also stimulates mast cells in connective tissue along the venule walls to release more histamine and eosinophil chemotactic factor of anaphylaxis. These substances produce disruptive lesions that weaken the venules. Red, itchy skin; wheals and swelling appear, and signs and symptoms worsen.

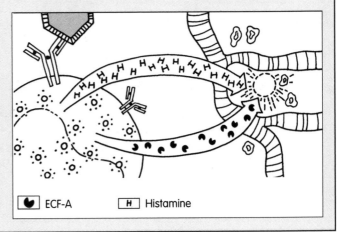

ECF-A   H Histamine

Understanding anaphylaxis *(continued)*

Distress

In the lungs, histamine causes endothelial cells to burst and endothelial tissue to tear away from surrounding tissue. Fluids leak into the alveoli, and leukotriene prevents the alveoli from expanding, thus reducing pulmonary compliance. Tachypnoea, stridor, use of accessory muscles and cyanosis signal respiratory distress. Resulting neurologic signs and symptoms include changes in level of consciousness, severe anxiety and, possibly, seizures.

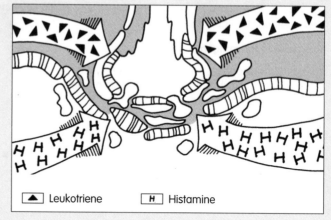

| ▲ | Leukotriene | H | Histamine |

Deterioration

Basophils and mast cells begin to release prostaglandins and bradykinin along with histamine and serotonin. These substances increase vascular permeability, causing fluids to leak from the vessels. Confusion; cool, pale skin; generalised oedema; tachycardia and hypotension signal rapid vascular collapse.

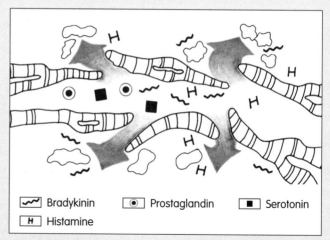

| ∿ | Bradykinin | ◉ | Prostaglandin | ■ | Serotonin |
| H | Histamine |

Failed compensatory mechanisms

Damage to the endothelial cells causes basophils and mast cells to release heparin. Additional substances are also released to neutralise the other mediators; eosinophils release arylsulfatase B to neutralise leukotriene, phospholipase D to neutralise heparin and cyclic adenosine monophosphate and the prostaglandins E_1 and E_2 to increase the metabolic rate. These events can't reverse anaphylaxis. The patient is at risk of progressing to DIC and cardiopulmonary arrest.

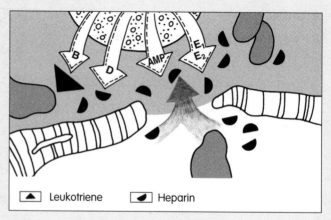

| ▲ | Leukotriene | ◢ | Heparin |

How it's treated – an ABCDE approach

- Establish a patent airway, ensuring adequate oxygenation with high-flow oxygen
- Immediate intramuscular administration of adrenaline 1:1,000 (500 μg [0.5 ml] for adults and children older than 12 years) to reverse bronchoconstriction and cause vasoconstriction. (I.V. adrenaline in anaphylaxis treatment must be given only by practitioners trained in its use). (See *Anaphylaxis algorithm*, page 80.)
- Be ready for ET or tracheostomy intubation and mechanical ventilation to maintain a patent airway
- Restore vascular volume with a fluid challenge using Hartmann's solution or 0.9% saline (500 to 1,000 ml for an adult and 20 ml/kg for a child). Monitor response and repeat as required. (Colloids are not recommended)
- After initial resuscitation – chlorphenamine (a antihistamine) and hydrocortisone (a steroid)
- May consider bronchodilators (if asthma-like symptoms) or cardiac drugs (vasopressors and inotropics) in specialised units when adrenaline and fluids have been proven unsuccessful.

Neurogenic shock

Neurogenic shock is the rarest of the shocks. It is caused by a loss of autonomic function below the level of a spinal cord injury caused by trauma to the spinal cord. Neurogenic shock is a type of distributive shock in which vasodilation causes a state of hypovolaemia. It occurs most commonly at the spinal level of T6 or above.

What causes it?

It may result from spinal cord injury: spinal anaesthesia, vasomotor centre depression, medications or hypoglycaemia.

How it happens

A loss of sympathetic vasoconstrictor tone in the vascular smooth muscle and reduced autonomic function lead to widespread arterial and venous vasodilation. Venous return is reduced as blood pools in the venous septum, leading to a drop in CO and hypotension.

What to look for

The neurogenic shock patient will display these signs and symptoms:
- Severe hypotension
- Bradycardia
- Warm, dry and flushed skin
- Hypothermia.

What tests tell you

Tests to determine neurogenic shock should include ABGs to determine the degree of cardiopulmonary compensation, ECG to determine cardiac arrhythmias and computed tomographic scan or magnetic resonance imaging to determine the extent of spinal injury.

How it's treated

Treatment goals include assessing ABCDE, treating hypothermia, administering fluid resuscitation and vasoconstrictors to increase BP, and administering agents such as atropine to block vagal effects that cause bradycardia.

What to do

- Speak to and reassure the patient and his family
- Assess the patient's LOC
- Assess the rate, depth and pattern of respirations, and auscultate breath sounds
- Palpate for peripheral pulses and auscultate the apical HR
- Assess the patient's vital signs, noting hypotension and bradycardia
- Observe the patient for warm, dry skin
- Obtain a blood sample for ABGs analysis
- Provide supplemental oxygen and prepare the patient for ET intubation and mechanical ventilation, as necessary
- Initiate cardiac and haemodynamic monitoring
- Treat hypothermia with a warming blanket
- You may be asked to insert an indwelling urinary catheter
- Initiate and administer I.V. fluid resuscitation such as normal saline solution or Hartmann's s solution to increase intravascular volume and BP
- Administer medications such as sympathomimetic drugs with alpha effects, such as noradrenaline, to cause vasoconstriction and increase BP
- Administer blood products to increase intravascular volume, an osmotic diuretic such as mannitol, if urine output is decreased to increase renal blood flow, and atropine or transcutaneous pacing to treat symptomatic bradycardia.

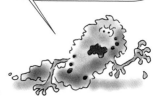

Gram-negative bacteria are the most common cause of septic shock.

Septic shock

Septic shock is caused by sepsis, also called 'bacteraemia (bacteria in the blood)', and is the result of circulating bacteria that cause the release of an endotoxin that causes vasodilatation and tissue hypoxia and so affects the normal distribution of blood flow. Bacteria, such as *Escherichia coli*, that enter the body by routes such as pneumonia, gut infections and I.V. lines. The disorder is thought to be a response to infections that release microbes or immune mediators, such as tumour necrosis factor (TNF) and interleukin-1.

It can occur in any person with impaired immunity, such as patients undergoing chemotherapy or HIV-positive patients or patients on long-term antibiotics, with children and older adults being at greatest risk. Low SVR leads to dry skin and warm peripheries (due to vasodilatation) and an elevated CO with a bounding pulse.

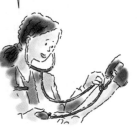

In a patient with chronic hypotension, mean arterial pressure may fall to less than 50 mm Hg before the patient exhibits signs of shock.

What causes it?

Any pathogenic organism can cause septic shock. Gram-negative bacteria, such as *E. coli*, *Klebsiella pneumoniae*, *Serratia*, *Enterobacter* and *Pseudomonas* rank as the most common causes and account for up to 70% of all cases. Opportunistic fungi cause about 3% of cases. Rare causative organisms include *Mycobacteria* and some viruses and protozoa.

How it happens

An immune response is triggered when bacteria release endotoxins. In response, macrophages secrete TNF and interleukins. These mediators in turn increase the release of platelet-activating factor, prostaglandins, leukotrienes, thromboxane A_2, kinins and complement.

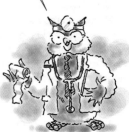

Any emergency nurse would be wise to look for these septic shock symptoms.

Truth about consequences

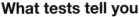

The consequences of this immune activity are vasodilation and vasoconstriction, increased capillary permeability, reduced SVR, microemboli and an elevated CO. Endotoxins also stimulate the release of histamine, further increasing capillary permeability.

Moreover, myocardial depressant factor, TNF, platelet-activating factor and other factors depress myocardial function. CO falls, resulting in systemic inflammatory response syndrome (SIRS) and multisystem organ dysfunction syndrome (MODS). (See *Understanding SIRS and MODS*, page 86.)

What tests tell you

• Blood cultures are usually positive for the offending organism
• FBC shows the presence or absence of anaemia and leukopenia, severe or absent neutropenia and (usually) the presence of thrombocytopenia
• ABG studies may reveal metabolic acidosis, hypoxemia and low $PaCO_2$ that progresses to increased $PaCO_2$ (indicating respiratory acidosis)
• U & Es are abnormal and creatinine clearance is decreased
• Prothrombin time, partial thromboplastin time and bleeding time increase, platelets decrease and fibrin split products increase
• CXRs reveal evidence of pneumonia (as the underlying infection) or acute respiratory distress syndrome (ARDS) (indicating progression of septic shock)
• ECG shows ST-segment depression and inverted T waves
• Amylase and lipase levels may show pancreatic insufficiency
• Hepatic enzyme levels are elevated because of liver ischaemia
• Blood glucose levels are initially elevated and then decreased
• Computed tomographic scan reveals abscesses or sources of possible infection.

How it's treated

Location and treatment of the underlying sepsis is essential to treating septic shock, including:
• Removal of the source of infection, such as I.V., intra-arterial or urinary drainage catheters
• Aggressive antimicrobial therapy appropriate for the causative organism
• Culture and sensitivity tests of urine and wound drainage
• Surgery, if appropriate
• Reduction or discontinuation of immunosuppressive drug therapy

Understanding SIRS and MODS

Systemic inflammatory response syndrome (SIRS)

SIRS is a systemic response to various initiators, of which infection is one. The diagnostic criteria are similar, requiring the presence of two or more of the following to define SIRS:
- Temperature – above 38.3°C or below 36.0°C
- HR – greater than 90 bpm
- Respiratory rate – greater than 20
- White blood cell count greater than 4 or less than $12 \times 10^9/L$
- Acutely altered mental status
- Hyperglycaemia – glucose greater than 8.3 mmol/L (unless diabetic).

Results such as indicated above should highlight to you that your patient is at risk of septic shock and an infection focus should be sought. It is, however, imperative that supportive measures are instigated immediately and not to wait for an infection source to be definitively identified.

The patient's history may include a disorder or treatment that causes immunosuppression, or a history of invasive tests or treatments, surgery or trauma. At onset, the patient may have fever and chills, although 20% of patients may be hypothermic. The patient's signs and symptoms will reflect the hyperdynamic (warm) phase of septic shock or the hypodynamic (cold) phase.

Multisystem organ dysfunction syndrome (MODS)

MODS is a condition that occurs when two or more organs or organ systems can't maintain homeostasis. Intervention is necessary to support and maintain organ function. MODS isn't an illness itself; rather, it's a manifestation of another progressive, underlying condition. MODS develops when widespread systemic inflammation overtaxes a patient's compensatory mechanisms. Infection, ischaemia, trauma of any sort, reperfusion injury or multisystem injury can trigger SIRS. If allowed to progress, SIRS can lead to organ inflammation and, ultimately, MODS.

Primary or secondary

Typically, MODS is classified as *primary* or *secondary*. In *primary MODS*, organ or organ system failure is due to a direct injury (such as trauma or a primary disorder) that usually involves the lungs, such as pneumonia, aspiration, near drowning and pulmonary embolism. The organ failure can be positively linked to the direct injury. Typically, ARDS develops and progresses, leading to encephalopathy and coagulopathy from hepatic involvement. As the syndrome continues, other organ systems are affected.

In *secondary MODS*, organ or organ system failure is due to sepsis. Typically, the infection source isn't associated with the lungs. The most common infection sources include intra-abdominal sepsis, extensive blood loss, pancreatitis or major vascular injuries. With secondary MODS, ARDS develops sooner and progressive involvement of other organs and organ systems occurs more rapidly.

Regardless of the type of MODS or triggering event, the overall underlying problem is inadequate perfusion.

- Possible granulocyte transfusions in patients with severe neutropenia
- Oxygen therapy and mechanical ventilation, if necessary
- Colloid or crystalloid infusions
- Administration of a vasopressor such as dopamine.

What to do
- Assess the patient's ABCDEs; monitor cardiopulmonary status closely
- Oximetry and administer supplemental oxygen to maintain target range
- ABGs values for evidence of hypoxemia and anticipate the need for ET intubation and mechanical ventilation if the patient's respiratory status deteriorates
- Place the patient in semi-recumbent position (Fowler's position) to maximise chest expansion and oxygenation (not if spinal injuries are suspected). Keep the patient as quiet and comfortable as possible to minimise oxygen demands
- Monitor the patient's vital signs continuously for changes. Observe his skin colour and check capillary refill. Notify the doctor if capillary refill is longer than 2 seconds.

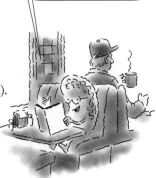

In a patient with septic shock, capillary refill shouldn't take longer than 2 seconds. I wish my 'coffee-lary' refills were that quick!

Ups and downs
- Keep in mind that the patient's temperature is usually elevated in the early stages of septic shock and that he frequently experiences shaking chills. As the shock progresses, the temperature usually drops and the patient experiences diaphoresis (sweating)
- If the patient's systolic BP drops below 80 mm Hg, you may need to increase the oxygen flow rate and you must notify the doctor immediately. Alert the doctor and increase the infusion rate if the patient experiences a progressive drop in BP accompanied by a thready pulse
- Remove I.V., intra-arterial or urinary drainage catheters and send them to the laboratory to culture for the presence of the causative organism (and prepare to reinsert or assist with reinsertion of new devices)
- Obtain blood cultures and begin antimicrobial therapy as ordered. Monitor the patient for possible adverse effects of therapy
- Institute continuous cardiac monitoring to evaluate for possible arrhythmias, myocardial ischaemia or adverse effects of treatment
- Monitor the patient's intake and output closely. Notify the doctor if the urine output is less than 0.5 ml/kg/hour
- Administer I.V. fluid therapy as ordered, usually normal saline or Hartmann's solution
- Monitor haemodynamic parameters to determine the patient's response to therapy.

Understanding DIC

DIC can occur as a complication of severe illness; 60% of cases are related to septic shock. As a result, accelerated clotting occurs, causing small vessel occlusion, organ necrosis, depletion of circulating clotting factors and platelets, activation of the fibrinolytic system and consequent severe haemorrhage. Mortality is high in acute severe DIC.

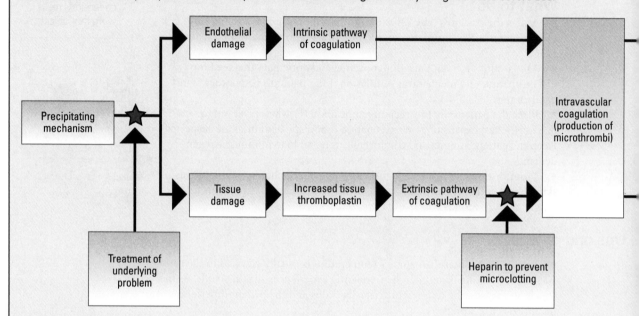

Overload alert!

- Be alert for signs and symptoms of possible fluid overload, such as dyspnoea, tachypnoea, crackles (crackles are caused by the sudden opening of small airways and alveoli collapsed by fluid, exudate or lack of aeration during expiration), peripheral oedema and jugular vein distension (indicating a raised CVP)
- Administer positive inotropic agents as ordered
- Institute infection control precautions; use strict aseptic technique for all invasive procedures
- Monitor laboratory test results, especially coagulation studies and hepatic enzyme levels, for changes indicative of DIC and hepatic failure, respectively
- Provide emotional support to the patient and his family
- Prepare the patient for surgery if appropriate.

Multi Organ Dysfunction (MOD)

Care for the patient with MODS is primarily supportive. Check whether your ED has a sepsis pathway protocol. The MODS patient is acutely ill and requires close, usually extensive monitoring. Emotional support is also crucial because mortality for a patient with MODS is directly proportional to the number of organs or organ systems affected. For example, mortality

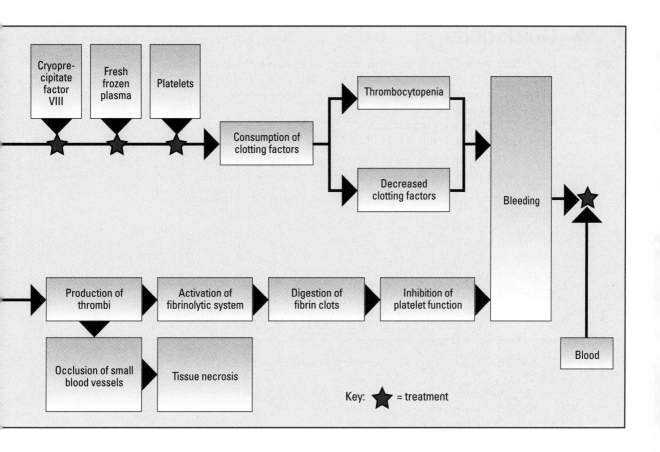

is 85% when three organs are involved; it jumps to 95% when four organs are involved and up to 99% with five-organ involvement. (See *Understanding SIRS and MODS*, page 86.)

Treatment focuses on supporting respiratory and circulatory function by using mechanical ventilation, supplemental oxygen, haemodynamic monitoring and fluid infusion to expand and maintain the intravascular compartment. Renal function is closely monitored, including hourly urine output measurements and serial laboratory tests to evaluate for trends indicating acute renal failure. Dialysis may ultimately be necessary.

Numerous drugs may be used such as:
• Antimicrobial agents to treat underlying infection
• Vasopressors, such as dopamine and noradrenaline
• Isotonic crystalloid solutions, such as normal saline and Hartmann's solution, to expand the intravascular fluid spaces
• Colloids, such as albumin, to help expand plasma volume without the added risk of causing fluid overload
• Some experimental agents, such as anti-TNF, endotoxin and anti-interleukin-1 antibodies. However, evidence supporting the effectiveness of these agents is currently unavailable.

Quick quiz

1. What's the highest priority when caring for a patient with hypovolaemic shock?

    A.   Assessing for dehydration.
    B.   Administering I.V. fluids.
    C.   Inserting a urinary catheter.
    D.   Obtaining a sample for FBC.

Answer: *B.* Hypovolaemic shock is an emergency that requires rapid infusion of I.V. fluids.

2. Which sign would lead you to suspect that a patient is experiencing septic shock?

    A.   Clear, watery sputum.
    B.   Severe hypertension.
    C.   Hypotension.
    D.   Polyuria.

Answer: *C.* Hypotension – along with pale, possibly cyanotic skin; mottling of extremities; decreased LOC; rapid, shallow respirations; decreased or absent urine output; absence of peripheral pulses or a rapid, weak pulse – is a sign of hypodynamic septic shock.

3. Which drug would you administer first to a patient with anaphylactic shock?

    A.   Adrenaline.
    B.   Hydrocortisone.
    C.   Chlorphenamine.

Answer: *A.* Immediate treatment of anaphylactic shock involves the administration of adrenaline to reverse bronchoconstriction. Later, corticosteroids, such as hydrocortisone, may be given.

4. Which of these formulae are correct?

    A. $CO = SV \times BP$.
    B. $BP = CO \times SVR$.
    C. $SV = CO \times SVR$.
    D. $CO = SV \times HR$.

Answer: *B* and *D* are correct.

Scoring

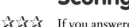   If you answered all four questions correctly, way to go! Your knowledge of this chapter's information is shockingly accurate!

    If you answered three questions correctly, nice job! Treat yourself to a multisystem-pleasing rest before going on to the next chapter.

    If you answered fewer than three questions correctly, don't be shocked! Just review the material and try again.

5 Trauma and musculoskeletal emergencies

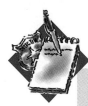

Just the facts

In this chapter, you'll learn:

♦ Assessment of the trauma patient

♦ Diagnostic tests and treatment procedures for trauma

♦ Common musculoskeletal emergencies, their causes and treatments

Multisystem trauma

Trauma is a physical injury or wound that's inflicted by an external or violent act; it may be intentional or unintentional, involving injuries to more than one body area or organ.

The type of trauma determines the extent of injury:

*   *Blunt trauma* – leaves the body surface intact
*   *Penetrating trauma* – disrupts the body surface
*   *Perforating trauma* – leaves entrance and exit wounds as an object passes through the body.

A patient experiencing multisystem trauma requires immediate action and a multidisciplinary team approach. The patient may have a head injury accompanied by chest and cardiac trauma. Or, he may have experienced a spinal cord injury along with numerous fractures and contusions to other body areas.

What causes it

Trauma may be caused by a physical injury, as from accidents, self-inflicted and other unnatural occurrence to the body.

How it happens

Trauma typically creates wounds. Traumatic wounds include:
- *Abrasion* – scraped skin, with partial loss of skin surface
- *Laceration* – torn skin, causing jagged, irregular edges (severity of which depends on size, depth and location)
- *Puncture wound* – skin penetrated by a pointed object, such as a knife or glass fragment
- *Incised would* – a sharp cut made by a sharp instrument
- *Traumatic amputation* – removal of part of the body (a limb or part of a limb).

What to look for

You should know your limitations when carrying out any assessment and if you are not competent or confident in carrying out a specific assessment you should seek senior help.

Initially, all trauma patients will be assessed and treated for life-threatening problems. This consists of a primary survey followed by a secondary survey when the patient is stabilised. A primary survey consists of a systematic assessment, ABCDE:
- A is for assessing and maintaining Airway and protecting the cervical spine (c-spine)
- B is for assessing and maintaining Breathing and adequate ventilation
- C is for assessing and maintaining Circulation and haemorrhage control
- D is for assessing Disability (level of consciousness)
- E is for Exposing the patient and rolling them to assess the posterior aspect

Whilst carrying out the assessment you need to be aware of keeping the patient comfortable (including analgesia, warmth and psychological comfort) and be alert to prepare the patient for transport and possible surgery.

What to do

- Assess the patient's ABCDEs and initiate emergency measures if necessary; administer supplemental oxygen as ordered
- Immobilise the patient's head and neck with an immobilisation device or sandbags, neck collar and tape (triple immobilisation)
- Assess and record the patient's breathing and assist with ventilation if required
- Assess record and monitor the patient for signs of hypovolaemic shock
- Monitor and record vital signs and note significant changes

- Depending on the patient's condition, insert two intravenous (I.V) large-bore catheters and infuse normal saline or Hartmann's solution as prescribed
- Obtain blood samples, including type and cross match
- Immobilise fractures
- Monitor the patient's oxygen saturation and cardiac rhythm
- Assess the patient's wounds and provide wound care as appropriate
Cover open wounds and control bleeding by applying pressure and elevating extremities
- Assess and record the patient's neurologic status, level of consciousness and pupillary and motor response
- Quickly and carefully assess the patient for multiple injuries
- Assess for increased abdominal distention and increased diameter of extremities
- Administer prescribed blood products as appropriate
- Provide prescribed pain medication as appropriate
- Reassurance the patient and his family.

All multisystem trauma patients require radiological images of c-spine, chest and pelvis to rule out any abnormalities and potential life-threatening conditions. Other images maybe performed depending on suspected injuries.

Is this secondary

After assessing and treating life-threatening conditions (primary survey) and when the patient is stable a secondary assessment needs to be performed, including reassessment and recording a full set of vital signs, taking a history and performing a physical head to toe examination. A thorough assessment helps systematically identify and correct problems and establishes a baseline for future comparison. If the patient deteriorates whilst the secondary survey is being carried out, the assessment needs to start from the beginning of the primary survey again.

Assessment findings vary according to the type and extent of trauma. A conscious patient with multiple injuries may be able to help focus the assessment on areas that need immediate attention, such as difficulty breathing and neurologic symptoms.

Out of time

During an emergency, you won't have time to obtain all of the patient's history. Focus on the most important information, including:
- Signs and symptoms related to the present condition
- Allergies to drugs, foods, latex or environmental factors
- Medication history, including prescription and over-the-counter medications, herbs and supplements
- Past medical history
- Last oral intake
- Events leading to the injury or condition.

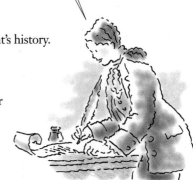

History – of the patient, that is – is always important, but in multisystem trauma emergency cases, you'll have to settle for the abridged version.

When the patient's condition is stabilised, fill in the other components of the normal health history. Always include a history of blood transfusions and tetanus immunisation, especially when the patient has an open wound. Additional diagnostic tests are performed based on the body system affected by the trauma. For example, a patient involved in a high speed road traffic collision will require X-rays such as chest, pelvis and c-spine as well as any other required X-rays. A patient with a blunt chest injury would require a chest X-ray to detect any rib, sternal fractures, pneumothorax, flail chest, pulmonary contusion and a lacerated or ruptured aorta. Admission to hospital for angiography studies would also be performed with suspected aortic laceration or rupture. Diagnostic tests for a patient with head trauma may include a CT scan of the brain and cervical spine. Someone with an asymptomatic head injury may still require cervical spine X-ray, depending on the examination and the mechanism of injury.

Some other diagnostic tests that may be performed on the patient with multisystem trauma include:
- Arterial Blood Gas (ABG) analysis to evaluate respiratory status and determine acidotic and alkalotic states
- Full Blood Count (FBC) to indicate the amount of blood loss
- Coagulation studies to evaluate clotting ability
- Serum electrolyte levels to indicate the presence of electrolyte imbalances.

All patients should be safely removed from a transfer board (spinal board) as soon as possible to relief the pain, discomfort and skin breakdown that can be potentially caused by prolonged immobilisation. This should be carried out by logrolling the patient and manually maintaining in line c-spine immobilisation. Until the c-spine is cleared of any injury; manual or triple immobilisation of the C-spine should be maintained.

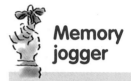

Memory jogger

To help remember what other useful information to obtain during assessment of the trauma patient, use the acronym SAMPLE.

S – Signs and symptoms
A – Allergies
M – Medications
P – Past medical history
L – Last meal
E – Events leading to injury

Understanding musculoskeletal emergencies

They may not be life-threatening, but musculoskeletal emergencies can sure mess up a patient's groove!

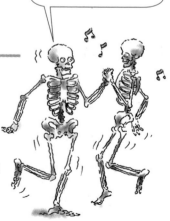

Musculoskeletal injuries are common in hospital emergency departments (EDs). The majority of these injuries aren't life threatening, but they do result in significant pain, long-term disability and possible disfigurement. These emergencies can involve the entire musculoskeletal system and include strains, sprains, contusions, fractures or traumatic amputation along with injuries to the muscles, tendons and ligaments.

Be prepared to call on your full range of nursing skills when providing orthopaedic care. While some musculoskeletal problems are subtle and difficult to assess, others are obvious or even traumatic and affect the patient physically and emotionally.

Assessment

Before you carry out any assessment of the human body you need to have the knowledge of surface anatomy, structure of the limbs and the surface landmarks of each joint.

Below is a brief outline:
- Bones – shape our structure
- Joints – bone, ligaments, cartilage, synovial membrane, synovial fluid and cavity
- Muscles – produce power and movement
- Tendons – connect muscle to bone
- Ligaments – connect bones to bones
- Nerves – communicate messages from the spinal cord or brain to organs or muscles
- Bursae – fluid filled sacs occurring at points of friction around joints
- Fibrocartilaginous discs – reduces friction between bones.

Your sharp assessment skills will help you uncover orthopaedic abnormalities and evaluate the patient's ability to perform activities of daily living (ADLs). However, because many musculoskeletal injuries are emergencies, you may have to rely on the patient's family for information about his history.

Health history

If possible, question the patient about his current and past illnesses and injuries, including allergies, medications and social history.

Current illness or injury

Question the patient about his chief complaint. Queries about the patient's pain level, factors and events came before the illness or injury and his capabilities after the illness or injury will help you decide how to initiate intervention.

Any ouchies?

For example, when a patient comes to the ED with hip pain, ask him: When did the pain start? Did he sustain an injury before the pain? If so, what type of injury – blunt trauma (a fall, a road traffic collision) or penetrating trauma (stabbing, puncture wound)?

How did it happen? For example, did he suffer hip injury after being hit by a car or did he fall from a ladder and land on his coccyx? This information will help guide your assessment and predict hidden trauma.

Out-of-joint, fractured or all muscle

Patients with joint injuries usually complain of pain, swelling or stiffness in the affected area. They may experience decreased range of movement (ROM) or be unable to bear weight. Patients with bone fractures have sharp pain when they move the affected area and will attempt to guard the affected area. Some swelling may be present. Patients with muscular injury commonly describe their pain as a burning sensation. Muscular injuries are commonly associated with swelling, bruising and weakness.

Ask the patient if his ability to carry out ADL's are affected. Has he noticed abnormal sounds (grating, crunching, clicking) when he moves certain parts of his body? Has he used ice, heat or other remedies to treat the problem?

Past illness or injury

Enquire whether the patient has ever had gout, arthritis, tuberculosis or cancer, which may cause bony metastases. Has he ever been diagnosed with osteoporosis or degenerative joint disease? Also, ask the patient whether he uses a walking aid, such as a stick, zimmer frame or brace. If so and if appropriate, watch him use the device to assess how he moves.

Medications

Question the patient about the medications he takes regularly because many drugs can affect the musculoskeletal system. Corticosteroids, for example, can cause muscle weakness, myopathy, osteoporosis, pathologic fractures and avascular necrosis of the heads of the femur and humerus. Also, ask whether he using alternative or complementary therapies.

Family history

Ask the patient if his family suffers from joint disease. Disorders with a hereditary component include:
• Gout
• Osteoarthritis of the interphalangeal joints
• Rheumatoid arthritis
• Spondyloarthropathies (such as ankylosing spondylitis, Reiter's syndrome, psoriatic arthritis and enteropathic arthritis).

Social history

Ask the patient about his dominant hand, job, hobbies and personal habits. DIY, playing football or tennis, working at a computer or doing building work can all cause repetitive stress injuries or injure the musculoskeletal system in other ways. Even carrying a heavy rucksack or bag can cause injury or increase muscle size.

What goes in

Ask about his social habits; smoking, drug or alcohol use and amount of caffeine consumed. (Caffeine can cause demineralisation of bones, causing bones to be more brittle.) Perform an abuse screen based on hospital policy. Most departments have general questions to ask all patients. These questions screen for potential abuse situations, especially intimate partner violence.

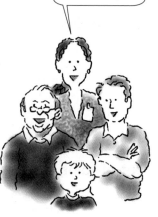

Without a doubt, gout is a hereditary disorder.

The five Ps of musculoskeletal injury

To swiftly assess a musculoskeletal injury, remember the five Ps: pain, paresthesia (sensation), paralysis (movement), pallor (colour) and pulse.

Pain

Ask the patient whether he feels pain and what increases the pain, followed by an assessment of its location, severity and quality.

Paresthesia

Evaluate the patient for loss of sensation by touching the injured area with a neurotip. Abnormal sensation or loss of sensation indicates neurovascular involvement.

Paralysis

Assess whether the patient can move the affected area. If he can't, he might have nerve or tendon damage.

Pallor

Paleness, discoloration and coolness on the injured side may indicate neurovascular compromise.

Pulse

Check all pulses distal to the injury site. A decreased or absent pulse means reduced blood supply to the area.

Physical assessment

Because the central nervous system and musculoskeletal system are interrelated, you should assess them together. To assess the musculoskeletal system, use look (inspect), feel (palpate) and move to test all the major bones, joints and muscles. Perform a whole examination if the patient has generalised symptoms, such as aching in several joints. Perform a brief examination if he has pain in only one body area, such as his ankle.

First things first

Always perform a primary survey and treat life threatening injuries first. Then perform a secondary survey, ensuring that you evaluate the neurovascular status of each injured limb. Because any patient experiencing trauma to an extremity risks neurovascular injuries and tissue ischaemia, use the 'Five Ps' to evaluate limb circulation (colour), motor function (movement) and sensation. (See *The five Ps of musculoskeletal injury*.)

After you've established the patient's airway, c-spine, breathing, circulation, disability and exposure (if needed), begin your physical assessment. As you do, ask questions that relate to the patient's history and the events leading to his injury.

A watchful eye

During inspection, be mindful of:
• Colour
• Disruption of skin integrity

- Position of the extremity
- Oedema, swelling or bruising
- Range of movement (ROM) or lack of ROM
- Symmetry, alignment, deformity.

With feeling

As you palpate, note:
- Skin temperature
- Pain and the point of tenderness
- Bony crepitus
- Joint instability
- Peripheral nerve function (sensory and motor).

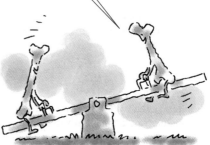

> Checking alignment isn't child's play, it's a vital part of musculoskeletal assessment.

Assessing the bones and joints

After finishing your primary survey, a secondary survey should be carried out, which includes, a head-to-toe evaluation using inspection and palpation, you can perform ROM exercises to determine whether the joints are healthy. Never force movement; ask the patient to tell you when he experiences pain. Also, watch his facial expressions for signs of pain or discomfort.

Check the neck

Before performing an examination of the neck, radiological studies of the cervical spine may be indicated to rule out injury. Spinal cord injury should be suspected whenever there is a history of significant trauma, such as a high-speed road traffic collision; fall from higher than 3 ft (1 m); significant trauma with loss of consciousness; loss or decrease of movement or sensation in the extremities; significant swelling, pain or tenderness to the neck; or penetrating trauma to the neck.

Before cervical spine clearance, the neck should be examined by manually immobilising the neck and removing the cervical collar. Inspect the front, back and sides of the patient's neck. Observe for obvious signs of injury to the cervical spine. Also assess the patient's ability to move his extremities and feel pain. Palpate the cervical area for pain, tenderness, deformity and crepitus. *Crepitus* is an abnormal grating sound, not the occasional crack we hear from our joints, and indicates fracture. Be sure to replace the collar when the neck examination is complete.

Secondly, inspect the patient's face for swelling, symmetry and evidence of trauma. The mandible should be in the midline, not shifted to the right or left.

Is the TMJ A-OK?

Next, evaluate ROM in the temporomandibular joint (TMJ). Place the tips of your first two or three fingers in front of the middle of the patient's ear and ask him to open and close his mouth. Then place your fingers into the depressed area over the joint, noting the motion of the mandible. The patient should be able to open and close his jaw and protract and retract his mandible easily, without pain or tenderness. If you hear or palpate a click as the patient's mouth opens, suspect an improperly aligned jaw. TMJ dysfunction may also lead to swelling of the area, crepitus or pain.

Head circles and chin-ups

Depending on local policy and when the doctor states that the cervical spine has been cleared of injury, you can remove the cervical collar. Now check ROM in the neck. Ask the patient to try touching his right ear to his right shoulder and his left ear to his left shoulder. The usual ROM is 40 degrees on each side. Next, ask him to touch his chin to his chest and then point his chin toward the ceiling. The neck should flex forward 45 degrees and extend backward 55 degrees.

To assess rotation, ask the patient to turn his head to each side without moving his trunk. His chin should be parallel to his shoulders. Lastly, ask him to move his head in a circle; normal rotation is 70 degrees.

Spine

Before performing an examination of the spine, radiologic studies may be indicated to rule out injury. As with cervical spine injury, injury to the spinal vertebrae should be suspected when there's significant trauma or clinical signs of injury.

The patient should be immobilised and logrolled with the assistance of four people. The remainder of the spine should be examined just as the cervical spine was. When the spine has been cleared of injury and the doctor states so, immobilisation can be discontinued. Observe the spine; it should be in midline position without deviation to either side.

Spine-tingling procedure

Palpate the spinal processes and the areas lateral to the spine. Have the patient bend at the waist and let his arms hang loosely at his sides; palpate the spine with your fingertips. Repeat the palpation using the side of your hand, lightly striking the lateral areas. Note tenderness, swelling or spasm.

Shoulders and elbows

Start by observing the patient's shoulders, noting asymmetry, muscle atrophy or deformity. Swelling or loss of normal, rounded shape could mean that one or more bones is dislocated or out of alignment. Remember, even if the patient seeks care for shoulder pain, the problem may not have started in the shoulder. Shoulder pain may come from other sources, including a heart attack, ruptured ectopic pregnancy, splenic/hepatic injury.

Palpate the shoulders with the palmar surfaces of your fingers to locate bony landmarks; note crepitus or tenderness. Using your entire hand, palpate the shoulder muscles for firmness and symmetry. Also palpate the elbow and the ulna for subcutaneous nodules that signal rheumatoid arthritis.

Lift and rotate

If the patient's shoulders are not dislocated, assess rotation. Start with the patient's arm straight at his side – the neutral position. Ask him to lift his arm straight up to shoulder level and then to bend his elbow horizontally until his forearm is at a 90-degree angle to his upper arm. His arm should be parallel to the floor and his fingers should be extended with palms down.

To assess external rotation, have him bring his forearm up until his fingers point toward the ceiling. To assess internal rotation, have him lower his forearm until his fingers point toward the floor. Normal ROM is 90 degrees in each direction.

Flex and extend

To assess flexion and extension, start with the patient's arm in the neutral position. To assess flexion, ask him to move his arm anteriorly over his head, as if reaching for the sky. Full flexion is 180 degrees. To assess extension, have him move his arm from the neutral position posteriorly as far as possible. Normal extension ranges from 30 to 50 degrees.

Swing into position

To assess abduction, ask the patient to move his arm from the neutral position laterally as far as possible. Normal ROM is 180 degrees. To assess adduction, have the patient move his arm from the neutral position across the front of his body as far as possible. Normal ROM is 50 degrees.

He up to his elbows

Next, assess the elbows for flexion and extension. Have the patient rest his arm at neutral position. Ask him to flex his elbow from this position and then extend it. Normal ROM is 90 degrees for flexion and extension.

To assess supination and pronation of the elbow, have the patient place the side of his hand on a flat surface with the thumb on top.
Ask him to rotate his palm down toward the table for pronation and upward for supination. The normal angle of elbow rotation is 90 degrees in each direction.

Wrists and hands

Inspect the wrists and hands for contour and compare them for symmetry. Also check for nodules, redness, swelling, deformities and webbing between fingers. Use your thumb and index finger to palpate both wrists and each finger joint. Note tenderness, nodules or bogginess. To avoid causing pain, be especially gentle with older adults and those with arthritis.

Rotate and flap

Assess ROM in the wrist. Ask the patient to rotate his wrist by moving his entire hand – first to the left and then to the right – as if he

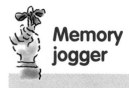

Memory jogger

Here's an easy way to keep adduction and abduction straight.

Adduction is moving a limb toward the body's midline; think of it as *adding* two things together.

Abduction is moving a limb away from the body's midline; think of it as taking something away, like *abducting* or kidnapping.

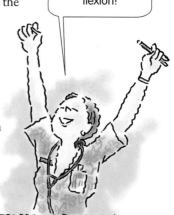

Reach for the sky – a good motto, and an even better way to check arm flexion!

waxing a car. Normal ROM is 55 degrees laterally and 20 degrees medially. Observe the wrist while the patient extends his fingers up toward the ceiling and down toward the floor, as if he flapping his hand. He should be able to extend his wrist 70 degrees and flex it 90 degrees.

Lift a finger; make a fist

To assess extension and flexion of the metacarpophalangeal joints, ask the patient to keep his wrist still and move only his fingers – first up toward the ceiling and then down toward the floor. Normal extension is 30 degrees; normal flexion, 90 degrees.

Next, ask the patient to touch his thumb to the little finger of the same hand. He should be able to fold or flex his thumb across his palm so that it touches or points toward the base of his little finger.

To assess flexion of all of the fingers, ask the patient to form a fist. Then have him spread his fingers apart to demonstrate abduction and draw them back together to demonstrate adduction.

Hips and knees

Inspect the hip area for contour and symmetry. Palpate each hip over the iliac crest and trochanteric area for tenderness or instability.

Hip, hip, hooray!

Assess ROM in the hip; these exercises are typically performed with the patient in a supine position. To assess hip flexion, place your hand under the patient's lower back and have him pull one knee as far as he can toward his abdomen and chest. You'll feel the patient's back touch your hand as the normal lumbar lordosis of the spine flattens. As the patient flexes his knee, the opposite hip and thigh should remain flat on the bed. Repeat on the opposite side.

To assess hip abduction, stand alongside the patient and press down on the superior iliac spine of the opposite hip with one hand to stabilise the pelvis. With your other hand, hold the patient's leg by the ankle and gently abduct the hip until you feel the iliac spine move. That movement indicates the limit of hip abduction. Then, while still stabilising the pelvis, move the ankle medially across the patient's body to assess hip adduction. Repeat on the other side. Normal ROM is about 45 degrees for abduction and 30 degrees for adduction.

To assess hip extension, have the patient lay prone (facedown) and gently extend the thigh upward. Repeat on the other thigh.

As the hip turns

To assess internal and external rotation of the hip, ask the patient to lift one leg up and, keeping his knee straight, turn his leg and foot medially and laterally. Normal ROM for internal rotation is 40 degrees; for external rotation, 45 degrees.

Assessing bulge sign

The bulge sign indicates excess fluid in the joint. To assess the patient for this sign, ask him to lie down so that you can palpate his knee. Then give the medial side of his knee two to four firm strokes, as shown top right, to displace excess fluid.

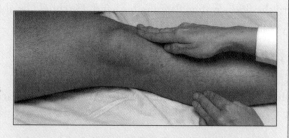

Lateral check

Next, tap the lateral aspect of his knee while checking for a fluid wave on the medial aspect, as shown bottom right.

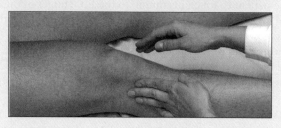

On bended knees

Inspect knee position, noting whether the patient is bowlegged (having knees that point out) or knock-kneed (having knees that turn in). Palpate both knees – they should feel smooth and the tissues should feel solid. (See *Assessing bulge sign*.)

Assess ROM in the knee. If the patient is standing, ask him to bend his knee as if he trying to touch his heel to his buttocks. Normal ROM for flexion is 120 to 130 degrees. If the patient is lying down, have him draw his knee up to his chest; his calf should touch his thigh.

Knee extension returns the knee to a neutral position of 0 degrees; however, some knees may normally be hyperextended 15 degrees. If the patient can't extend his leg fully or if his knee pops audibly and painfully, consider the response abnormal.

Other abnormalities include pronounced crepitus, which may signal a chronic disease of the knee and sudden buckling, which may indicate a ligament injury.

Ankles and feet

Inspect the ankles and feet for swelling, redness, nodules and other deformities. Check the arch of the foot and look for toe deformities. Also note oedema, calluses, bunions, corns, ingrown toenails, plantar warts, trophic ulcers, hair loss or unusual pigmentation.

Use your fingertips to palpate the bony and muscular structures of the ankles and feet. Palpate each toe joint by compressing it with your thumb and fingers.

Pop in a glass? Absolutely! But pop in a knee? Abnormal!

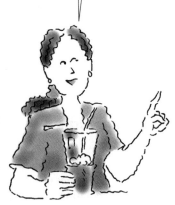

The ankle angle

To examine the ankle, have the patient sit in a chair or on the side of a bed. To test plantar flexion, ask him to point his toes toward the floor. Test dorsiflexion by asking him to point his toes toward the ceiling. Normal ROM for plantar flexion is about 45 degrees; for dorsiflexion, 20 degrees.

Next, assess ROM in the ankle. Ask the patient to demonstrate inversion by turning his feet inward and eversion by turning his feet outward. Normal ROM for inversion is 45 degrees; for eversion, 30 degrees.

To assess the metatarsophalangeal joints, ask the patient to flex his toes and then straighten them.

Assessing the muscles

When assessing the muscles, start by inspecting all major muscle groups for tone, strength and symmetry. If a muscle appears atrophied or hypertrophied, measure it by wrapping a tape measure around the largest circumference of the muscle on each side of the body and comparing the two numbers.

Other abnormalities of muscle appearance include contracture and abnormal movements, such as spasms, tics, tremors and fasciculation (fine movements of a small area of muscle).

Tuning in to muscle tone

Muscle tone describes muscular resistance to passive stretching. To test the patient's arm muscle tone, move his shoulder through passive ROM exercises. You should feel a slight resistance. Then let his arm drop. It should fall easily to his side.

Test leg muscle tone by putting the patient's hip through passive ROM exercises and then letting the leg fall to the examination table or bed. Like the arm, the leg should fall easily.

Abnormal findings include muscle rigidity and flaccidity. Rigidity indicates increased muscle tone, possibly caused by an upper motor neuron lesion after a stroke. Flaccidity may result from a lower motor neuron lesion.

Wrestling with muscle strength

Observe the patient's gait and movement to judge his general muscle strength. Grade muscle strength on a scale of 0 to 5, with 0 representing no strength and 5 representing maximum strength. Document the results as a fraction, with the score as the numerator and maximum strength as the denominator. (See *Grading muscle strength*, page 104.)

To test specific muscle groups, asks the patient to move the muscles while you apply resistance; then compare the contralateral muscle groups. (See *Testing muscle strength*, page 104.)

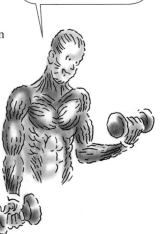

Nurses can't resist me, but I have to resist them pretty often. I tell them it's for the sake of muscle tone.

Grading muscle strength

Grade muscle strength on a scale of 0 to 5:
- 5/5 = Normal – Patient moves joint through full range of motion (ROM) and against gravity with full resistance
- 4/5 = Good – Patient completes ROM against gravity with moderate resistance
- 3/5 = Fair – Patient completes ROM against gravity only
- 2/5 = Poor – Patient completes full ROM with gravity eliminated (passive motion)
- 1/5 = Trace – Patient's attempt at muscle contraction is palpable but without joint movement
- 0/5 = Zero – There is no evidence of muscle contraction.

Testing muscle strength

To test the muscle strength of your patient's arm and ankle muscles, use the techniques shown here.

Biceps strength

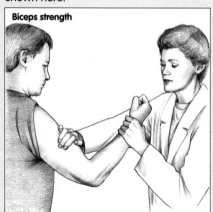

Ankle strength: Plantar flexion

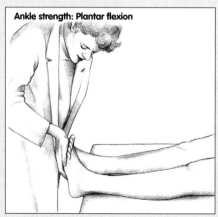

Triceps strength

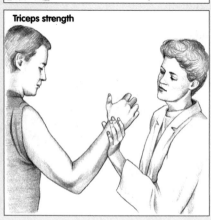

Ankle strength: Dorsiflexion

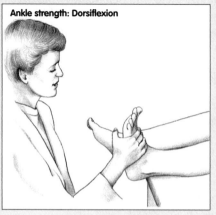

Shoulder, arm, wrist and hand strength

Test the strength of the patient's shoulder girdle by asking him to extend his arms with the palms up and hold this position for 30 seconds. If he can't lift both arms equally and keep his palms up or if one arm drifts down, he probably has shoulder girdle weakness on that side. If he passes the first part of the test, gauge his strength by placing your hands on his arms and applying downward pressure as he resists you.

Testing the bi's and tri's

Next, ask the patient to hold his arm in front of him with the elbow bent. To test bicep strength, pull down on the flexor surface of his forearm as he resists. To test triceps strength, have him try to straighten his arm as you push upward against the extensor surface of his forearm.

Forcing his hand

Assess the strength of the patient's flexed wrist by pushing against it. Test the strength of the extended wrist by pushing down on it. Test the strength of finger abduction, thumb opposition and handgrip the same way. (See *Testing handgrip strength*.)

Leg strength

Ask the patient to lie in a supine position on the examining table or bed and lift both legs at the same time. Note whether he lifts both legs at the same time and to the same distance. To test quadricep strength, have him lower his legs and raise them again while you press down on his anterior thighs.

Then ask the patient to flex his knees and put his feet flat on the bed. Assess lower-leg strength by pulling his lower leg forward as he resists and then pushing it backward as he extends his knee.

Lastly, assess ankle strength by having the patient push his foot down against your resistance and then pull his foot up as you try to hold it down.

Testing handgrip strength
When testing handgrip strength, face the patient, extend the first and second fingers of each hand and ask him to grasp your fingers and squeeze. Don't extend fingers with rings on them; a strong handgrip on those fingers can be painful.

Diagnostic tests

Diagnostic tests help confirm the diagnosis and identify the underlying cause of musculoskeletal emergencies. Common procedures include X-ray, arthrocentesis, computed tomography (CT) scan and magnetic resonance imaging (MRI).

X-rays

Anteroposterior, posteroanterior and lateral X-rays allow three-dimensional visualisation. They help diagnose:
- Fractures and dislocations
- Bone disease, including solitary lesions, multiple focal lesions in one bone or generalised lesions involving all bones

• Joint disease (such as arthritis), infection, degenerative changes, synoviosarcoma, osteochondromatosis, avascular necrosis, slipped femoral epiphysis and inflamed tendons and bursae around a joint
• Masses and calcifications.
    If the doctor needs further clarification of standard X-rays, he may order a CT scan or an MRI.

Shall or shan't I

To assist the assessment of whether an X-ray is required, Ottawa ankle and knee rules can be used. The **Ottawa Ankle Rules,** are a set of guidelines to help practitioners decide whether a patient with foot or ankle pain should be offered X-rays to diagnose a possible bone fracture. The following guidelines will help you establish the appropriateness of ordering an X-ray.
    An ankle X-ray is required only if there is any pain in the malleolar zone and any of these findings:
• Bone tenderness at the posterior edge or tip of the lateral malleolus
• Bone tenderness at the posterior edge or tip of medial malleolus.
    A foot X-ray is required if there is any pain in the midfoot zone and any of these findings:
• Bone tenderness at the base of 5th metatarsal

> Sure, X-rays help diagnose fractures, but did you know they can also point out joint disease, bone disease, and masses?

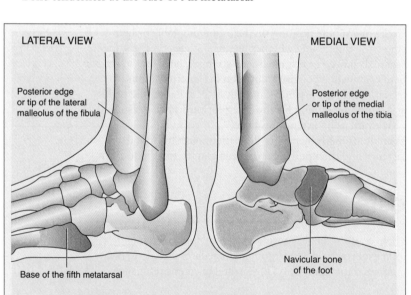

OTTAWA GUIDELINES FOR THE ANKLE & FOOT (Demonstrated on the left foot)

Drawing by: Frances Thornton, medical animator, College of Human & Health Sciences Swansea University. Reproduced from, a study to develop clinical decision rules for the use of radiography in acute ankle injuries Ian G Stiell, et al. (1992) (21):384–390. Copyright with permission from Annals of Emergency Medicine, Elsevier Ltd.

- Bone tenderness at the navicular
- Inability to weight bears both immediately and in the emergency department.

Ottawa knee rules

A knee X-ray is only required for knee injury patients with any of these findings:
- Age 55 or over
- Tenderness of the patella (no bone tenderness of the knee other than the patella)
- Tenderness at the head of the fibula
- Inability to flex to 90 degrees
- Inability to weight bear both immediately and in the emergency department (4 steps – unable to transfer weight twice onto each lower limb regardless of limping).

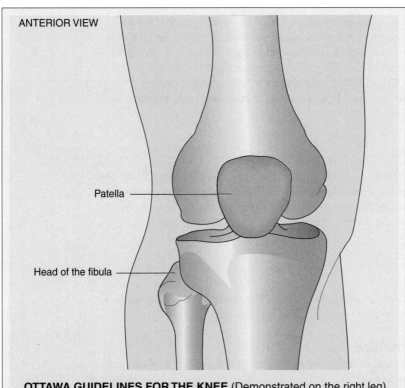

OTTAWA GUIDELINES FOR THE KNEE (Demonstrated on the right leg)

Drawing by: Frances Thornton, medical animator College of Human & Health Sciences Swansea University. Reproduced from Stiell IG, et al. (1997) Implementation of the Ottawa knee rule for the use of radiography in acute knee injuries, 278:2075–2079. Copyright with permission from Journal of the American Medical Association.

Practice pointers for an X-ray

- Explain the procedure to the patient
- Make sure the patient removes all jewellery from the area to be X-rayed
- Verify that the X-ray order includes pertinent recent history such as trauma and identifies the point tenderness site. It should also include past fractures, dislocations or surgery involving the affected area
- Medicate patients for pain before radiography. Radiography can involve movement of the affected area, increasing the patient's level of discomfort, which can lead to an uncooperative patient, poor radiography quality and an inaccurate diagnosis.

Arthrocentesis

Arthrocentesis is a joint aspiration that's used to collect synovial fluid for analysis to identify the cause of pain and swelling, to assess for infection and to distinguish forms of arthritis, such as pseudogout and infectious arthritis. The practitioner will probably choose the knee for this procedure, but he may tap synovial fluid from the wrist, ankle, elbow or first metatarsophalangeal joint. It is important that aseptic technique is crucial for this procedure.

Telltale findings

In joint infection, synovial fluid looks cloudy and contains more white blood cells (WBCs) and less glucose than normal. When trauma causes bleeding into a joint, synovial fluid contains red blood cells. In specific types of arthritis, crystals can confirm the diagnosis, such as urate crystals indicating gout.

Doing double duty

Arthrocentesis also has therapeutic value. For example, in symptomatic joint effusion, removing excess synovial fluid relieves pain.

Practice pointers

- Gain consent and describe the procedure to the patient. Explain that he'll be asked to assume a certain position, depending on the joint being aspirated and that he'll need to remain still
- After the test, the doctor may ask you to apply ice or cold packs to the joint to reduce pain and swelling
- If the doctor removed a large amount of fluid, tell the patient that he may need to wear an elastic bandage.

CT scan

A CT scan aids diagnosis of bone tumours and other abnormalities. It helps assess questionable fractures, fracture fragments, bone lesions and intra-articular loose bodies.

Beam me up

A computerised body scanner directs multiple X-ray beams at the body from different angles. The beams pass through the body and strike radiation detectors, producing electrical impulses. A computer then converts these impulses into digital information, which is displayed as a three-dimensional image on a visual display monitor.

Practice pointers
- Verify patient allergies and hypersensitivities
- The patient should be in a hospital gown and instructed to remove all jewellery and hairpins
- Inform the patient that he won't be in an enclosed space, that the machine isn't enclosed and that it's shaped like a doughnut. Let him know that he'll hear a low-pitched spinning sound
- Tell him there will be no pain involved
- Instruct him to remain still during the test. Although he'll be alone in the room, assure him that he can communicate with the technician through an intercom system.

MRI

MRI can show irregularities of soft tissue (such as brain tissue), bone and muscle.

The MRI scanner uses a powerful magnetic field and radiofrequency energy to produce images based on the hydrogen content of body tissues. The computer processes signals and displays the resulting high-resolution image on a video monitor. The patient can't feel the magnetic fields and no harmful effects have been observed.

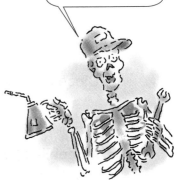

Metal and magnets don't mix! Make sure patients remove all metal objects before entering the MRI.

Practice pointers
- Make sure the patient is in a hospital gown and has removed all metal objects, including jewellery, piercings, watches, eyeglasses, hearing aids and dental appliances. He should also secure his belongings – including credit, bank and parking cards – because the scan could erase their magnetic codes

- Explain the patient that he'll be positioned on a narrow bed that slides into a large cylinder housing the MRI magnets. Ask if claustrophobia has ever been a problem for him. If so, sedation may help him tolerate the scan
- Tell the patient he'll hear soft thumping noises during the test
- Instruct him to remain still during the test. Although he'll be alone in the room, assure him that he can communicate with the technician through an intercom system.

Treatments

Pain and impaired mobility are good motivators for obtaining medical care. Consequently, most patients with musculoskeletal problems eagerly seek treatment.

Get up and go again

To restore a patient's mobility, several treatments are used alone or in combination:
- Drug therapy to control pain, inflammation or muscle spasticity
- Nonsurgical treatments, including closed reduction or immobilisation
- Surgery with subsequent immobilisation in a cast, brace or other device.

Drug therapy

Salicylates are the first line of defence against arthropathies. Other drug therapy includes analgesics, nonsteroidal anti-inflammatory drugs, corticosteroids and skeletal muscle relaxants.

Nonsurgical treatments

Some patients with musculoskeletal emergencies require nonsurgical treatment. Treatment options include closed reduction of a fracture or immobilisation.

Closed reduction

Closed reduction involves external manipulation of fracture fragments or dislocated joints to restore their normal position and alignment. It may be done under conscious sedation or local, regional or general anaesthesia.

Immobilisation/spintage

Immobilisation devices are commonly used to maintain proper alignment, limit movement and help relieve pain and pressure.

Don't move a muscle!

Immobilisation devices include:
- Plaster and synthetic casts applied after closed or open reduction of fractures or after other severe injuries
- Splints to immobilise fractures, dislocations or subluxations

Education edge

Teaching about immobilisation devices

While discharging a patient with a musculoskeletal injury that has been prescribed an immobilisation device, be sure to include these points:

- Tell him to promptly report signs of complications, including increased pain, drainage or swelling in the involved area
- Stress the need for strict compliance with activity restrictions while the immobilisation device is in place
- If the patient was given a walking frame or crutches to use with a leg or ankle cast, splint or knee immobiliser, make sure he able to demonstrate correct ambulation using the device
- If the patient has a removable device, such as a knee immobiliser, make sure he/she knows how to apply it correctly
- Advise the patient to keep scheduled medical appointments to evaluate healing.

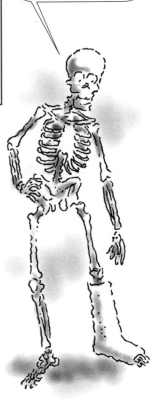

Casts can be applied after severe injuries for closed or open fracture reductions.

- Slings to support and immobilise an injured arm, wrist or hand or to support the weight of a splint or hold dressings in place
- Skin or skeletal traction, using a system of weights and pulleys to reduce fractures, treat dislocations, correct deformities or decrease muscle spasms
- Braces to support weakened or deformed joints
- Cervical collars to immobilise the cervical spine, decrease muscle spasms and, possibly, relieve pain. Remember, a person with a cervical spine injury needs triple immobilisation
- Long spine boards with cervical immobilisation devices to fully immobilise the entire spine. (See *Teaching about immobilisation devices*.)

Surgery

The patient could be admitted to hospital for surgical procedures that involves open reduction and internal fixation. During open reduction, the surgeon restores the normal position and alignment of fracture fragments or dislocated joints, then inserts internal fixation devices – such as pins, screws, wires, nails, rods or plates – to maintain alignment until healing begins.

Common disorders

In any musculoskeletal emergency, neurologic and vascular status must be evaluated carefully because a patient with a musculoskeletal illness or injury is in danger of potential neurovascular injuries and tissue ischaemia. Musculoskeletal emergencies may include many ailments, some of which are:

Dislocations and fractures

A *dislocation* is an injury that occurs at the articulation of two or more bones, causing to move out of their anatomically correct position. Dislocations may also include associative soft tissue and vascular or nerve injury. (See *Types of dislocations*.)

A *fracture* is an interruption in the continuity and stability of the bone. Fractures however, painful and temporarily debilitating, don't cause fatalities. If not recognised and treated, the complications of a fracture can lead to permanent disability and even death. They are classified by five general divisions:

 Anatomic location

 Direction of fracture lines

 Relationship of fragments to each other

 Stability

Associated soft tissue injury.

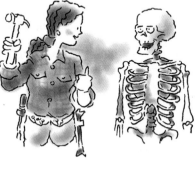

Can you pick up more screws and nails at the store? I need them for home repair, and you need them for bone repair.

Trauma and force

Direct trauma is an injury caused by a force directly impacted or caused the damage, while *indirect trauma* is caused by the transmission of force from one area to another.

Location and direction

Anatomic location describes exactly the location of fracture in a bone. A long bone is divided into sections:
- Proximal
- Middle or distal
- Head, shaft or base.
  The *direction* of the fracture line is categorised as:
- *transverse* – when the fracture is perpendicular to the bone
- *oblique* – when the line runs across the bone at a 45- to 60-degree angle
- *spiral* – when the direction of the fracture line looks twisted
- *comminuted* – when the bone is broken into more than two fragments
- *impacted* – when the ends of the fracture are compressed together.
(See *Classifying fractures*, page 115.)

Transverse, oblique or comminuted fractures generally occur as a result of direct force. Avulsion, spiral and stress fractures are typically caused by indirect force.

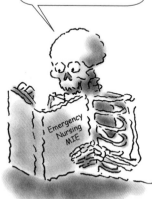

Interruption of stability, relationship of fragments – this fracture stuff sounds awfully emotional.

Types of dislocations

This chart lists the common sites of dislocations, causes, common signs and symptoms and treatments for each type.

Location	Causes	Signs and symptoms	Treatments
Acromioclavicular separation	• Common athletic injury • Fall or direct blow to the point of the shoulder	• Severe pain in the joint area • Inability to raise the arm or adduct the arm across the chest • Deformity • Point tenderness	• Depends on the degree of dislocation • Reduction, which should take place as soon as possible to avoid complications • Post reduction treatment of minor injuries, including splinting in position of comfort with sling, which the patient should maintain for approximately 7 to 10 days • Open reduction or having the patient wear the splint for a longer period for more severe injuries
Shoulder	*Anterior* • Usually an athletic injury resulting from a fall on an extended arm which is externally rotated and abducted *Posterior* • Rare but may be seen when the arm has been forcefully abducted and internally rotated	• Decreased or limited range of motion (ROM) • Decreased function • Deformity	• Closed reduction after associative fracture is ruled out • Reduction, which should occur immediately if neurovascular compromise is present • Operative interventions when indicated, as when there's soft-tissue interposition, displaced greater tuberosity fracture and Glenoid rim fracture measuring greater than 5 mm • Surgery, possibly the treatment of choice for athletes
Elbow	• Fall on an extended arm	• Pain that increases with movement • Neuro-vascular deficits • Decreased or limited ROM • Decreased function • Deformity	• Varied, based on direction of dislocation, but usually closed reduction followed by splint application • Surgical repair for a dislocation that's irreducible or one that has associative neurovascular compromise
Wrist	• Fall on an outstretched hand (FOOSH)	• Pain, especially with movement • Deformity	• Support in position of comfort • Closed reduction • Surgical intervention
Hand or finger	• Fall on an outstretched hand (FOOSH) • Direct blow to the fingertip or a jamming force to the fingertip	• Pain • Swelling • Deformity • Inability to move the joint	• Support in position of comfort • Reduction

(continued)

Types of dislocations (Continued)

Location	Causes	Signs and symptoms	Treatments
Hip	• Major trauma such as frontal road traffic collision (foot on brake pedal or knee hits dashboard). A significant force required and therefore considers other injuries.	• Hip pain • Knee pain • Pain that may radiate to groin • Hip flexed, adducted and internally rotated (posterior dislocation) • Hip slightly flexed, abducted and externally rotated (anterior dislocation [rare]) • Patient complaints of joint feeling locked • Inability to move the leg	• Support in position of comfort • Surgical reduction • For postsurgical dislocation, closed reduction under moderate sedation or, if unsuccessful, completed under general anaesthesia
Knee	• Major trauma • High-speed road traffic collision • Sports injury	• Severe pain • Deformity • Gross swelling • Inability to move the joint	• Splint in position of comfort • Immediate reduction (within 24 hours) • Admission or transfer to the operating room
Patella	• History of spontaneous dislocation • Direct trauma • Rotation of a planted foot	• Knee in flexed position • Pain • Loss of function • Swelling • Tenderness	• Possible spontaneous reduction into place • Splint or cast • Crutches
Ankle	• Commonly associated with a road traffic collision (foot on pedal) • Commonly associated with a fracture	• Swelling • Neurovascular deficits • Deformity • Pain • Inability to move the joint	• Possible surgical reduction • Splint or cast • Crutches

Relationship and stability

The relationship of the fracture fragments to each other is described by *alignment* and *apposition*. *Alignment* tells about the position and placement of bones. *Apposition* describes the contact between the fracture surfaces.

Stability describes the tendency of a fracture to displace after reduction. A *stable* fracture doesn't displace; an *unstable* fracture does.

Don't go soft on us now

Associated soft tissue injury is divided into:
• *Simple* – when there's no break in the skin
• *Compound* – when overlying skin is broken, but there's no direct communication between open skin and the fracture
• *Complicated* – when there's associative neurovascular, visceral, ligament or muscular damage. (Intra-articular fractures are also categorised as complicated.)

Classifying fractures

One of the best-known systems for classifying fractures uses a combination of terms – such as *simple*, *nondisplaced* and *oblique* – to describe them.

General classification of fractures
- *Simple (closed)* – Bone fragments don't penetrate the skin
- *Compound (open)* – Bone penetrating through the skin
- *Incomplete (partial)* – Bone continuity isn't completely interrupted
- *Complete* – Bone continuity is completely interrupted.

Classification by fragment position
- *Comminuted* – The bone breaks into small pieces
- *Impacted* – One bone fragment is forced into another
- *Angulated* – Fragments lie at an angle to each other
- *Displaced* – Fracture fragments separate and are deformed
- *Nondisplaced* – The two sections of bone maintain essentially normal alignment
- *Overriding* – Fragments overlap, shortening the total bone length
- *Segmental* – Fractures occur in two adjacent areas with an isolated central segment
- *Avulsed* – Fragments are pulled from normal position by muscle contractions or ligament resistance.

Classification by fracture line
- *Linear* – The fracture line runs parallel to the bone's axis
- *Longitudinal* – The fracture line extends in a longitudinal (but not parallel) direction along the bone's axis
- *Oblique* – The fracture line crosses the bone at roughly a 45-degree angle to the bone's axis
- *Spiral* – The fracture line crosses the bone at an oblique angle, creating a spiral pattern
- *Transverse* – The fracture line forms a right angle with the bone's axis.

> Soft tissue injuries are like good stories; some are simple, and some are complicated.

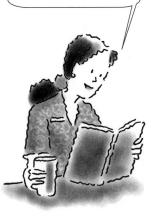

What causes it
Direct or indirect trauma is the root cause of most of dislocations and fractures, although some have different causes. Stress fractures result from repetitive use or motion. Pathologic fractures occur in a bone weakened by a pre-existing disease. They can be preceded by injury or occur during normal activity. Regardless of underlying disease, the mechanism of injury plays an important role. (See *understanding fractures*, pages 116–121.)

How it happens
The degree and severity of dislocations or fractures depends on outside factors: amount, direction and duration of force, and the frequency of the injury-causing act.

(Text continues on page 120.)

Understanding fractures

Fractures can occur in almost every part of every limb. Depending on where and how they occur, each brings with it specific complications and therapeutic interventions to be alert for. The chart below describes common fractures, their causes, signs and symptoms, interventions and the possible complications associated with each type.

Fracture	Causes	Signs and symptoms
Clavicle	• Most common in paediatric patients • Fall on extended arm or shoulder • Contact sports • Direct blow to shoulder	• Pain in clavicle area • Swelling • Deformity • Bony crepitus • Patient can't or won't raise arm
Shoulder and humerus	• Fall on outstretched arm • Direct shoulder trauma from a fall or a blunt instrument	• Pain in shoulder area • Point tenderness • Posterior rotation • Inability to move affected arm • Adduction of the humerus • Abduction of humerus • Gross oedema and discoloration that can extend to chest wall
Scapula	• Direct trauma; penetrating or blunt. Significant force required, therefore need to look for underlying lung/cardiac injury	• Pain on shoulder movement • Point tenderness • Arm held in adduction with resistance to abduction • Bruising • Palpable bony displacement • Swelling
Upper arm	• Fall on arm or direct blow • Twisting or throwing of the arm	• Bony crepitus • Bruising • Inability to move arm • Pain • Point tenderness • Severe deformity • Swelling
Elbow	• Fall on extended arm • Fall on flexed elbow	• Severe pain • Point tenderness • Rapid swelling • Shortening of the arm • Delayed capillary refill
Radius or ulna	• Fall on extended arm • Direct blow • Forced pronation of the forearm	• Pain • Point tenderness • Swelling • Deformity • Angulation • Shortening

Interventions	Possible complications
• Shoulder immobilisation	• Brachial plexus injury • Ligament damage • Malunion • Subclavian vascular injury
• Immobilisation of arm in a sling, shoulder immobiliser or collar and cuff • Surgery if fracture is impacted, comminuted or displaced	• Laceration of the axillary artery • Brachial plexus injury • Avascular necrosis of the humeral head • Frozen shoulder syndrome • Nonunion
• Immobilisation of arm in a sling, shoulder immobiliser or collar and cuff • Padding the axilla to avoid injury to the brachial plexus and artery	• Injury to the ribs • Pneumorthorax • Haemothorax • Compression fractures of the spine
• Immobilisation of arm in a sling, shoulder immobiliser or collar and cuff • Surgical intervention (for fracture that extends below the elbow, spiral fractures or shaft fractures)	• Laceration or stretching of the radial nerve resulting in neuropraxia
• Splint the arm "as it lies" • Orthopaedic consult • Assess for vascular compromise	• Brachial artery laceration • Nerve damage • Volkmann's ischemic contracture
• Closed reduction • Casting • Referral to orthopaedic surgeon • Open reduction and internal fixation	• Paralysis of the radial nerve • Malunion • Volkmann's ischemic contracture

(continued)

Understanding fractures *(Continued)*

Fracture	Causes	Signs and symptoms
Wrist	• Dorsiflexion, usually following a fall on an extended arm or open hand	• Pain • Snuff box tenderness (Scaphoid) • Swelling • Deformity • Limited range of motion • Numbness • Weakness
Hand and finger	• Forceful hyperextension • Direct trauma • Crush injury	• Pain • Point tenderness • Severe swelling • Deformity • Inability to use hand
Pelvis	• Road traffic collision • Fall from a height • Crush injury • Direct trauma	• Tenderness when iliac wings are compressed • Paraspinous muscle spasms • Sacroiliac joint tenderness • Haematuria • Pelvic bruising • Groin pain • Blood at the urethral meatus • Perineal haematomas • Prostate displacement and loss of sphincter tone
Hip (acetabulum, greater trochanter, femoral head)	• Direct blow or fall • Common older adult injury • Axial transmission of force from knees as in knee-to-dashboard injuries	• Pain in hip or groin area • Severe pain with movement • Inability to bear weight • External rotation of the affected hip and leg • Shortening of the affected limb
Femur	• Indirect force upward through a flexed knee • Direct trauma • Falls • Road traffic collision (especially vehicle-pedestrian collision)	• Angulation • Shortening of the limb • Severe muscle spasm • Bony crepitus • Severe pain • Swelling of the thigh • Haematoma in the thigh • Inability to bear weight on the affected leg
Knee	• High-velocity trauma • Pedestrian trauma (such as from a bumper) • Fall from a height onto a flexed knee • Hyperabduction	• Bony crepitus • Tense swelling in the popliteal area • Haemarthrosis, swelling around the joint • Knee pain and tenderness • Inability to straighten or bend the knee

Interventions	Possible complications
• Closed reduction • Rigid splint or a thumb spica cast • Referral to orthopaedic surgeon	• Rare aseptic necrosis
• Closed reduction • Finger traction • Splinting distal phalanges with a padded aluminium guard • Neighbour strapping an injured finger to an uninjured one • Antibiotics for open fractures	• Malunion • Osteomyelitis • Subungual haematoma
• Aggressive resuscitation (oxygen, crystalloids, blood transfusion) • Immobilisation of the spine and legs • Pelvic stabilisation (internal or external fixation) • Pelvic computed tomography (CT) scan • Abdominal CT scan • Antibiotics	• Haemorrhage, shock, death • Bladder, genital or lumbosacral trauma • Ruptured internal organs • Osteomyelitis • Compartment syndrome • Chronic pain • GI tract injury • Pulmonary or fat emboli
• Immobilisation in a comfortable position • Traction • Referral to an orthopaedic surgeon • Surgical intervention	• Avascular necrosis of the femoral head • Phlebitis of the femoral vein • Osteoarthritis • Sciatic nerve injury • Hypovolaemic shock • Fat embolism syndrome
• Aggressive resuscitation (oxygen, crystalloids, blood transfusion) • Immobilisation of the thigh with a traction splint • Referral to an orthopaedic surgeon • Open reduction with internal fixation	• Haemorrhage • Severe muscle damage • Knee trauma (commonly overlooked)
• Non-weight bearing cast • Traction • Crutches • Referral to an orthopaedic surgeon • Open reduction and internal fixation	• Popliteal nerve or artery injury • Fat emboli • Rotational deformities • Traumatic arthrosis

(continued)

Understanding fractures (Continued)

Fracture	Causes	Signs and symptoms
Patella	• Direct trauma (dashboard impact) or a fall • Indirect trauma (after quadriceps muscle pull or contraction)	• Knee pain • Haemarthrosis • Inability to extend the knee
Tibia and fibula	• Twisting or rotating forces • Direct trauma • Fall with compression forces • Fall with foot fixed in place such as in a ski injury	• Pain • Point tenderness • Swelling • Deformity • Bony crepitus
Ankle	• Direct trauma • Indirect trauma • Torsion, eversion or inversion	• Popping sound at time of injury (torn ligaments) • Bruising • Bony crepitus • Pain on ambulation or altered gait • Inability to bear weight if injury is unstable
Foot	• Similar to ankle injury • Athletic injuries • Direct trauma	• Deep pain • Point tenderness • Bruising • Swelling • Subungual haematoma • Inability to bear weight • Deformity
Heel	• Fall from a height. Need to look for coexisting lower spinal injury	• Increased pain with hyperflexion • Point tenderness • Pain in hind foot • Soft tissue bruising • Superficial skin blistering • Deformity
Toe	• Direct trauma (stubbing or kicking) • Crush injuries • Athletic injuries	• Subungual haematoma • Pain • Deformity • Discoloration

Dislocation

A dislocation occurs when there's a disruption in the relationship of the bones at their junction. Reduction of dislocations must be completed as soon as possible to restrict the injury from progressing to adjacent vasculature and nerves.

Fracture

A fracture occurs when the stress applied to the bone exceeds its plasticity. The bone's strength is directly related to its density. An underlying disease process, specific medication regimens and some congenital anomalies,

Interventions	Possible complications
• Surgery for quadriceps repair	• Avascular necrosis
• Assessment for puncture wound associated with tibia (open fracture) • Wound debridement and irrigation • Casting • Crutches • Open reduction and internal fixation	• Compartment syndrome • Infection • Osteomyelitis • Nonunion
• Closed reduction • Posterior splint • Possible open reduction and internal fixation • Casting • Crutches	• Nonunion • Infection • Posttrauma arthritis
• Bulky dressing • Orthopaedic shoe • Posterior splint • Crutches	• Avascular necrosis • Malunion • Gait abnormalities
• Bulky and compression dressings • Ensuring non-weight-bearing or partial-weight-bearing • Crutches • Surgery (usually not scheduled for 2 days to 2 weeks following injury) • Closed reduction for displaced fractures • Assessment for associated trauma	• Chronic pain • Nerve entrapment
• Compression bandage • Neighbour taping/strapping • Orthopaedic shoe • Crutches as needed	• None

affect the density of bony structure. Immediately after a fracture, the bone body initiates its own healing process. This process occurs in three phases:

Inflammatory phase

Reparative phase

Remodelling phase.

It's a haematoma!

Because the periosteum is torn, a haematoma forms between the two separated areas of bone. In the *inflammatory phase*, the haematoma begins to clot and deprives the osteocytes at the bones' ends of oxygen and nutrients, which causes them to die. A significant inflammatory response ensues, including vasodilation, causing release of inflammatory cells, leukocytes and macrophages.

Organisation is key

Next, in the *reparative phase*, cells within the haematoma (mesenchymal cells) organise, localise and begin to form bone. Osteoblasts move from inside the bone toward the damaged ends and assist in the healing process.

I'm brand new!

New bone is formed from trabeculae organisation – causing the reconnection of the previously separated bone edges – in the *remodelling phase* of healing.

What to look for

The most common signs and symptoms of dislocations and fractures include:
- Pain
- Swelling
- Bruising
- Point tenderness.

What's more...

Deformity may also be present and can be associated with a loss of normal function ranging from minimal to complete, depending on the injury. Associative blood loss shouldn't be overlooked during patient care; blood loss volumes can be minimal to shock-inducing. Estimated blood loss can be up to 3 L (in conjunction with a pelvic fracture), leading to hypovolaemia and shock.

A pathologic fracture can produce painless swelling and generalised bone pain without swelling.

Signs and symptoms of stress fractures can vary depending on the area of injury. However, the patient's chief complaint is of pain that has been getting progressively worse over time during an activity.

What tests tell you

These tests help determine dislocation or fracture:
- MRIs are most helpful with the diagnosis of tendon, ligament and soft tissue injuries
- CT scans to evaluate a bone for a fracture, especially when serial radiography has been discomforting but the patient complains of persistent pain

- X-rays provide evidence of most fractures. Some fractures will only show up after a long time, so follow-up radiography is an important part of fracture management.

How it's treated

Fracture management is based on evaluation of the type and classification of the injury and practitioner preference based on experience and evidence based practice:
- Pain management is a primary concern for all dislocations and fractures
- Splinting is the initial treatment for most fractures and is applied in the ED. Splints are used to prevent further soft tissue injury from fracture fragments, to decrease pain by providing support and position of comfort and to lower the risk of clinical fat emboli. (See *Common splint types*)
- General indications for surgical treatment of fractures include displaced intra-articular fractures, associated arterial injury, when closed methods of treatment have failed, fractures through metastatic lesions or for patients who can't be confined to bed. Postoperatively, a splint or cast is applied to maintain correct alignment
- Closed reduction should be performed within 6 to 12 hours of the time of injury because swelling makes the procedure difficult.

Inspired casting

- Indications for applying a cast include pain relief, immobilisation of a fracture for healing and stabilisation of an unstable fracture. Casts are individually moulded for the patient using plaster or fibreglass casting material. As a therapy, casts are generally reserved for application until swelling has resolved – approximately 3 to 5 days after the injury or surgery
- Pathologic fractures are treated with immobilisation, rest as well as pain control. They need to be referred to further investigation of the cause of the fracture
- Stress fracture treatment varies depending on severity and location and is similar to the treatment of a sprain or strain. The injuring activity is limited or eliminated. Rest is one of the most important interventions for recovery. Treatment for stress fracture in the lower extremity involves crutches. The healing time frame is approximately 4 to 6 weeks. The few cases in which casting treatment is preferred over splinting are usually managed by a orthopaedic doctor
- Unstable fractures are treated surgically.

What to do

- Assess the patient's ABCDEs and ensure that the cervical spine has been cleared before addressing secondary findings
- Assess for paresthesia
- Assess the injured area for vascular stability, capillary refill and pulses distal to the injury
- Remove jewellery from or distal to affected area because it can act as a tourniquet if left in place

Common splint types

Examples of commonly used splints include:
- Thomas's splint for shaft of femur fractures preoperatively
- Futuro splints for immobilisation and support of the wrist or ankle
- Box splints for immobilisation and support of the ankle or foot
- Vacuum splints used in the pre-hospital environment to provide immobilisation to extremities
- Fibreglass and plaster of paris splinting material in a variety of widths and lengths.

- Evaluate the patient's tetanus status. Administer a booster if the patient is not fully immunised (a total of 5 doses of a tetanus-containing vaccine)
- Apply ice for 20-minute intervals to decrease swelling
- Assist with splinting as appropriate
- Cover open fractures with a moist, sterile dressing
- Request and provide analgesia
- Prepare the patient for admission if appropriate
- Prepare the patient for the operating room if appropriate.

Pelvic plan

If the patient has a suspected pelvic fracture, follow these steps:
- Wrap the pelvis with an external fixator (the policy varies in different departments) to reduce bleeding
- If not contraindicated, decrease pain by having the patient flex his knees
- Prepare for and assist with analgesia
- Monitor vital signs, including neurovascular assessment, every 5 minutes
- Administer prescribed fluids and antibiotics via a large-bore I.V. line and administer supplemental oxygen
- Administer prescribed blood products as ordered
- Prepare the patient for the operating room to receive definitive care.

Puncture wounds

A *puncture wound* is a piercing of the skin by a foreign object, causing a hole in the skin and underlying tissues. Puncture wounds can be superficial and only involve the skin or can extend through tissue and into the bone, depending on the mechanism of injury.

What causes it

Puncture wounds are caused by direct trauma. The possible mechanisms of injury are endless, but some examples include bites and foreign objects, such as nails, needles, pins and knives. The length of the offending object may not realistically relate to the depth of the wound as the skin and tissues depress, therefore, the wound maybe deeper than the length of the object.

What to look for

Assess the wound for signs and symptoms of infection and obvious presence of a retained foreign body.

What tests tell you

X-rays should be completed if the wound is near a joint or bone to rule out underlying fracture and presence of some types of foreign bodies.

How it's treated

If the wound is simple and the patient is healthy, prophylactic antibiotics may not help; in fact, they may predispose the patient to superinfection of *Pseudomonas*. In many cases, cleaning and irrigating the wound is all that's necessary.

What to do

- Assess the patient's ABCDEs and ensure cervical spine clearance before addressing secondary findings
- Control bleeding with direct pressure and elevation; note the amount of blood loss from the wound. Take help from a senior if bleeding doesn't stop within 10 minutes of applying pressure
- Evaluate the patient's tetanus status
- Irrigate the wound if it isn't associated with an underlying fracture
- If the wound contains foreign matter, is associated with a fracture or is more than 8 hours old, there may be need to administer oral or I.V. antibiotics
- Perform wound care, such as, necessary dressings, immobilisation devices and potentially wound closure (see Chapter 12, *Environmental emergencies*).

Strains and sprains

Strain is used to describe a pulling apart of muscle fibres, while a *sprain* describes a pulling apart of the fibres within a ligament. Both can result from direct or indirect trauma.

What causes it

The most common cause of strains and sprains is sports-related trauma. Other common causes include road traffic collisions and falls.

How it happens

A strain is classified by degree and location of the muscle:
- A *first-degree* strain is caused by a forcible overstretching of a muscle
- A *second-degree* strain is a disruption of more muscle fibres (more forceful contraction or stretch) than a first-degree strain
- A *third-degree* strain entails a complete disruption of the muscle fibres and may be accompanied by a rupture of the overlying fascia or an avulsion fracture of the underlying bone.

Sprain, sprain, go away!

A sprain is also diagnosed by degree and location, but of ligaments (not muscle).
- In a *first-degree* sprain, the involved ligament stretches without tearing – the joint remains stable and joint function remains normal
- A *second-degree* sprain involves stretching and tearing of the involved ligament, causing moderate function loss and mild to moderate joint instability
- A *third-degree* sprain is the most painful and physically limiting. It involves a complete disruption of the

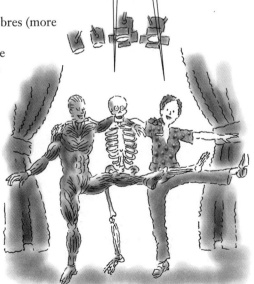

I'm glad you let me be in the show, but I didn't have time to stretch.

Then, Skelly, you got some sprainin' to do!

ligament, causing profound joint instability, moderate to severe loss of function and an inability to hold an object (if located in the upper extremity) or weight bear (if located in the lower extremity).

What to look for

First- and second-degree strains are similar in presentation, therefore differentiation is based on the degree of loss of function and level of swelling. Characteristics of first- and second-degree strains include:
- Mild localised swelling
- Bruising
- Mild spasms
- Localised discomfort, possibly aggravated by movement or pressure
- Minimal but transient loss of function and strength.
 Characteristics of a third-degree strain include:
- Moderate to severe swelling with bruising
- Moderate to severe pain
- Muscle spasm
- Moderate to complete loss of function
- Knotlike protrusion on the muscle at the injury site.

Sprain symptoms

Patients with a first-degree sprain demonstrate:
- Minimal swelling
- Little or no joint instability
- Mild discomfort.
Symptoms of a second-degree sprain are more pronounced. They include:
- Moderate to severe swelling
- Bruising
- Moderate functional loss
- Mild to moderate joint instability.
A third-degree sprain causes:
- Patient's inability to bear weight or hold an object
- Moderate to severe swelling
- Bruising
- Joint instability.

Any good chef will tell you that presentation is everything. That goes double when you're diagnosing strains and sprains.

What tests tell you

Just like contusions, strains and sprains are diagnosed by clinical presentation. X-rays will only verify the lack of an underlying fracture. Thus, radiography isn't always needed before diagnosis. For example, if a patient has lower back pain and mild spasms but denies recent trauma such as a fall, then radiography isn't necessarily indicated.

Stress test

To test the severity of a strain a stress test can be performed. This involves a method of applying tension to a joint to estimate the integrity of a ligament.

What to do

- Position the patient in a relaxed position
- Take hold of the proximal end of the injury
- Take hold of the distal end of the injury
- Position the limb in the correct position
- Apply a force in the suitable direction to stretch the ligament.

The greater the positive result the greater the injury.

How it's treated

Treatment depends on the extent of the injury extent. All strains and sprains are treated with analgesia, ice, elevation and immobilisation on arrival at the ED. When a differential diagnosis has been made, treatment methods and recovery periods vary:

- *First-degree* strains and sprains are treated with ice and rest over a couple of days. Mild analgesics may be prescribed. Activity can be gradually resumed as tolerated
- In addition to analgesia, rest, ice and elevation, a *second-degree* strain or sprain is immobilised and all patient activity is restricted until swelling and pain subside. Use of immobilisers (for upper-extremity injuries) and crutches (for lower-extremity injuries) is common. Ice is applied for the first 24 to 48 hours, after which the use of heat is prescribed. Use of the injured muscle is gradual and stopped if pain is experienced. Slow and steady progression is the key to recovery. Returning to normal activity too soon will cause re-injury
- *A third-degree* strain or sprain is initially treated in the same way as a second-degree strain: with analgesia, ice, elevation and immobilisation. After these interventions, the patient is referred to a specialist for further evaluation and treatment, which may include surgical repair. A more substantial analgesia medication may be required by these patients because of the injury's extent.

What to do

- Assess the patient's ABCDEs and manage life-threatening concerns The patient's ABCDEs and cervical spine should be cleared before addressing secondary findings.
- Request and administer analgesics
- Immediately apply ice, provide support with a splint or other immobilisation device and elevate the area for comfort
- Obtain a thorough history of the present illness, including precipitating factors. For example, a patient may have ankle pain as his chief complaint because that's what is bothering him now, but asking when the pain and swelling began may reveal that he fell down the steps. Further questioning may reveal that he actually had an episode of syncope while using the steps to get to his sublingual nitro-glycerine medication
- Remove jewellery from or distal to the affected area because it can act as a tourniquet if left in place
- Assist the patient into a wheelchair or onto a stretcher, if appropriate, to prevent further injury from weight-bearing activity
- Provide patient education. (See *Teaching about strains and sprains*, page 128.)

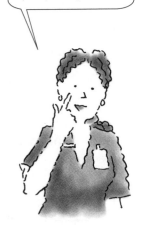

There's often a lot more to a strain or sprain than meets the eye. Be sure to ask about precipitating factors.

Education edge

Teaching about strains and sprains

Teaching about strains and sprains should include:
- Explanation of the diagnosis
- Information regarding prescribed medications
- Instruction on use of supportive, immobilisation and assistive devices.
  In addition, follow these guidelines:
- The patient should be able to demonstrate his understanding of the use of the assistive devices provided
- Emphasise applying ice and elevating and resting the affected area
- Stress that use of the affected area shouldn't be initiated until all swelling and pain have subsided. When this occurs, the patient should begin progressively active exercises and perform them to the limit of pain
- Instruct the patient to follow up or return to the emergency department as directed
- Explain the importance of follow-up care and the risks if follow-up care isn't completed.

Compartment syndrome

Compartment syndrome is a condition in which increased pressure within a closed-tissue space compromises circulation to the capillaries, muscles and nerves within that space. It is one of the few true orthopaedic emergencies which occur in the ED. The key to a positive patient outcome is early recognition, diagnosis and intervention. If left untreated, it can be one of the most devastating and debilitating injuries a patient can experience.

What causes it
Compartment syndrome can result from external or internal causes.

External
- Casts
- Tight dressing
- Splints
- Skeletal traction.

Internal
- Frostbite
- Snakebite
- Fractures or contusions
- Bleeding into a muscle
- I.V. infiltration or extravasation.

How it happens

Compartments are composed of arteries, veins, nerves, muscles and bones. Compartment syndrome occurs when an increase of pressure within the compartment leading ischaemia to its contents. This ischaemia causes severe pain but, because the cause isn't readily observed, it will seem out of proportion to the injury. Compartment syndrome can occur immediately or as long as 4 days after the injury.

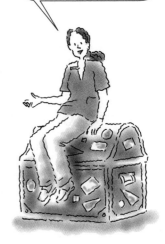

Increased pressure within a small space? Compartment syndrome sounds a lot like my packing strategy!

What to look for

Signs and symptoms of compartment syndrome include:
- Swelling
- Paresthesia
- Pain out of proportion to injury (especially on passive movement)
- Diminished pulse (a late sign).

What tests tell you

These tests are used to diagnose compartment syndrome:
- X-rays will help rule out other diagnoses
- Obtaining a compartment pressure can be accomplished quickly and easily using a commercially available battery-powered monitor
- Normal pressure is approximately zero but always less than 10 mmHg
- Compromise of capillary blood flow occurs at a pressure greater than 20 mmHg and pressure above 30 to 40 mmHg indicates an immediate risk because muscle and nerve tissue necrosis will occur if pressure isn't alleviated
- Laboratory studies should include FBC to evaluate haemoglobin level, haematocrit, WBC and platelet count; and chemistry for analysis of metabolic stability and renal function. Myoglobinuria is a common adverse effect of compartment syndrome, so close observation of renal function is imperative for a positive patient outcome.

How it's treated

- Mild cases are treated with immediate application of ice and elevation of the affected area to help decrease swelling. When the compartment pressures are over 40 mmHg, surgical decompression by fasciotomy is required
- Constant observation, assessment and reassessment in conjunction with frequent monitoring of compartment pressures is key to management of compartment syndrome
- Cases that aren't diagnosed expeditiously require a surgical procedure known as a fasciotomy. This procedure involves surgically opening the fascia through the entire length of both compartments of the affected limb. Opening both compartments prevents swelling and ischemia in a lateral area. The surgical site is left open until all the swelling has resolved (approximately 3 to 5 days) and is then closed by skin grafting.

What to do
- Assess the patient's ABCDEs and manage his life-threatening concerns. The patient's ABCDEs and cervical spine should be cleared before addressing secondary findings
- Obtain a thorough history of the present illness
- Immediately apply ice and elevation to any traumatic injury to stop the pressure of swelling
- Remove any constrictive or restrictive clothing, dressings or devices (especially jewellery)
- Request and administer analgesia
- Obtain I.V. access
- Administer tetanus toxoid.

Contusions

A *contusion* is an injury resulting from a direct blow to the affected area.

What causes it
The causes of contusion vary but can include road traffic collisions, falls, being struck by a blunt object or striking an immovable object with a part of the body.

How it happens
A contusion results from minor haemorrhaging underneath unbroken skin. Following the injury, blood extravasates into the surrounding tissue, causing swelling or bruising. This 'black-and-blue' mark will change to a yellowish-green colour after approximately 2 days as the healing process progresses. The patient may experience minor discomfort from the initial injury but it will subside as swelling decreases and the blood is reabsorbed by the body.

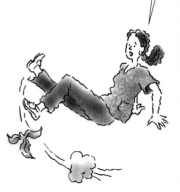

Whoops! I sense a contusion – and a lot of laughter – coming on.

What to look for
- Report of recent trauma to the area causing discomfort
- Bruising or swelling to the injured area. (If the patient reports pain that seems out of proportion to the observed injury, you must consider the possibility of compartment syndrome.)

What tests tell you
The diagnosis of a contusion is based on clinical findings. Diagnostic tests are performed based on the mechanism of injury only to rule out underlying pathologic conditions such as a fracture.

How it's treated
Treatment is supportive and is based on symptoms:
- Ice helps decrease swelling and prevent further complications
- A mild analgesia may be prescribed if appropriate

- Observation may be necessary depending on the location and severity of the contusion
- If symptoms progress further, evaluation and consultation may be warranted.

What to do
- Assess the patient's ABCDEs and manage his life-threatening concerns. The patient's ABCDEs and cervical spine should be cleared before addressing secondary findings
- Obtain a thorough patient history, including mechanism of injury, time and treatment performed before the patient's arrival.

History of violence

- Be alert when obtaining the patient's history for any red flags indicating abuse. (See *Abuse alerts*)
- Provide physical care, including ice application and, if appropriate, immobilisation to decrease pain
- Mild analgesia, such as ibuprofen should be effective; if these drugs provide no decrease in pain, you should attempt to rule out compartment syndrome
- Patient education should include trauma prevention and early signs and symptoms of compartment syndrome. The patient should follow up with his primary care doctor or return to the ED if he experiences worsening symptoms or his condition doesn't improve.

Stay on the ball

Abuse alerts

Red flags indicating abuse might include:
- A delay in presentation
- Multiple bruises in various stages of healing
- Impatience with treatment times
- Desire to leave by a specific time
- Lack of direct eye contact when describing what happened
- Conflicting stories from patient and caregiver.

   If the patient arrives with a significant other, observe their interaction. The patient should be interviewed privately and specifically asked about abuse. If he reports being an abuse victim, take appropriate measures to ensure both his and the medical staff's safety. Contact a social services representative as soon as possible after patient presentation. This representative will provide emotional support during hospitalisation and assist the patient with legal processes and aftercare.

Amputations (traumatic)

Amputation is the removal of a part of the body by traumatic means. Two common types of amputations are the complete (guillotine) or incomplete (crush or tear). A *complete amputation* occurs when the appendage has been completely severed from the body. An *incomplete amputation* occurs when an attachment of the appendage to the body is still present, even if minute in size.

What causes it

Amputation is traumatic and it can originate from human or mechanical error. Potential for traumatic amputations exists anywhere there are humans working around machinery or hand tools.

How it happens

Complete and incomplete amputations occur with equal frequency. Incomplete amputations acquire greater tissue damage because of the distortion and destruction of the involved and surrounding structures, especially the vasculature. Tissue damage in complete amputations is minor because there's a precise cut between the body and affected part.

What to look for

- Observe the extent and location of the injury. Some amputations will require the patient to go immediately to the operating room
- Assess what's missing and how much, if any, of the appendage is left intact
- Determine the amount and colour of the blood. Dark blood indicates a venous injury, while bright red blood indicates an arterial injury
- Palpate pulses distal to the injury. If the pulses aren't palpable, immediate intervention is warranted
- Capillary refill should be less than 2 seconds to indicate adequate perfusion
- Pain may be present depending on the extent of nerve involvement and damage
- Determine the underlying physiological or psychological pathology prompting the injury. For example, did the patient get dizzy and fall into machinery? Or, was his leg amputated by a train as he was trying to kill himself?

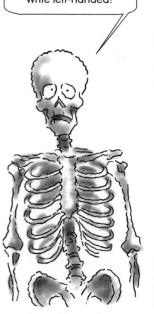

Traumatic is right! One minute my arm is attached, the next minute I'm learning to write left-handed!

What tests tell you

- X-rays will evaluate the extent to which underlying bony structures are involved or damaged and also determine the level of injury and suitability for replantation
- Vascular studies, such as arteriograms, determine the extent of vascular compromise caused by the injury
- Laboratory tests requested for initial management and preoperative screening may include full blood count (FBC) with differential, chemistry, type and screen; prothrombin time; partial thromboplastin time; International Normalized Ratio level; urine drug screen; and urinalysis.

These studies reveal infections and evaluate blood loss, electrolyte balance and kidney function. Bleeding times and clotting times are important factors for patient management

• An electrocardiogram evaluates cardiac activity and can identify disease processes that cause complications from fluid resuscitation or anaesthesia. These studies can also give clues about the injury's cause – for example, whether the patient had a syncopal episode while using the circular saw, which in turn caused the amputation of his finger.

How it's treated

Treatment for amputation may include surgical replantation. Antibiotics are administered before surgery and postoperatively.

What to do

• Assess the patient's ABCDEs and manage his life-threatening concerns. The patient's ABCDEs and cervical spine should be cleared before addressing secondary findings
• Administer oxygen
• Control bleeding
• Insert two large-bore I.V. lines; depending on the site of amputation, the patient may require central access
• Administer analgesics and antibiotics
• Clean the site using normal saline solution irrigation only; don't scrub or use cleaning solution on the stump
• Administer tetanus prophylaxis
• Apply sterile dressings
• Prepare the patient for transfer to an appropriate facility or the operating room
• Provide a psychosocial report for the patient and his family
• Don't apply a tourniquet to the affected limb
• Immobilise the limb in its correct anatomical position
• Take care to preserve the amputated part for possible reimplantation by wrapping it in saline-moistened gauze and placing it in a sealed plastic bag. The bag should then be placed in a bath of ice water. Make sure that the part doesn't freeze. Don't allow the part to be submerged directly in the ice.

Quick quiz

1. If your patient can't move his right arm away from his side, you should document this as impaired:

    A. supination.
    B. abduction.
    C. eversion.
    D. adduction.

Answer: *B.* Abduction is the ability to move a limb away from the midline.

2. A condition in which increased pressure within a closed-tissue space compromises circulation to the capillaries, muscles and nerves within that space is the definition of:
   A. sprain.
   B. strain.
   C. compression fracture.
   D. compartment syndrome.

Answer: D. Compartment syndrome is characterised by increased pressure within a closed-tissue space compromising circulation to its contents.

3. An injury that occurs at the articulation of two or more bones and causes the bones involved to be moved out of the anatomically correct position is the definition of a:
   A. fracture.
   B. sprain.
   C. strain.
   D. dislocation.

Answer: D. A dislocation is defined as an injury that occurs at the articulation of two or more bones, causing the bones involved to be moved out of the anatomically correct position.

4. You suspect a cervical spine injury in a patient. Which action is most appropriate?
   A. Remove the cervical collar before attempting to open the airway.
   B. Use the head-tilt chin-lift manoeuvre to open the airway.
   C. Turn the patient on his side to prevent aspiration.
   D. Use the jaw-thrust manoeuvre to open the airway.

Answer: D. In a patient with a suspected cervical spine injury, the most appropriate way to open the airway is to use the jaw-thrust manoeuvre.

Scoring

☆☆☆   If you answered all four questions correctly, way to go! You're a bred-in-the-bone musculoskeletal maven!

☆☆   If you answered three questions correctly, impressive! Make no bones about it, you have a mastery of musculoskeletal matters!

☆   If you answered fewer than three questions correctly, don't become unhinged! Just bone up a bit and you'll be playing ball and socket with the big boys soon.

6 Cardiac emergencies

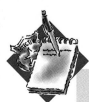

Just the facts

In this chapter, you'll learn:

♦ Emergency assessment of the cardiovascular system

♦ Diagnostic tests and procedures for cardiovascular emergencies

♦ Cardiovascular disorders in the emergency department (ED) and their treatments

♦ How to deal with a cardiac arrest situation

Understanding cardiac emergencies

The cardiovascular system is a major control system in the body, playing a key role in cellular nutrition and circulation. It's responsible for the provision and the carrying of life-sustaining oxygen and nutrients to the cells and the removal of cellular waste products via the blood. When faced with an emergency involving the cardiovascular system, you must assess the patient thoroughly, always being alert for subtle changes that might indicate a potential deterioration in the patient's condition. A thorough nursing assessment forms the basis for your interventions that must be instituted quickly to minimise potentially life-threatening risks to the patient.

Assessment

Assessment of a patient's cardiovascular system includes a health history and physical examination. If you can't interview the patient because of his condition, you may gather history information from the patient's family members, the patient's general practitioner, the paramedic or other health care providers. Remember the ABCDE assessment discussed in Chapter 3, and be aware that you may need to commence resuscitative measures at anytime.

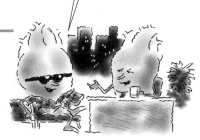

I don't wanna brag here, Bob, but my system happens to be one of the body's major players.

Health history

To obtain the health history of a patient's cardiovascular system, begin by introducing yourself and then obtain information on the patient's presenting complaint, personal and family health and chest pain, if any. The patient's medical history is important, especially any history of angina or myocardial infarction (MI) and health risk factors, such as diabetes or hypertension.

Presenting complaint

Use the seven attributes of a symptom, as listed below, to obtain details about the patient's presenting complaint:

Location (Where is it? Does it radiate?)

Quality (What's it like?)

Quantity or severity (How bad is it on a 1–10 scale?)

Timing (When does it start? How long does it last? How often does it occur?)

Setting or environmental factors, including personal activities and contributing factors, such as climbing stairs and exercising

Factors that make it better or worse

Associated manifestations. (See *Cardiac questions*.)

Personal and family health

Ask the patient for details about his family history, especially any family history of cardiovascular disease and medical history. Also ask about:
• Health affecting habits, such as smoking, alcohol intake, caffeine intake, exercise and high dietary intake of fat and sodium
• Stressors in the patient's life and coping strategies he uses to deal with them
• Environmental or occupational factors
• Activities of daily living
• Drugs the patient is taking, including prescription drugs, over-the-counter drugs and herbal preparations. Question the patient about any complementary therapies that he may be or has been having
• Menopause (if applicable)
• Previous surgery.

Complaints of chest pain

Many patients with cardiovascular problems complain of chest pain. Use the seven attributes of a symptom to get a complete picture of the patient's pain.

Cardiac questions

To thoroughly assess your patient's cardiac function, be sure to ask the following questions:
- Are you in pain?
- Where's the pain located?
- Does the pain feel like a burning, tight or squeezing sensation?
- Does the pain radiate to your arm, neck, back or jaw?

- When did the pain begin?
- What relieves or aggravates it?
- Are you experiencing nausea, dizziness or sweating?
- Do you feel short of breath? Has breathing trouble ever awakened you from sleep?
- Does your heart ever pound or skip a beat? When?

- Do you ever get dizzy or faint? When?
- Do you experience swelling in your ankles or feet? When? Does anything relieve the swelling?
- Do you urinate frequently at night?
- Have you had to limit your activities?

Where, what and why

If the patient isn't in distress, ask questions that require more than a yes-or-no response. Use familiar expressions rather than medical terms whenever possible.

In his own words

Let the patient describe his condition in his own words. Ask him to describe the location, radiation, intensity and duration of pain and precipitating, exacerbating or relieving factors to obtain an accurate description of chest pain. (See *Differentiating chest pain*, page 138.)

Physical examination

Cardiac emergencies affect people of all ages, ethnicities and cultures and can take many forms. To best identify abnormalities, use a consistent, methodological approach to the physical examination. Because of the emergency nature of the patient's condition, there may be a need to limit the examination to specific problem areas or to stop the examination entirely to intervene if the patient exhibits signs or symptoms that indicate his condition is deteriorating. If initial screening indicates a cardiac problem, then a more detailed assessment may need to be conducted.

The heart of it

When performing an assessment of a patient's heart health, this is the order to proceed:

 Inspection

Palpation

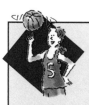

Stay on the ball

Differentiating chest pain

Use this table to help you more accurately assess chest pain.

What it feels like	Where it's located	What makes it worse	What causes it	What makes it better
Aching, squeezing, pressure, heaviness, burning pain; usually subsides within 10 minutes	Substernal; may radiate to jaw, neck, arms and back	Eating, physical effort, smoking, cold weather, stress, anger, hunger, lying down	Angina pectoris	Rest, nitroglycerin (GTN) (*Note:* Unstable angina appears even at rest)
Tightness or pressure; burning, aching pain, possibly accompanied by shortness of breath, sweating, weakness, anxiety or nausea; sudden onset; lasts ½ hour to 2 hours	Typically across chest but may radiate to jaw, neck, arms or back	Exertion, anxiety	Acute MI	GTN and opioid analgesics such as morphine
Sharp and continuous; may be accompanied by friction rub; sudden onset	Substernal; may radiate to neck or left arm	Deep breathing, supine position	Pericarditis Costochondritis	Sitting up, leaning forward, anti-inflammatory drugs
Excruciating, tearing pain; may be accompanied by blood pressure (BP) difference between right and left arm; sudden onset	Retrosternal, upper abdominal or epigastric; may radiate to back, neck or shoulders	Not applicable	Dissecting aortic aneurysm	Analgesics, surgery
Sudden, stabbing pain; may be accompanied by cyanosis, dyspnoea, or cough with haemoptysis	Over lung area	Inspiration	Pulmonary embolus	Analgesics
Sudden, severe pain; sometimes accompanied by dyspnoea, increased pulse rate, decreased breath sounds, or deviated trachea	Lateral thorax	Normal respiration	Pneumothorax	Analgesics, chest tube insertion

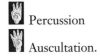 Percussion

Auscultation.

Inspection
First, take a moment to assess the patient's general appearance.

First impressions

Is the patient too thin or obese? Is he alert? Does he appear anxious? Note the patient's skin colour. Are his fingers clubbed? (Clubbing is a sign of chronic hypoxia caused by a lengthy cardiovascular or respiratory disorder.) If the patient is dark-skinned, inspect his mucous membranes for pallor.

Check the chest

Next, the chest is inspected. Landmarks are noted so the examiner can describe findings as well as the structures underlying the chest wall. Pulsations, symmetry of movement, recessions or heaves (strong outward thrusts of the chest wall that display during systole) are looked for.

Arms and legs, too

The patient's arms or legs are inspected, noting colour, hair distribution and lesions, ulcers or oedema.

The point of maximum impulse

The location of the apical impulse is noted. This location is also usually the point of maximum impulse (PMI) and should be located in the fifth intercostal space (ICS) medial to the left midclavicular line. The apical impulse indicates how well the left ventricle is working because it corresponds to the apex of the heart. To find the apical impulse in a woman with large breasts, the breasts are displaced during the examination.

Checking the pulse

When checking the pulse you will note the presence, the location, the quality, the rate and the rhythm of the pulses. This simple test will give you important information on cardiac output and perfusion. Compare distal and proximal pulses and note results. All pulses should be regular in rhythm and equal in strength.

Neck next

Carotid artery pulsations (noted by looking at the arteries in the neck) should be brisk and localised and don't decrease when the patient is upright, when he inhales, or when palpated. The jugular veins are inspected. The internal jugular vein has a softer, undulating pulsation, which changes in response to position, breathing and palpation. In children younger than 1 year finding their carotid pulse can be difficult so the brachial artery can be used.

Then go for the jugular

The jugular venous pressure (JVP) can be checked by asking the patient to lie on his back with the head of the bed elevated to 30 to 45 degrees, the patient then turns his head away slightly. Normally, the highest pulsation takes place no more than 3.8 cm above the sternal notch. If pulsations appear higher, it indicates elevation in central venous pressure (CVP) and jugular vein distension.

Abnormal findings

Here are some of the abnormal findings that may be noted on inspection and what these findings indicate:

- Cyanosis, pallor or cool or cold skin may indicate poor cardiac output and tissue perfusion
- Skin may be flushed if the patient has a fever
- Absence of body hair on the arms or legs may indicate diminished arterial blood flow to those areas
- Swelling, or *oedema*, may indicate heart failure or venous insufficiency. It may also be caused by varicosities or thrombophlebitis
- Chronic right-sided heart failure (*Cor Pulmonale*) may cause ascites and generalised oedema
- Inspection may reveal barrel chest (rounded thoracic cage caused by chronic obstructive pulmonary disease), scoliosis (lateral curvature of the spine) or kyphosis (convex curvature of the thoracic spine). If severe enough, these conditions can impair cardiac output by preventing chest expansion and inhibiting heart muscle movement
- Recessions (visible indentations of the soft tissue covering the chest wall) or the use of accessory muscles to breathe typically result from a respiratory disorder, but a congenital heart defect or heart failure may also cause them.

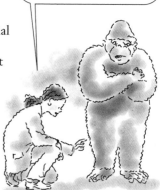

Hmmm … well, since diminished arterial blood flow is usually signaled by lack of arm or leg hair, I think you're probably safe.

Palpation

Skin temperature, elasticity and texture should be examined. Gentle palpitation over the precordium using the ball of the hand and then fingertips, finds the apical impulse. Heaves or thrills (fine vibrations that feel like the purring of a cat) are noted.

Palpate the potentials

Palpitation of the sternoclavicular, aortic, pulmonic, tricuspid and epigastric areas may detect abnormal pulsations. Pulsations aren't usually felt in these areas. However, an aortic arch pulsation in the sternoclavicular area or an abdominal aorta pulsation in the epigastric area may be a normal finding in a thin patient.

Refill, please

Capillary refill time (CRT) is checked by assessing the nail beds on the fingers and toes. Refill time should be no more than seconds, or long enough to say 'capillary refill'. If you are unable to obtain CRT because of patient injuries or disease, firmly press in the sternal area and assess for blanching in 2 seconds.

And compare

Palpate for the pulse on each side of the neck, comparing pulse volume and symmetry. *DO NOT* palpate both carotid arteries at the same time or press too firmly. If you do so the patient may faint or become bradycardic due to baroreceptor stimulation.

Abnormal findings

Abnormal findings on palpation may reveal:
• Weak pulse, indicating low cardiac output or increased peripheral vascular resistance, such as in arterial atherosclerotic disease (note that older adults commonly have weak pedal pulses)
• Strong bounding pulse, commonly found in hypertension and in high cardiac output states, such as exercise, pregnancy, anaemia and thyrotoxicosis
• Apical impulse that exerts unusual force and lasts longer than one-third of the cardiac cycle – a possible indication of increased cardiac output
• Displaced or diffuse impulse, possibly indicating left ventricular hypertrophy
• Pulsation in the aortic, pulmonic or right ventricular area, which is a sign of chamber enlargement or valvular disease
• Pulsation in the sternoclavicular or epigastric area, which is a sign of an aortic aneurysm.

What a thrill!

• A palpable thrill is an indication of blood flow turbulence and is usually related to valvular dysfunction

Auscultation – a developing nursing skill

You can learn a great deal about the heart by auscultating for heart sounds, and this investigation is increasingly being incorporated into the clinical skills repertoire of nurses in the UK. Cardiac auscultation requires a methodical approach. However, you will need to check the policies regarding undertaking auscultation and the scope of nursing practice in your department. To undertake effective auscultation the nurse must have excellent knowledge of the anatomy and physiology of the heart (*Anatomy and Physiology Made Incredibly Easy* (2004); Lippincott Williams & Wilkins, in the same series as this book gives a good overview). Heart sounds can

Heart sound sites

When auscultating for heart sounds, the stethoscope is placed over the four different sites illustrated here.

Auscultation sites are identified by the names of heart valves but aren't located directly over the valves. Rather, these sites are located along the pathway blood takes as it flows through the heart's chambers and valves.

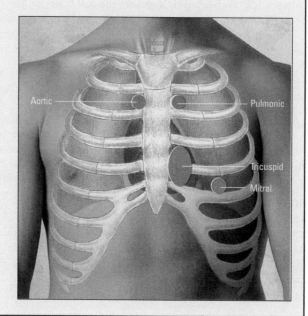

Aortic — Pulmonic

Tricuspid

Mitral

be heard on web sites such as: http://depts.washington.edu/physdx/heart/demo.html.

Erb and friends

First, identify the auscultation sites, including the sites over the four cardiac valves. Locate the best site to hear S1 (the first heart sound) at 'Erb's point' (found at the third ICS, on the left sternal border between the pulmonic and tricuspid valve areas). Use the bell to hear low-pitched sounds and the diaphragm to hear high-pitched sounds. (See *Heart sound sites*.)

Auscultate for heart sounds with the patient in three positions:

Lying on his back with the head of the bed raised 30 to 45 degrees

Sitting up

Lying on his left side.

Upward, downward, zigward, zagward

Use a zigzag pattern over the precordium. Start at the apex and work upward, or at the base and work downward. Whichever approach you use, be consistent. Use the diaphragm to listen as you go in one direction; use the bell as you come back in the other direction.

Be sure to listen over the entire precordium, not just over the valves. Note the patient's heart rate and rhythm.

1, 2, 3, 4 and more

Systole is the period of ventricular contraction:
- As pressure in the ventricles increases, the mitral and tricuspid valves snap closed. The closure produces the first heart sound, S_1
- At the end of ventricular contraction, the aortic and pulmonic valves snap shut. This snap produces the second heart sound, S_2
- S_1 and S_2 should be identified and then adventitious (extra or additional) sounds, such as the third and fourth heart sounds (S_3 and S_4) listened for
- Also listen for murmurs (vibrating, blowing or rumbling sounds) and rubs (harsh, scratchy, scraping or squeaking sounds).

Listen for the 'dub'

Start auscultating at the aortic area where the S_2 is loudest. An S_2 is best heard at the base of the heart at the end of ventricular systole. It occurs when the pulmonic and aortic valves close and is generally described as sounding like 'dub'. Its sound is shorter, higher-pitched and louder than S_1. When the pulmonic valve closes later than the aortic valve during inspiration, you hear a split S_2.

Rub-a-'dub'-'lub'! The S_2 sound is high-pitched and loud, whereas the S_1 sound is low-pitched and dull.

Listen for the 'lub'

From the base of the heart, move to the pulmonic area and then down to the tricuspid area. Then move to the mitral area, where S_1 is the loudest.

An S_1 is best heard at the apex of the heart. It results from closure of the mitral and tricuspid valves and is generally described as sounding like 'lub'. It's low-pitched and dull. An S_1 occurs at the beginning of ventricular systole. It may be split if the mitral valve closes just before the tricuspid valve.

Major auscultation, man!

Also auscultate the major arteries, such as the carotid, femoral and popliteal arteries, using the bell of the stethoscope to assess for bruits.

Bruits

Sounds aren't normally heard over the carotid arteries. A bruit – which sounds like buzzing or blowing – could indicate arteriosclerotic plaque formation. When you auscultate for the femoral and popliteal pulses, check for a bruit or other abnormal sounds. A bruit over the femoral or popliteal artery usually indicates narrowed vessels.

Bothersome bruits

During auscultation of the central and peripheral arteries, you may notice a continuous bruit caused by turbulent blood flow. A bruit over the abdominal aorta usually indicates an aneurysm (weakness in the arterial wall that allows a sac to form) or a dissection (a tear in the layers of the arterial wall).

Abnormal findings

On auscultation, you may detect S_1 and S_2 heart sounds that are accentuated, diminished or inaudible. Other abnormal heart sounds – such as S_3, S_4 and murmurs – may result from pressure changes, valvular dysfunctions and conduction defects. (See *Interpreting abnormal heart sounds*.)

Third heart sound

The third heart sound – known as S_3, or *ventricular gallop* – is a low-pitched noise best heard by placing the bell of the stethoscope at the apex of the heart. This can sometimes be present in young people and during pregnancy; however, its presence usually indicates abnormal filling pressures in the atria secondary to heart failure.

Hearing a gallop

Its rhythm resembles a horse galloping, and its cadence resembles the word 'Ken-tuc-ky' (lub-dub-by). Listen for S_3 with the patient in a supine or left-lateral lying position.

An S_3 usually sounds during early diastole to mid-diastole, at the end of the passive-filling phase of either ventricle. Listen for this sound immediately after S_2. It may signify that the ventricle isn't compliant enough to accept the filling volume without additional force.

Fourth heart sound

The fourth heart sound, or S_4, is always an abnormal finding and occurs late in diastole, just before the pulse upstroke. It immediately precedes the S_1 of the next cycle. Known as the *atrial* or *presystolic gallop*, it occurs during atrial contraction. This sound indicates either increased pressure in the atria or decreased compliance (stretching) of the left ventricle.

Tennessee walker

An S_4 shares the same cadence as the word 'Ten-nes-see' (le-lub-dub). It's heard best with the bell of the stethoscope and with the patient in the supine position.

What S_4 says

An S_4 may indicate cardiovascular disease, such as:
- Acute MI
- Anaemia

Ages and stages

Interpreting abnormal heart sounds

An S_3 may occur normally in a child or young adult. In a patient older than age 30, however, it usually indicates a disorder, such as:
- Right-sided heart failure
- Left-sided heart failure
- Pulmonary congestion
- Intracardiac blood shunting
- MI
- Anaemia
- Thyrotoxicosis.

Common S4

S_4 commonly appears in older adults with age-related systolic hypertension and aortic stenosis.

Identifying heart murmurs

To identify a heart murmur, first listen closely to determine its timing in the cardiac cycle. Then determine its other characteristics, including quality, pitch and location, as well as possible causes.

Timing	Quality and pitch	Location	Possible causes
Midsystolic (systolic ejection)	Harsh and rough with medium to high pitch	Pulmonic	Pulmonic stenosis
	Harsh and rough with medium to high pitch	Aortic and suprasternal notch	Aortic stenosis
Holosystolic (pansystolic)	Harsh with high pitch	Tricuspid	Ventricular septal defect
	Blowing with high pitch	Mitral, lower left sternal border	Mitral insufficiency
	Blowing with high pitch	Tricuspid	Tricuspid insufficiency
Early diastolic	Blowing with high pitch	Mid-left sternal edge (not aortic area)	Aortic insufficiency
	Blowing with high pitch	Pulmonic	Pulmonic insufficiency
Mid-diastolic to late diastolic	Rumbling with low pitch	Apex	Mitral stenosis
	Rumbling with low pitch	Tricuspid, lower right sternal border	Tricuspid stenosis

- Angina
- Aortic stenosis
- Cardiomyopathy
- Coronary artery disease (CAD)
- Elevated left ventricular pressure
- Hypertension.

If the S_4 sound persists, it may indicate impaired ventricular compliance or volume overload.

Murmurs

A murmur that is longer than a heart sound makes a vibrating, blowing or rumbling noise. Just as turbulent water in a stream babbles as it passes through a narrow point, turbulent blood flow produces a murmur. Patients may have normal, physiological murmurs or a murmur can indicate a pathological finding.

If you detect a murmur, identify where it's loudest, pinpoint when it sounds during the cardiac cycle and describe its pitch, pattern, quality and intensity. (See *Identifying heart murmurs*.)

Location, location and . . . timing

Murmurs can start in any cardiac auscultatory site and may radiate from one site to another. To identify the radiation area, auscultate from the site where the murmur seems loudest to the farthest site where it's still heard. Note the anatomic landmark of this farthest site.

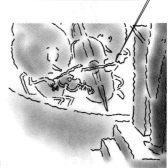

Just for fun, let's keep this piece down to a murmur and see if the audience can identify it. Ready?

Pinpoint its presence

Determine whether the murmur happens during systole (between S_1 and S_2) or diastole (between S_2 and the next S_1). Then pinpoint when in the cardiac cycle the murmur takes place – for example, during mid-diastole or late systole. A murmur heard throughout systole is called a *holosystolic* (or *pansystolic*) *murmur*, and a murmur heard throughout diastole is called a *pandiastolic murmur*. Occasionally, murmurs run through both portions of the cycle (continuous murmur).

Pitch

Depending on the rate and pressure of blood flow, pitch may be high, medium or low. You can best hear a low-pitched murmur with the bell of the stethoscope, a high-pitched murmur with the diaphragm and a medium-pitched murmur with both.

Pattern

Crescendo is produced when the velocity of blood flow increases and the murmur becomes louder. Decrescendo is produced when velocity decreases and the murmur becomes quieter. A crescendo-decrescendo pattern describes a murmur with increasing loudness followed by increasing softness.

Quality

The volume of blood flow, the force of the contraction and the degree of valve compromise all contribute to murmur quality. Terms used to describe quality include *musical, blowing, harsh, rasping, rumbling* or *machinelike*.

Intensity

Use a standard, six-level grading scale to describe the intensity of the murmur:

Grade I – extremely faint; barely audible even to the trained ear

Grade II – soft and low; easily audible to the trained ear

Grade III – moderately loud; about equal to the intensity of normal heart sounds

Grade IV – loud with a palpable thrill at the murmur site

Grade V – very loud with a palpable thrill; audible with the stethoscope in partial contact with the chest

Grade VI – extremely loud, with a palpable thrill; audible with the stethoscope over, but not in contact with the chest.

Rubs

To detect a pericardial friction rub, use the diaphragm of the stethoscope to auscultate in the third left ICS along the lower left sternal border.

Rubbed the wrong way

Listen for a harsh, scratchy, scraping or squeaking sound throughout systole, diastole or both. To enhance the sound, have the patient sit upright and lean forward or exhale. A rub usually indicates pericarditis.

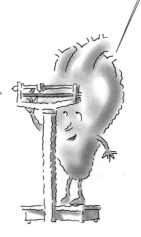

Just like using a regular scale, the heart murmur scale involves a lot of intensity.

Diagnostic tests

Advances in diagnostic testing allow for earlier and easier diagnosis and treatment of cardiac emergencies in the ED.

Cardiac monitoring

Cardiac monitoring is a form of electrocardiography (ECG) that enables continuous observation of the heart's electrical activity. It's an essential assessment tool in the ED and is used to continually monitor the patient's cardiac status to enable rapid identification and treatment of abnormalities in rate, rhythm or conduction. The monitor screen must be seen (if it is behind a curtain it won't be) and the alarms set correctly. The usual monitor view is of Lead II.

Practice pointers

• Always explain to the patient what you are doing before attaching a cardiac monitor (or undertaking a 12-lead ECG) and seek their consent
• Explain that they won't feel anything apart from the electrodes or the electrode cream feeling cold!
• Make sure the patient (and his family) understands that the monitor isn't part of the treatment and isn't keeping the heart beating
• You may need to shave the patient so that the electrodes can make contact and remain in place
• Clean skin with a sterile wipe before attaching electrodes
• If the patient is an amputee place both electrodes on the same leg and note on the ECG recording where placed
• Ask the patient to lie still, with his arms at his side and his legs not touching if a 12-lead ECG is being recorded
• Make sure any recording is correctly labelled and time taken noted (if not done so automatically).

A test with 12 views

The 12-lead ECG measures the heart's electrical activity and records it as waveforms. It's one of the most valuable and commonly used diagnostic tools and is used in conjunction with other tests. The standard 12-lead ECG uses a series of electrodes placed on the patient's extremities and chest wall to assess the heart from 12 different views (leads). The 12 leads include three bipolar limb leads (I, II and III), three unipolar augmented limb leads (aV_R, aV_L and aV_F) and six unipolar precordial limb leads (V_1 to V_6). The limb leads and augmented leads show the heart from the frontal plane. The precordial leads show the heart from the horizontal plane. (See *Precordial lead placement*.)

> A 12-lead ECG lets you assess the heart from the vantage of 12 different views.

Up, down and across. . .

Scanning up, down and across the heart, each lead transmits information about a different area. The waveforms obtained from each lead vary depending on the location of the lead in relation to the wave of electrical stimulus, or *depolarisation*, passing through the myocardium.

. . .from top to bottom. . .

The six limb leads record electrical activity in the heart's frontal plane. This plane is a view through the middle of the heart from top to bottom. Electrical activity is recorded from the anterior to the posterior axis.

. . .and, finally, horizontal

The six precordial leads provide information on electrical activity in the heart's horizontal plane, a transverse view through the middle of the heart, dividing it into upper and lower portions. Electrical activity is recorded from a superior or an inferior approach.

Practice pointers

• A systematic approach is needed to interpret the ECG recording. Ideally, one would compare a previous ECG with the patient's current one to help identify changes
• P waves should be upright; however, they may be inverted in lead aV_R or biphasic or inverted in leads III, aV_L and V_1
• PR intervals should always be constant, just like QRS-complex durations
• QRS-complex deflections vary in different leads. Observe for pathologic Q waves
• ST segments should be isoelectric or have minimal deviation
• ST-segment elevation >1 mm above the baseline and ST-segment depression >0.5 mm below the baseline are considered abnormal. Leads facing an injured area have ST-segment elevations, and leads facing away show ST-segment depressions
• The T wave normally deflects upwards in leads I, II and V_3 through V_6. It's inverted in lead aV_R and variable in the other leads. T-wave changes have many

Precordial lead placement

To record a 12-lead ECG, place electrodes on the patient's arms and left leg (LL) and place a ground lead on the patient's right leg. The three standard limb leads (I, II and III) and the three augmented leads (aV_R, aV_L and aV_F) are recorded using these electrodes. Then, to record the precordial chest leads, place electrodes as follows:

- V_1 – fourth ICS, right sternal border
- V_2 – fourth ICS, left sternal border
- V_3 – midway between V_2 and V_4
- V_4 – fifth ICS, left midclavicular line
- V_5 – fifth ICS, left anterior axillary line
- V_6 – fifth ICS, left midaxillary line.

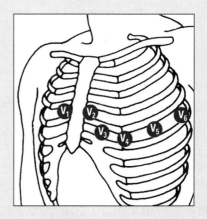

Right precordial lead placement

Right precordial leads can provide specific information about the function of the right ventricle. Place the six leads on the right side of the chest in a mirror image of the standard precordial lead placement, as follows:

- V_{1R} – fourth ICS, left sternal border
- V_{2R} – fourth ICS, right sternal border
- V_{3R} – halfway between V_{2R} and V_{4R}
- V_{4R} – fifth ICS, right midclavicular line
- V_{5R} – fifth ICS, right anterior axillary line
- V_{6R} – fifth ICS, right midaxillary line.

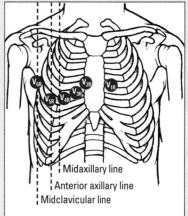

Midaxillary line
Anterior axillary line
Midclavicular line

Posterior lead placement

Posterior leads can be used to assess the posterior side of the heart although this is rarely use in the ED setting. To ensure an accurate reading, make sure the posterior electrodes V_7, V_8 and V_9 are placed at the same horizontal level as the V_6 lead at the fifth ICS. Place lead V_7 at the posterior axillary line, lead V_9 at the paraspinal line and lead V_8 halfway between leads V_7 and V_9.

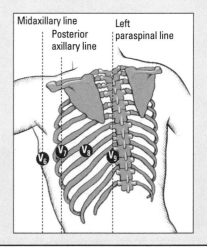

Midaxillary line
Posterior axillary line
Left paraspinal line

causes and aren't always a reason for alarm. Excessively tall, flat or inverted T waves accompanying such symptoms as chest pain may indicate ischaemia
• A normal Q wave generally has duration of less than 0.04 second. An abnormal Q wave has duration of 0.04 second or more, a depth >4 mm or a height one-fourth of the R wave. Abnormal Q waves indicate myocardial necrosis, developing when depolarisation can't follow its normal path because of damaged tissue in the area
• Remember that aV_R normally has a large Q wave, so disregard this lead when searching for abnormal Q waves.

Cardiac arrhythmias

In cardiac arrhythmia, abnormal electrical conduction or automaticity changes heart rate and rhythm.

Asymptomatic to catastrophic

Cardiac arrhythmias vary in severity, from those that are mild, asymptomatic and require no treatment (such as sinus arrhythmia, in which heart rate increases and decreases with respiration) to catastrophic pulseless ventricular tachycardia (VT), ventricular fibrillation (VF) or asystole, all of which require immediate resuscitation.

Cardiac arrhythmias: organised by origin and effects

Cardiac arrhythmias are generally classified according to their origin (ventricular or supraventricular). Their effect on cardiac output and BP, partially influenced by the site of origin, determines their clinical significance. Lethal arrhythmias, such as VT and VF, are a major cause of sudden cardiac death.

What causes it

Common causes of cardiac arrhythmias include:
• Emotional stress
• Drug toxicity
• Congenital defects
• Acid–base imbalances
• Electrolyte imbalances
• Cellular hypoxia
• Connective tissue disorders
• Degeneration of the conductive tissue
• Hypertrophy of the heart muscle
• Myocardial ischaemia or infarction
• Organic heart disease.

How it happens

Cardiac arrhythmias may result from:
• Abnormal electrical conduction
• Escape beats (additional abnormal heart beats resulting from a very slow heart rate)

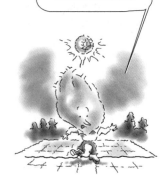

Boy, having this cardiac arrhythmia change my rhythm sure does make it harder to dance.

- Enhanced automaticity
- Re-entry.

What to look for

When a patient presents with a history of symptoms suggesting cardiac arrhythmias or has been treated for a cardiac arrhythmia, be alert for:
- Reports of precipitating factors, such as exercise, smoking, sleep patterns, emotional stress, exposure to heat or cold, caffeine intake, position changes or recent illnesses
- Attempts to alleviate the symptoms, such as coughing, rest, medications or deep breathing
- Reports of sensing the heart's rhythm, such as palpitations, irregular beating, skipped beats or rapid or slow heart rate.

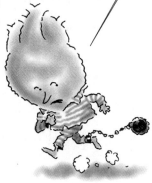

Look out! Escape beats are a major cause of arrhythmias!

A matter of degree

Physical examination findings vary depending on the arrhythmia and the degree of haemodynamic compromise. Circulatory failure, along with an absence of pulse and respirations, is found with asystole, VF and sometimes VT. (See *Understanding Cardiac arrhythmias.*)

That's not all

Additional findings may include:
- Dizziness
- Weakness
- Chest pains
- Cold and clammy extremities
- Hypotension
- Dyspnoea
- Pallor
- Reduced urine output
- Syncope (with severely impaired cerebral circulation).

What tests tell you

- A 12-lead ECG is the standard test for identifying cardiac arrhythmias. A 15-lead ECG (in which additional leads are applied to the right side of the chest) or an 18-lead ECG (in which additional leads are also added to the posterior scapular area) may be done to provide more definitive information about the patient's right ventricle and posterior wall of the left ventricle. (See *Understanding cardiac arrhythmias*, pages 152–159.)
- Laboratory testing may reveal electrolyte abnormalities, hypoxaemia or acid–base abnormalities (with arterial blood gases (ABG) analysis) or drug toxicities as the cause of arrhythmias
- Exclude accidental or deliberate drug toxicities as the cause of arrhythmias – consider contacting the poisons centre
- Electrophysiologic testing may be used to identify the mechanism of an arrhythmia and location of accessory pathways and to assess the effectiveness of antiarrhythmic drugs. *(Text continues on page 158.)*

Understanding cardiac arrhythmias

Here's an outline of many common cardiac arrhythmias and their features, causes and treatments. Use a normal electrocardiogram strip, if available, to compare normal cardiac rhythm configurations with the rhythm strips shown here. Characteristics of normal sinus rhythm include:

- Ventricular and atrial rates of 60 to 100 beats/minute
- Regular and uniform QRS complexes and P waves
- PR interval of 0.12 to 0.20 second
- QRS duration <0.12 second
- Identical atrial and ventricular rates, with constant PR intervals.

Arrhythmia and features

Sinus tachycardia

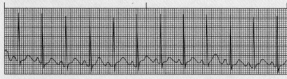

- Atrial and ventricular rhythms regular
- Rate >100 beats/minute; rarely, >160 beats/minute
- Normal P waves preceding each QRS complex

Sinus bradycardia

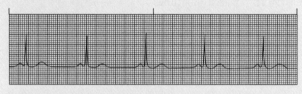

- Atrial and ventricular rhythms regular
- Rate <60 beats/minute
- Normal P waves preceding each QRS complex

Paroxysmal supraventricular tachycardia

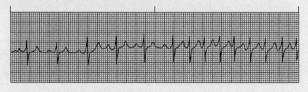

- Atrial and ventricular rhythms regular
- Heart rate >160 beats/minute; rarely exceeds 250 beats/minute
- P waves regular but aberrant; difficult to differentiate from preceding T waves
- P waves preceding each QRS complex
- Sudden onset and termination of arrhythmia

Atrial flutter

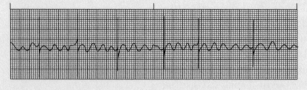

- Atrial rhythm regular; rate 250 to 400 beats/minute
- Ventricular rate variable, depending on degree of AV block (usually 60 to 100 beats/minute)
- No P waves; atrial activity appears as flutter waves (F waves); saw-tooth configuration common in lead II
- QRS complexes are uniform in shape but commonly irregular in rhythm

Causes	Treatment
• Normal physiologic response to fever, exercise, anxiety, pain, dehydration; may also accompany shock, left-sided heart failure, cardiac tamponade, hyperthyroidism, anaemia, hypovolaemia, pulmonary embolism (PE) and anterior wall MI • May also occur with atropine, adrenaline, isoproterenol, quinidine, caffeine, alcohol, cocaine, amphetamine and nicotine use	• Correction of underlying cause • Beta-adrenergic blockers or calcium channel blocker
• Normal in a well-conditioned heart, as in an athlete • Increased intracranial pressure; increased vagal tone due to straining during defecation, vomiting, intubation, or mechanical ventilation; sick sinus syndrome (SSS); hypothyroidism; and inferior-wall MI • May also occur with anticholinesterase, beta-adrenergic blocker, digoxin and morphine use	• Correction of underlying cause • For low cardiac output, dizziness, weakness, altered level of consciousness, or low BP, advanced cardiac life support (ACLS) protocol for administration of atropine • Transcutaneous or permanent pacemaker • Dopamine or adrenaline infusion
• Intrinsic abnormality of AV conduction system • Physical or psychological stress, hypoxia, hypokalaemia, cardiomyopathy, congenital heart disease, MI, valvular disease, Wolff-Parkinson-White syndrome, cor pulmonale, hyperthyroidism and systemic hypertension • Digoxin toxicity; use of caffeine, marijuana or central nervous system stimulants	• If patient is unstable, perform immediate cardioversion • If QRS complex is narrow and regular and patient is stable, perform vagal manoeuvres or administer adenosine • If QRS complex is narrow and irregular, control the rate using calcium channel blockers or beta-adrenergic blockers • If QRS complex is wide and irregular, administer antiarrhythmics such as amiodarone; if ineffective, then magnesium
• Heart failure, tricuspid or mitral valve disease, PE, cor pulmonale, inferior-wall MI and pericarditis • Digoxin toxicity	• If patient is unstable with a ventricular rate >150 beats/minute, immediate cardioversion • If patient is stable, follow ACLS protocol for cardioversion and drug therapy, which may include calcium channel blockers, beta-adrenergic blockers, amiodarone or digoxin • Anticoagulation therapy possibly also needed • Radiofrequency ablation to control rhythm

(continued)

Understanding cardiac arrhythmias (Continued)

Arrhythmia and features (Continued)

Atrial fibrillation

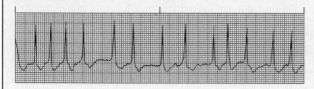

- Atrial rhythm grossly irregular; rate >400 beats/minute
- Ventricular rhythm grossly irregular
- QRS complexes of uniform configuration and duration
- PR interval indiscernible
- No P waves; atrial activity appears as erratic, irregular, baseline fibrillatory waves (F waves)

Junctional rhythm

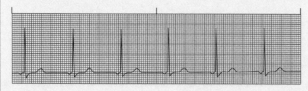

- Atrial and ventricular rhythms regular; atrial rate 40 to 60 beats/minute; ventricular rate usually 40 to 60 beats/minute (60 to 100 beats/minute is accelerated junctional rhythm)
- P waves preceding, hidden within (absent), or after QRS complex; usually inverted if visible
- PR interval (when present) <0.12 second
- QRS complex configuration and duration normal, except in aberrant conduction

First-degree AV block

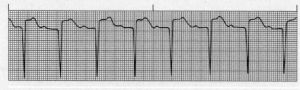

- Atrial and ventricular rhythms regular
- PR interval > 0.20 second
- P wave precedes QRS complex
- QRS complex normal

Second-degree AV block Mobitz I (Wenckebach)

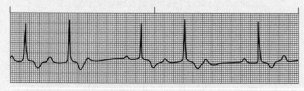

- Atrial rhythm regular
- Ventricular rhythm irregular
- Atrial rate exceeds ventricular rate
- PR interval progressively longer with each cycle until QRS complex disappears (dropped beat); PR interval shorter after dropped beat

Second-degree AV block (Mobitz II)

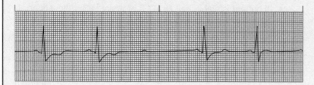

- Atrial rhythm regular
- Ventricular rhythm regular or irregular, with varying degree of block
- PR interval constant for conducted beats
- P waves normal size and shape, but some aren't followed by a QRS complex

Causes	Treatment
• Heart failure, chronic obstructive pulmonary disease, thyrotoxicosis, constrictive pericarditis, ischaemia heart disease, sepsis, PE, rheumatic heart disease, hypertension, mitral stenosis, atrial irritation or complication of coronary bypass or valve replacement surgery • Nifedipine and digoxin use	• If patient is unstable with a ventricular rate >150 beats/minute, immediate cardioversion • If patient is stable, follow ACLS protocol and drug therapy, which may include calcium channel blockers, beta-adrenergic blockers, amiodarone or digoxin • Anticoagulation therapy possibly also needed • In some patients with refractory atrial fibrillation uncontrolled by drugs, radiofrequency catheter ablation
• Inferior-wall MI or ischaemia, hypoxia, vagal stimulation and SSS • Acute rheumatic fever • Valve surgery • Digoxin toxicity	• Correction of underlying cause • Atropine for symptomatic slow rate • Pacemaker insertion if patient doesn't respond to drugs • Discontinuation of digoxin, if appropriate
• Possible in healthy persons • Inferior-wall MI or ischaemia, hypothyroidism, hypokalaemia and hyperkalemia • Digoxin toxicity; use of quinidine, procainamide, beta-adrenergic blockers, calcium channel blockers, or amiodarone	• Correction of underlying cause • Possibly atropine if severe symptomatic bradycardia develops • Cautious use of digoxin, calcium channel blockers and beta-adrenergic blockers
• Inferior-wall MI, cardiac surgery, acute rheumatic fever and vagal stimulation • Digoxin toxicity; use of propranolol, quinidine or procainamide	• Treatment of underlying cause • Atropine or transcutaneous pacemaker for symptomatic bradycardia • Discontinuation of digoxin, if appropriate
• Severe CAD, anterior-wall MI and acute myocarditis • Digoxin toxicity	• Temporary or permanent pacemaker • Atropine, dopamine, or adrenaline for symptomatic bradycardia • Discontinuation of digoxin, if appropriate

(continued)

Understanding cardiac arrhythmias *(Continued)*

Arrhythmia and features *(Continued)*

Third-degree AV block (complete heart block)

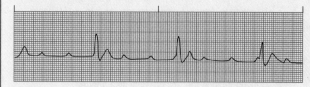

- Atrial rhythm regular
- Ventricular rhythm regular and rate slower than atrial rate
- No relation between P waves and QRS complexes
- No constant PR interval
- QRS duration normal (junctional pacemaker) or wide and bizarre (ventricular pacemaker)

Premature ventricular contraction (PVC)

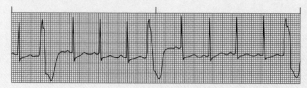

- Atrial rhythm regular
- Ventricular rhythm irregular
- QRS complex premature, usually followed by a complete compensatory pause
- QRS complex wide and distorted, usually >0.12 second
- Premature QRS complexes occurring alone, in pairs, or in threes, alternating with normal beats; focus from one or more sites
- Ominous when clustered, multifocal, with R-wave-on-T pattern

Ventricular tachycardia

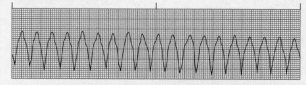

- Ventricular rate 100 to 220 beats/minute; rhythm usually regular
- QRS complexes wide, bizarre and independent of P waves
- P waves not discernible
- May start and stop suddenly

Causes	Treatment
• Inferior-or anterior-wall MI, congenital abnormality, rheumatic fever, hypoxia, postoperative complication of mitral valve replacement, postprocedure complication of radiofrequency ablation in or near AV nodal tissue, Lev's disease (fibrosis and calcification that spreads from cardiac structures to the conductive tissue) and Lenégre's disease (conductive tissue fibrosis) • Digoxin toxicity	• Atropine, dopamine, or adrenaline for symptomatic bradycardia • Transcutaneous or permanent pacemaker
• Heart failure; old or acute MI, ischaemia or contusion; myocardial irritation by ventricular catheter or a pacemaker,; hypercapnia, hypokalaemia, hypocalcemia and hypomagnesemia • Drug toxicity (digoxin, aminophylline, tricyclic antidepressants, beta-adrenergic blockers, isoproterenol or dopamine) • Caffeine, tobacco or alcohol use • Psychological stress, anxiety, pain or exercise	• If warranted, procainamide, amiodarone or lidocaine I.V. • Treatment of underlying cause • Discontinuation of drug causing toxicity • Potassium chloride I.V. if PVC induced by hypokalaemia • Magnesium sulphate I.V. if PVC induced by hypomagnesemia
• Myocardial ischaemia, MI or aneurysm; CAD, rheumatic heart disease, mitral valve prolapse, heart failure, cardiomyopathy, ventricular catheters, hypokalaemia, hypercalcemia, hypomagnesemia and PE • Digoxin, procainamide, adrenaline or quinidine toxicity • Anxiety	• If regular QRS rhythm (monomorphic), administer amiodarone (follow ACLS protocol); if drug is unsuccessful, cardioversion • If irregular QRS rhythm (polymorphic) and QT interval is prolonged, stop medications that may prolong QT interval; correct electrolyte imbalance and administer magnesium; if ineffective, cardioversion • If irregular QRS rhythm (polymorphic) and QT interval is normal, stop medications that may prolong QT interval; correct electrolyte balance; administer amiodarone; if ineffective, cardioversion • If the patient with monomorphic or polymorphic QRS complexes becomes unstable, immediate defibrillation • If pulseless, initiate CPR; follow ACLS protocol for defibrillation, endotracheal (ET) intubation and administration of adrenaline or vasopressin, followed by amiodarone or lidocaine and, if ineffective, magnesium sulphate or procainamide • ICD if recurrent VT

(continued)

Understanding cardiac arrhythmias *(Continued)*

Arrhythmia and features *(Continued)*

Ventricular fibrillation

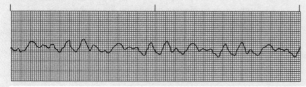

- Ventricular rhythm and rate chaotic and rapid
- QRS complexes wide and irregular; no visible P waves

Asystole

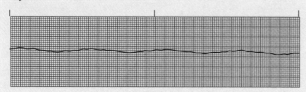

- No atrial or ventricular rate or rhythm
- No discernible P waves, QRS complexes or T waves

How it's treated

The goals of treatment for cardiac arrhythmias are to return pacer function to the sinus node, increase or decrease ventricular rate to normal, regain atrioventricular (AV) synchrony and maintain normal sinus rhythm. Treatments to correct abnormal rhythms include therapy with:
- Antiarrhythmic drugs
- Electrical conversion with defibrillation and cardioversion
- Management of the underlying disorder, such as correction of hypoxia
- Temporary or permanent placement of a pacemaker to maintain heart rate
- Valsalva's manoeuvre
- Implantable cardioverter-defibrillator (ICD), if indicated
- Surgical removal or cryotherapy of an irritable ectopic focus to prevent recurring arrhythmias.

What to do

- Evaluate the patient's ECG frequently for arrhythmia and assess haemodynamic parameters as indicated. Document arrhythmias and notify the practitioner immediately
- When life-threatening arrhythmias develop, rapidly assess the patient's level of consciousness (LOC), pulse and respiratory rates and haemodynamic parameters. Monitor his ECG continuously. Be prepared to initiate CPR, if indicated. Follow ALS protocol to treat specific life-threatening arrhythmias
- Assess the patient for predisposing factors, such as fluid and electrolyte imbalance, and signs of drug toxicity, especially with Digoxin
- Administer medications as ordered; monitor for adverse effects and monitor vital signs, haemodynamic parameters (as appropriate)

Causes	Treatment
• Myocardial ischaemia, MI, untreated VT, R-on-T phenomenon, hypokalaemia, hyperkalemia, hypercalcemia, hypoxemia, alkalosis, electric shock and hypothermia • Digoxin, adrenaline or quinidine toxicity	• CPR; follow ACLS protocol for defibrillation, ET intubation and administration of adrenaline or vasopressin, amiodarone or lidocaine and, if ineffective, magnesium sulphate or procainamide • ICD if risk of recurrent VF
• Myocardial ischaemia, MI, aortic valve disease, heart failure, hypoxia, hypokalaemia, severe acidosis, electric shock, ventricular arrhythmia, AV block, PE, heart rupture, cardiac tamponade, hyperkalemia and electromechanical dissociation • Cocaine overdose	• Continue CPR; follow ACLS protocol for ET intubation, temporary pacing and administration of adrenaline or vasopressin and atropine

and appropriate laboratory studies. Prepare to assist with or perform cardioversion or defibrillation, if indicated
•   If you suspect drug toxicity, report it to the doctor or senior nurse immediately and withhold the next dose
•   Prepare the patient for cardioversion, transcutaneous or transvenous pacing, if appropriate
•   If a temporary pacemaker must be inserted, monitor the patient's pulse rate regularly after insertion and watch for signs of pacemaker failure and decreased cardiac output.

Prepare the patient for transfer to undergo electrophysiology studies, an angiogram, an internal cardiac defibrillator placement or pacemaker placement.

Echocardiography

Echocardiography is used to examine the size, shape and motion of cardiac structures. It's done using a transducer placed at an acoustic window (an area where bone and lung tissue are absent) on the patient's chest. The transducer directs sound waves towards cardiac structures, which reflect these waves.

Echo, echo

The transducer picks up the echoes, converts them to electrical impulses and relays them to an echocardiography machine for display on a screen and for recording on a strip chart or videotape. The most commonly used echocardiography techniques are motion mode (M-mode) and two-dimensional.

Echo abnormalities

The echocardiogram may detect mitral stenosis, mitral valve prolapse, aortic insufficiency, wall motion abnormalities and pericardial effusion (excess pericardial fluid).

Practice pointers
- Explain the procedure to the patient, and advise him to remain still during the test because movement can distort results
- Tell the patient that conductive gel is applied to the chest (and it will be cold) and that a quarter-sized transducer is placed directly over it. Because pressure is exerted to keep the transducer in contact with the skin, warn the patient that he may feel minor discomfort
- After the procedure, remove the conductive gel from the skin.

Haemodynamic monitoring

Haemodynamic monitoring is an invasive procedure used to assess cardiac function and determine the effectiveness of therapy by measuring:
- BP
- Cardiac output
- Intracardiac pressures
- Mixed oxygen saturation. (See *Putting haemodynamic monitoring to use.*)

Getting involved

Haemodynamic monitoring involves insertion of a catheter into the vascular system. The types of haemodynamic monitoring include:
- Arterial BP monitoring
- Pulmonary artery pressure monitoring (PAP), using the internal and external jugular and subclavian veins. (Femoral and antecubital veins may be used but aren't the sites of choice.)

Controversial contraindications

As an invasive procedure, haemodynamic monitoring remains controversial in some EDs because of the risks involved, including sepsis, pneumothorax, air embolism and pulmonary artery (PA) infarction.

Arterial BP monitoring
In arterial BP monitoring, the practitioner inserts a catheter into the radial or femoral artery to measure BP or obtain samples of arterial blood for diagnostic tests such as ABG studies. A transducer transforms the flow of blood during systole and diastole into a waveform, which appears on an oscilloscope.

Putting haemodynamic monitoring to use

Haemodynamic monitoring provides information on intracardiac pressures, arterial pressure and cardiac output. To understand intracardiac pressures, picture the heart and vascular system as a continuous loop with constantly changing pressure gradients that keep the blood moving. Haemodynamic monitoring records the gradients within the vessels and heart chambers. Cardiac output indicates the amount of blood ejected by the heart each minute.

Pressure and description	Normal values	Causes of increased pressure	Causes of decreased pressure
Central venous pressure or right atrial pressure The CVP or right atrial pressure shows right ventricular function and end-diastolic pressure.	Normal mean pressure ranges from 1 to 6 mm Hg (1.34 cm to 8 cm H_2O).	• Right-sided heart failure • Volume overload • Tricuspid valve stenosis or insufficiency • Constrictive pericarditis • Pulmonary hypertension • Cardiac tamponade • Right ventricular infarction	• Reduced circulating blood volume
Right ventricular pressure Typically, the doctor measures right ventricular pressure only when initially inserting a pulmonary artery catheter. Right ventricular systolic pressure normally equals PA systolic pressure; right ventricular end-diastolic pressure, which reflects right ventricular function, equals right atrial pressure.	Normal systolic pressure ranges from 20 to 30 mm Hg; normal diastolic pressure, from 0 to 5 mm Hg.	• Mitral stenosis or insufficiency • Pulmonary disease • Hypoxemia • Constrictive pericarditis • Chronic heart failure • Atrial and ventricular septal defects • Patent ductus arteriosus	• Reduced circulating blood volume
Pulmonary artery pressure Pulmonary artery Systolic PAP shows right ventricular function and pulmonary circulation pressures. PA diastolic pressure reflects left ventricular pressures, specifically left ventricular end-diastolic pressure, in a patient without significant pulmonary disease.	Systolic pressure normally ranges from 20 to 30 mm Hg. The mean pressure usually ranges from 10 to 15 mm Hg.	• Left-sided heart failure • Increased pulmonary blood flow (left or right shunting, as in atrial or ventricular septal defects) • Any condition causing increased pulmonary arteriolar resistance (such as pulmonary hypertension, volume overload, mitral stenosis or hypoxia)	• Reduced circulating blood volume
Pulmonary artery wedge pressure PAWP reflects left atrial and left ventricular pressures, unless the patient has mitral stenosis. Changes in PAWP reflect changes in left ventricular filling pressure.	The mean pressure normally ranges from 6 to 12 mm Hg.	• Left-sided heart failure • Mitral stenosis or insufficiency • Pericardial tamponade	• Reduced circulating blood volume

PAP monitoring

Continuous PAP and intermittent pulmonary artery wedge pressure (PAWP) measurements provide important information about left ventricular function and preload. This information is used for monitoring, aiding diagnosis, refining assessment, guiding interventions and projecting patient outcomes.

PAP purposes

PAP monitoring is indicated for patients who:
- Are haemodynamically unstable
- Need fluid management or continuous cardiopulmonary assessment
- Are receiving multiple or frequently administered cardioactive drugs
- Are experiencing shock, trauma, pulmonary or cardiac disease or multiple organ dysfunction syndrome.

PAP's parts

A PA catheter has up to six lumens that gather haemodynamic information. In addition to distal and proximal lumens used to measure pressures, a PA catheter has a balloon inflation lumen that inflates the balloon for PAWP measurement and a thermistor connector lumen that allows cardiac output measurement. Some catheters also have a pacemaker wire lumen that provides a port for pacemaker electrodes and measures continuous mixed venous oxygen saturation.

PAP and PAWP procedures

In PAP or PAWP measurement, the practitioner inserts the balloon-tipped, multilumen catheter into the patient's internal jugular or subclavian vein. When the catheter reaches the right atrium, the balloon is inflated to float the catheter through the right ventricle into the PA. When the catheter is in the PA, PAWP measurement is possible through an opening at the catheter's tip. The catheter is then deflated and rests in the PA, allowing diastolic and systolic PAP readings.

The balloon should be totally deflated except when taking a PAWP reading because prolonged wedging can cause pulmonary infarction.

Practice pointers
Arterial BP monitoring
- Explain the procedure to the patient and his family, if possible
- After catheter insertion, observe the pressure waveform to assess arterial pressure
- Assess the insertion site for signs of infection, such as redness and swelling. Notify the practitioner immediately if you note such signs
- Document the date and time of catheter insertion, catheter insertion site, type of flush solution used, type of dressing applied and patient's tolerance of the procedure.

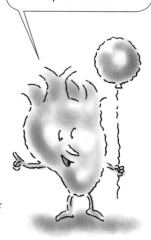

Careful … over inflating a PA catheter balloon can distend the pulmonary artery and rupture vessels.

Better assessor

Cardiac output is better assessed by calculating cardiac index, which takes body size into account. To calculate the patient's cardiac index, divide his cardiac output by his body surface area, a function of height and weight. The normal cardiac index ranges from 2.5 to 4.2 L/minute/m^2 for adults or 3.5 to 6.5 L/minute/m^2 for pregnant women.

Physiologic changes can affect the cardiac output and the cardiac index; they include:
- Decreased preload
- Increased preload
- Vasoconstriction (changes in afterload)
- Vasodilatation (changes in afterload)
- Hypothermia.

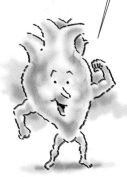

Lucky for me, cardiac index takes body size into account!

Treatments

Many treatments are available for patients with cardiac emergencies. Commonly used treatment measures include drug therapy, surgery and other treatments, such as defibrillation, synchronised cardioversion and pacemaker insertion.

Drug therapy

Types of drugs used to improve cardiovascular function include adrenergics, adrenergic blockers, antianginals, antiarrhythmics, anticoagulants, antihypertensives, cardiac glycosides and phosphodiesterase (PDE) inhibitors, diuretics and thrombolytics.

Adrenergics

Adrenergic drugs are also called *sympathomimetics* because they produce effects similar to those produced by the sympathetic nervous system. Adrenergic drugs are classified in two groups based on their chemical structure – catecholamines (naturally occurring and synthetic) and noncatecholamines. (See *Understanding adrenergics*, page 164.)

Which receptor

Therapeutic use of adrenergic drugs depends on which receptors they stimulate and to what degree. Adrenergic drugs can affect:
- alpha-adrenergic receptors
- beta-adrenergic receptors
- dopamine receptors.

Understanding adrenergics

Adrenergic drugs produce effects similar to those produced by the sympathetic nervous system. They can affect alpha-adrenergic receptors, beta-adrenergic receptors or dopamine receptors. However, most of the drugs stimulate the alpha- and beta-receptors, mimicking the effects of noradrenaline and adrenaline. Dopaminergic drugs act on receptors typically stimulated by dopamine. Use this table to learn about the indications and adverse reactions associated with these drugs.

Drugs	Indications	Adverse reactions
Catecholamines		
Dobutamine	• Increase cardiac output in short-term treatment of cardiac decompensation from depressed contractility	• Headache • Tachycardia • Cardiac arrhythmias (PVCs) • Hypertension
Dopamine	• Adjunct in shock to increase cardiac output, BP and urine flow	• Dyspnoea • Bradycardia • Palpitations • Tachycardia • Cardiac arrhythmias (ventricular) • Hypotension • Widened QRS • Angina
Adrenaline	• Anaphylaxis • Bronchospasm • Hypersensitivity reactions • Restoration of cardiac rhythm in cardiac arrest	• Restlessness • Anxiety • Headache • Tachycardia • Palpitations • Cardiac arrhythmias (VF) • Precordial pain (in patients with ischaemic heart disease)
Noradrenaline	• GI bleeding • Maintain BP in acute hypotensive states	• Headache • Bradycardia • Hypertension
Noncatecholamines		
Ephedrine hydrochloride	• Maintain BP in acute hypotensive states, especially with spinal anesthesia • Treatment of orthostatic hypotension and bronchospasm	• Restlessness • Anxiety • Dizziness • Headache • Cardiac arrhythmias (VF) • Nausea
Phenylephrine hydrochloride	• Maintain BP in hypotensive states, especially hypotensive emergencies with spinal anesthesia	• Restlessness • Anxiety • Dizziness • Headache • Palpitations • Cardiac arrhythmias

Mimicking noradrenaline and adrenaline

Most of the adrenergic drugs produce their effects by stimulating alpha- and beta-adrenergic receptors. These drugs mimic the action of noradrenaline or adrenaline.

Doing it like dopamine

Dopaminergic drugs act primarily on receptors in the sympathetic nervous system that are stimulated by dopamine.

Catecholamines
Because of their common basic chemical structure, catecholamines share certain properties. They stimulate the nervous system, constrict peripheral blood vessels, increase heart rate and dilate the bronchi. They can be manufactured in the body or in a laboratory.

Excitatory or inhibitory

Catecholamines primarily act directly. When catecholamines combine with alpha- or beta-receptors, they cause an excitatory or inhibitory effect. Typically, activation of alpha-receptors generates an excitatory response except for intestinal relaxation. Activation of the beta-receptors mostly produces an inhibitory response except in the cells of the heart, where noradrenaline produces excitatory effects.

How heartening

The clinical effects of catecholamines depend on the dosage and the route of administration. Catecholamines are potent inotropes, meaning they make the heart contract more forcefully. As a result, the ventricles empty more completely with each heartbeat, increasing the workload of the heart and the amount of oxygen it needs to do this harder work.

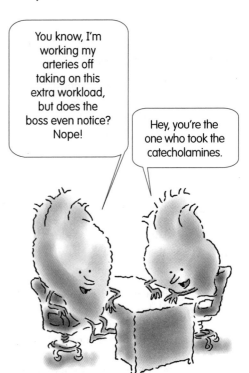

You know, I'm working my arteries off taking on this extra workload, but does the boss even notice? Nope!

Hey, you're the one who took the catecholamines.

Rapid rates

Catecholamines also produce a positive chronotropic effect, which means they cause the heart to beat faster. The heart beats faster because catecholamines increase the depolarisation rate of pacemaker cells in the sinoatrial (SA) node of the heart. As catecholamines cause blood vessels to constrict and BP to increase, the heart rate decreases as the body tries to prevent an excessive increase in BP.

Fascinating rhythm

Catecholamines can cause the Purkinje fibres (an intricate web of fibres that carry electrical impulses into the ventricles of the heart) to fire spontaneously, possibly producing abnormal heart rhythms, such as PVCs and fibrillation. Adrenaline is likelier than noradrenaline to produce this spontaneous firing.

Noncatecholamines
Noncatecholamine adrenergic drugs have a variety of therapeutic uses because of the many effects these drugs can have on the body, such as the local or systemic constriction of blood vessels by phenylephrine.

Alpha active

Direct-acting noncatecholamines that stimulate alpha activity include phenylephrine hydrochloride. Those that selectively exert beta$_2$ activity include:
- salbutamol
- orciprenaline sulphate.

Adrenergic blockers
Adrenergic blocking drugs, also called *sympatholytic drugs*, are used to disrupt sympathetic nervous system function. (See *Understanding adrenergic blockers*.)

Impending impulses

Adrenergic blockers work by blocking impulse transmission (and thus sympathetic nervous system stimulation) at adrenergic neurons or adrenergic receptor sites. The action of the drugs at these sites can be exerted by:
- Interrupting the action of sympathomimetic (adrenergic) drugs
- Reducing available noradrenaline
- Preventing the action of cholinergic drugs.

Classified information

Adrenergic blockers are classified according to their site of action as alpha-adrenergic blockers or beta-adrenergic blockers.

Alpha-adrenergic blockers
Alpha-adrenergic blockers work by interrupting the actions of sympathomimetic drugs at alpha-adrenergic receptors. This interruption results in:
- Relaxation of the smooth muscle in the blood vessels
- Increased dilation of blood vessels
- Decreased BP.
  Drugs in this class include:
- Phentolamine
- Prazosin.

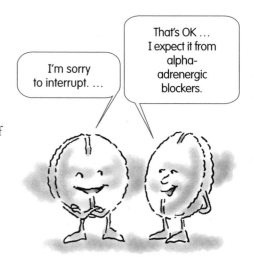

Understanding adrenergic blockers

Adrenergic blockers block impulse transmission at adrenergic receptor sites by interrupting the action of adrenergic drugs, reducing the amount of noradrenaline available and blocking the action of cholinergics. Use this table to learn the indications and adverse reactions associated with these drugs.

Drugs	Indications	Adverse reactions
Alpha-adrenergic blockers		
Phentolamine and Prazosin	• Hypertension • Peripheral vascular disorders • Pheochromocytoma	• Orthostatic hypotension • Severe hypertension • Bradycardia • Tachycardia • Oedema • Difficulty breathing • Lightheadedness • Flushing • Arrhythmias • Angina • Heart attack • Shock
Beta-adrenergic blockers		
Nonselective Carvedilol, Labetalol, Nadolol, Pindolol Propranolol, Sotalol and Timolol	• Prevention of complications after MI, angina, hypertension, supraventricular arrhythmias, anxiety, essential tremor, cardiovascular symptoms associated with thyrotoxicosis, migraine headaches, pheochromocytoma	• Hypotension • Bradycardia • Peripheral vascular insufficiency • Heart failure • Bronchospasm • Sore throat • AV block
Selective Acebutolol, Atenolol Betaxolol, Bisoprolol, Esmolol and Metoprolol		

Not very discriminating

Alpha receptor sites are either alpha$_1$ or alpha$_2$ receptors. Alpha-adrenergic blockers include drugs that block stimulation of alpha$_1$ receptors and that may block alpha$_2$ stimulation.

Reducing resistance

Alpha-adrenergic blockers occupy alpha receptor sites on the smooth muscle of blood vessels, which prevents catecholamines from occupying and stimulating the receptor sites. As a result, blood vessels dilate, increasing local blood flow to the skin and other organs. The decreased peripheral vascular resistance (resistance to blood flow) helps to decrease BP.

Beta-adrenergic blockers

Beta-adrenergic blockers are the most widely used adrenergic blockers. They prevent stimulation of the sympathetic nervous system by inhibiting the action of catecholamines and other sympathomimetic drugs at beta-adrenergic receptors.

Selective (or not)

Beta-adrenergic drugs are selective or nonselective. Nonselective beta-adrenergic drugs affect:
- Beta$_1$-receptor sites (located mainly in the heart)
- Beta$_2$-receptor sites (located in the bronchi, blood vessels and uterus).
  Nonselective beta-adrenergic drugs include Carvedilol, Timolol, Nadolol, Penbutolol, Labetalol, Pindolol, Sotalol and Propranolol.

Highly discriminating

Selective beta-adrenergic drugs primarily affect the beta$_1$-adrenergic sites. They include Atenolol, Esmolol, Acebutolol and Metoprolol.

Intrinsically sympathetic

Some beta-adrenergic blockers, such as Pindolol and Acebutolol, have intrinsic sympathetic activity. This sympathetic activity means that, instead of attaching to beta-receptors and blocking them, these beta-adrenergic blockers attach to beta-receptors and stimulate them. These drugs are sometimes classified as *partial agonists*.

Widely effective

Beta-adrenergic blockers have widespread effects in the body because they produce their blocking action not only at the adrenergic nerve endings but also in the adrenal medulla. Effects on the heart include:
- Increased peripheral vascular resistance
- Decreased BP
- Decreased force of contractions of the heart
- Decreased oxygen consumption by the heart
- Slowed conduction of impulses between the atria and ventricles
- Decreased cardiac output.

Selective or nonselective

Some of the effects of beta-adrenergic blocking drugs depend on whether the drug is classified as selective or nonselective. Selective beta-adrenergic blockers, which preferentially block beta$_1$ receptor sites, reduce stimulation of the heart. They're commonly called *cardioselective beta-adrenergic blockers*.

Nonselective beta-adrenergic blockers, which block beta$_1$ and beta$_2$ receptor sites, reduce stimulation of the heart and cause the bronchioles of the lungs to constrict. This constriction causes bronchospasm in patients with chronic obstructive lung disorders.

Antianginals

When the oxygen demands of the heart exceed the amount of oxygen being supplied, areas of heart muscle become ischaemic (not receiving enough oxygen). When the heart muscle is ischaemic the individual then experiences chest pain. This condition is known as *angina* or *angina pectoris*.

Reduce demand, increase supply

Although angina's cardinal symptom is chest pain, the drugs used to treat angina aren't typically analgesics. Instead, antianginal drugs correct angina by reducing myocardial oxygen demand (the amount of oxygen the heart needs to do its work), increasing the supply of oxygen to the heart, or both.

The top three

The three classes of commonly used antianginal drugs include:

Nitrates (for acute angina)

Beta-adrenergic blockers (for long-term prevention of angina)

Calcium channel blockers (used when other drugs fail to prevent angina). (See *Understanding antianginal drugs*, page 170.)

Nitrates

Nitrates are the drug of choice for relieving acute angina.

Anti-angina effect

Nitrates cause the smooth muscle of the veins and, to a lesser extent, the arteries to relax and dilate. Here's what happens:
• When the veins dilate less blood returns to the heart
• Decreased blood return reduces the amount of blood in the ventricles at the end of diastole, when the ventricles are full. (This blood volume in the ventricles just before contraction is called *preload*)
• By reducing preload, nitrates reduce ventricular size and ventricular wall tension so the left ventricle doesn't have to stretch as much to pump blood. This reduction in size and tension in turn reduces the oxygen requirements of the heart
• As the coronary arteries dilate, more blood is delivered to the myocardium, improving oxygenation of the ischaemic tissue.

Understanding antianginal drugs

Antianginal drugs are effective in treating patients with angina because they reduce myocardial oxygen demand, increase the supply of oxygen to the heart, or both. Use this table to learn about the indications and adverse reactions associated with these drugs.

Drugs	Indications	Adverse reactions
Nitrates		
Isosorbide dinitrate isosorbide mononitrate and GTN	• Relief and prevention of angina	• Dizziness • Headache • Hypotension • Increased heart rate
Beta-adrenergic blockers		
Atenolol, metoprolol, nadolol and propranolol	• First-line therapy for hypertension • Long-term prevention of angina	• Angina • Arrhythmias • Bradycardia • Bronchial constriction • Diarrhea • Fainting • Fluid retention • Heart failure • Nausea • Shock • Vomiting
Calcium channel blockers		
Amlodipine, diltiazem, nicardipine, nifedipine and verapamil	• Long-term prevention of angina (especially Prinzmetal's variant angina)	• Arrhythmias • Dizziness • Flushing • Headache • Heart failure • Hypotension • Orthostatic hypotension • Persistent peripheral oedema • Weakness

Reducing resistance

The arterioles provide the most resistance to the blood pumped by the left ventricle (called *systemic vascular resistance*). Nitrates decrease afterload by dilating the arterioles, reducing resistance, easing the heart's workload and easing oxygen demand.

Beta-adrenergic blockers

Beta-adrenergic blockers are used for long-term prevention of angina and are one of the main types of drugs used to treat hypertension.

Down with everything

Beta-adrenergic blockers decrease BP and block beta-adrenergic receptor sites in the heart muscle and conduction system. These actions decrease the heart rate and reduce the force of the heart's contractions, resulting in lower demand for oxygen.

Calcium channel blockers

Calcium channel blockers are commonly used to prevent angina that doesn't respond to nitrates or beta-adrenergic blockers. Some calcium channel blockers are also used as antiarrhythmics.

Preventing passage

Calcium channel blockers prevent the passage of calcium ions across the myocardial cell membrane and vascular smooth-muscle cells, causing dilation of the coronary and peripheral arteries. This dilation in turn decreases the force of the heart's contractions and reduces the workload of the heart.

Rate reduction

By preventing arterioles from constricting, calcium channel blockers also reduce afterload. In addition, decreasing afterload decreases oxygen demands of the heart.

Conduction reduction

Calcium channel blockers also reduce the heart rate by slowing conduction through the SA and AV nodes. A slower heart rate reduces the heart's need for oxygen.

Antiarrhythmics

Antiarrhythmics are used to treat arrhythmias, which are disturbances of the normal heart rhythm.

Benefits vs. risks

Unfortunately, many antiarrhythmic drugs can worsen or cause arrhythmias, too. In any case, the benefits of antiarrhythmic therapy must be weighed against its risks.

Anticoagulants

Anticoagulants are used to reduce the ability of the blood to clot. (See *Understanding anticoagulants*, page 172.) Major categories of anticoagulants include antiplatelet drugs, heparin and oral anticoagulants. Antiplatelet drugs are used to prevent arterial thromboembolism, especially in patients at risk for MI, stroke and arteriosclerosis (hardening of the arteries). They interfere with platelet activity in different drug-specific and dose-related ways.

Understanding anticoagulants

Anticoagulants reduce the blood's ability to clot and are included in the treatment plans for many patients with cardiovascular disorders. Use this table to learn about the indications and adverse reactions associated with these drugs.

Drugs	Indications	Adverse reactions
Heparins		
Heparin and low-molecular-weight heparins	• Deep vein thrombosis • Disseminated intravascular coagulation • Embolism prophylaxis • Prevention of complications after MI	• Bleeding
Oral anticoagulants		
Warfarin	• Atrial arrhythmias • Deep vein thrombosis prophylaxis • Prevention of complications of prosthetic heart valves or diseased mitral valves	• Bleeding (may be severe)
Antiplatelet drugs		
Aspirin, Dipyridamole and Clopidogrel	• Decreases the risk of death after MI • Patients at risk for ischaemia events (clopidogrel) • Patients with acute coronary syndrome (clopidogrel) • Prevention of complications of prosthetic heart valves	• Bleeding • GI distress • Headache (clopidogrel)

Low is good

Low dosages of aspirin (usually 75 mg/day) appear to inhibit clot formation by blocking the synthesis of prostaglandin, which in turn prevents formation of the platelet-aggregating substance thromboxane A_2. There is, however, an increased risk of gastrointestinal bleeding. Dipyridamole may inhibit platelet aggregation.

Anticlumping

Clopidogrel inhibits platelet aggregation by blocking adenosine diphosphate receptors on platelets, thereby preventing the clumping of platelets.

Heparin

Heparin, prepared commercially from animal tissue, is used to prevent clot formation. Low-molecular-weight heparin, such as dalteparin and enoxaparin, prevents deep vein thrombosis (usually in the legs) in surgical patients. Be aware, however, that a patient placed on any form of heparin is at risk for developing heparin-induced thrombocytopenia.

No new clots

Because it doesn't affect the synthesis of clotting factors, heparin can't dissolve already formed clots. It does prevent the formation of new thrombi. Here's how it works:
• Heparin inhibits the formation of thrombin and fibrin by activating antithrombin III
• Antithrombin III then inactivates factors IXa, Xa, XIa and XIIa in the intrinsic and common pathways. The end result is prevention of a stable fibrin clot
• In low doses, heparin increases the activity of antithrombin III against factor Xa and thrombin and inhibits clot formation. Much larger doses are necessary to inhibit fibrin formation after a clot has formed. This relationship between dose and effect is the rationale for using low-dose heparin to prevent clotting
• Whole blood-clotting time, thrombin time and partial thromboplastin time are prolonged during heparin therapy. However, these times may be only slightly prolonged with low or ultra-low preventive doses.

Circulate freely

Heparin can be used to prevent clotting when a patient's blood must circulate outside the body through a machine, such as a cardiopulmonary bypass machine or haemodialysis machine.

Oral anticoagulants

Oral anticoagulants alter the ability of the liver to synthesise vitamin K-dependent clotting factors, including prothrombin and factors VII, IX and X. Clotting factors already in the bloodstream continue to coagulate blood until they become depleted, so anticoagulation doesn't begin immediately.

Warfarin vs. coagulation

The major oral anticoagulant used in the UK is Warfarin. It is important when history-taking to identify if a patient is taking Warfarin, as a minor injury may lead to concealed bleeding resulting in major blood loss. This is of particular relevance with head injury patients.

Treating Hypertension

Hypertension, a disorder characterised by high systolic BP and a high diastolic BP, or both.
• The normal adult BP is a reading between 90 to 120 mm Hg systolic and 60 to 80 mm Hg diastolic
• A pre-high BP reading is between 120 and 140 mm Hg systolic and 80 to 90 mm Hg diastolic
• A patient is hypertension once his BP is over 140 mm Hg systolic and 90 mm Hg diastolic
• A severe elevation in BP of over 200 mm Hg systolic and 120 mm Hg diastolic is defined as a hypertensive crisis. (See *What happens in hypertensive crisis*, page 214.)

Know the programme

Although treatment for hypertension begins with beta-adrenergic blockers and diuretics, antihypertensives are used if those drugs aren't effective. Antihypertensive therapy includes the use of sympatholytics (other than beta-adrenergic blockers), vasodilators, angiotensin-converting enzyme (ACE) inhibitors and angiotensin receptor blockers alone or in combination. It is dangerous to reduce the BP too rapidly (aim to reduce the diastolic BP to 100 to 110 mm Hg within 2 to 4 hours) and ideally oral drugs are utilised. IV drugs are only used in specific circumstances.

Sympatholytics

Sympatholytic drugs include several different types of drugs. However, all of these drugs work by inhibiting or blocking the sympathetic nervous system, which causes dilation of the peripheral blood vessels or decreases cardiac output, thereby reducing BP.

Where and how

Sympatholytic drugs are classified by their site or mechanism of action and include:
- Central-acting sympathetic nervous system inhibitors, such as clonidine and methyldopa
- Alpha blockers, such as Doxazosin, Prazosin and Terazosin
- Mixed alpha- and beta-adrenergic blockers, such as Labetalol
- Noradrenaline depletors, such as Guanethidine.

Vasodilators

The two types of vasodilating drugs include calcium channel blockers and direct vasodilators. These drugs decrease systolic and diastolic BP.

Calcium stoppers

Calcium channel blockers produce arteriolar relaxation by preventing the entry of calcium into the cells. This relaxation prevents the contraction of vascular smooth muscle.

Direct dial

Direct vasodilators act on arteries, veins or both. They work by relaxing peripheral vascular smooth muscles, causing the blood vessels to dilate. This dilation decreases BP by increasing the diameter of the blood vessels, reducing total peripheral resistance.

Hydralazine and Minoxidil are usually used to treat patients with resistant or refractory hypertension. Diazoxide and Nitroprusside are reserved for use in hypertensive crisis.

ACE inhibitors

ACE inhibitors reduce BP by interrupting the renin–angiotensin–aldosterone system.

Without ACE inhibition

Here's how the renin–angiotensin–aldosterone system works:
- Normally, the kidneys maintain BP by releasing the hormone renin
- Renin acts on the plasma protein angiotensinogen to form angiotensin I
- Angiotensin I is then converted to angiotensin II
- Angiotensin II, a potent vasoconstrictor, increases peripheral resistance and promotes the excretion of aldosterone
- Aldosterone, in turn, promotes the retention of sodium and water, increasing the volume of blood the heart needs to pump.

With ACE inhibition

ACE inhibitors work by preventing the conversion of angiotensin I to angiotensin II. As angiotensin II is reduced, arterioles dilate, reducing peripheral vascular resistance. By reducing aldosterone secretion, ACE inhibitors promote the excretion of sodium and water. Less sodium and water reduces the amount of blood the heart needs to pump, resulting in lower BP.

Angiotensin II receptor antagonists

Unlike ACE inhibitors, which prevent production of angiotensin, angiotensin II receptor antagonists block the action of angiotensin II, a major culprit in the development of hypertension, by attaching to tissue-binding receptor sites.

Cardiac glycosides and PDE inhibitors

Cardiac glycosides and phosphodiesterase (PDE) inhibitors increase the force of the heart's contractions. Increasing the force of contractions is known as a *positive inotropic effect*, so these drugs are also called *inotropic agents* (effecting the force or energy of muscular contractions). (See *Understanding cardiac glycosides and PDE inhibitors*, page 176.)

Slower rate

Cardiac glycosides, such as Digoxin, also slow the heart rate (called a *negative chronotropic effect*) and slow electrical impulse conduction through the AV node (called a *negative dromotropic effect*.)

Boosting output

PDE inhibitors, such as Milrinone, are typically used for short-term management of heart failure or long-term management in patients awaiting heart transplant surgery and can provide a sustained haemodynamic benefit. PDE inhibitors improve cardiac output by strengthening contractions. These drugs are thought to help move calcium into the cardiac cell or to increase calcium storage in the sarcoplasmic reticulum. By directly relaxing vascular smooth muscle, they also decrease peripheral vascular resistance (afterload) and the amount of blood returning to the heart (preload). There is, however, no evidence of any beneficial effect in survival rate with PDE inhibitors.

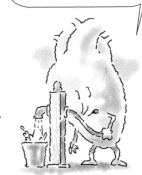

The more water and sodium excreted thanks to ACE inhibitors, the less blood I need to pump. Thank goodness – my arm is killing me!

Understanding cardiac glycosides and PDE inhibitors

Cardiac glycosides and PDE inhibitors have a positive inotropic effect on the heart, meaning they increase the force of contraction. Use this table to learn about the indications and adverse reactions associated with these drugs.

Drugs	Indications	Adverse reactions
Cardiac glycoside		
Digoxin	• Heart failure, supraventricular arrhythmias	• Digoxin toxicity (abdominal pain, arrhythmias, depression, headache, insomnia, irritability, nausea, vision disturbances)
PDE inhibitors		
Milrinone	• Heart failure refractory to digoxin, diuretics and vasodilators • Not to be used immediately after MI	• Arrhythmias • Chest pain • Fever • Headache • Hypokalaemia • Mild increase in heart rate • Nausea • Thrombocytopenia • Vomiting

Diuretics

Diuretics are used to promote the excretion of water and electrolytes by the kidneys. By doing so, diuretics play a major role in treating hypertension and other cardiovascular conditions. (See *Understanding diuretics*.)

The major diuretics used as cardiovascular drugs include:
• Loop diuretics
• Potassium-sparing diuretics
• Thiazide and thiazide-like diuretics.

Loop diuretics
Loop diuretics are highly potent drugs.

High potency, big risk

Loop diuretics are the most potent diuretics available, producing the greatest volume of diuresis (urine production). They also carry a high potential for causing severe adverse reactions.

In the loop

Loop diuretics receive their name because they act primarily on the thick ascending Loop of Henle (the part of the nephron responsible for concentrating urine) to increase the secretion of sodium, chloride

Understanding diuretics

Diuretics are used to treat patients with various cardiovascular conditions. They work by promoting the excretion of water and electrolytes by the kidneys. Use this table to learn about the indications and adverse reactions associated with these drugs.

Drugs	Indications	Adverse reactions
Thiazide and thiazide-like diuretics		
Bendroflumethiazide chlorthalidone Hydrochlorothiazide and Hydroflumethiazide	• Oedema • Hypertension	• Hypokalaemia • Hyponatremia • Orthostatic hypotension
Loop diuretics		
Bumetanide and Frusemide	• Oedema • Heart failure • Hypertension	• Dehydration • Hyperuricaemia • Hypocalcaemia • Hypochloraemia • Hypokalaemia • Hypomagnesaemia • Hyponatraemia • Orthostatic hypotension
Potassium-sparing diuretics		
Amiloride, Spironolactone and Triamterene	• Cirrhosis • Diuretic-induced hypokalaemia in patients with heart failure • Oedema • Hypertension • Nephrotic syndrome	• Hyperkalaemia

and water. These drugs may also inhibit sodium, chloride and water reabsorption.

Potassium-sparing diuretics

Potassium-sparing diuretics have weaker diuretic and antihypertensive effects than other diuretics, but they have the advantage of conserving potassium.

Potassium-sparing effects

The direct action of the potassium-sparing diuretics on the distal tubule of the kidneys produces:
• Increased urinary excretion of sodium and water
• Increased excretion of chloride and calcium ions
• Decreased excretion of potassium and hydrogen ions.
  These effects lead to reduced BP and increased serum potassium levels.

Thiazide and thiazide-like diuretics
Thiazide and thiazide-like diuretics are sulfonamide derivatives.

Sodium stoppers

Thiazide and thiazide-like diuretics work by preventing sodium from being reabsorbed in the kidney. As sodium is excreted, it pulls water along with it. Thiazide and thiazide-like diuretics also increase the excretion of chloride, potassium and bicarbonate, which can result in electrolyte imbalances.

Stability with time

Initially, these drugs decrease circulating blood volume, leading to a reduced cardiac output. However, if therapy is maintained, cardiac output stabilises but plasma fluid volume decreases.

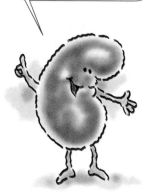

Sodium once, shame on you; sodium twice, shame on me! Thiazide diuretics prevent me from reabsorbing the stuff.

Surgery

Types of surgery used to treat cardiovascular system disorders include coronary artery bypass graft (CABG), vascular repair and insertion of a ventricular assist device (VAD). Percutaneous transluminal coronary angioplasty (PTCA) is a nonsurgical way to open coronary vessels narrowed by arteriosclerosis. It's usually used with cardiac catheterisation to assess the stenosis and efficacy of angioplasty. It can also be used as a visual tool to direct the balloon-tipped catheter through a vessel's area of stenosis. These procedures are performed within cardiac catheterisation laboratories within regional centres.

Other treatments

Other treatments for cardiovascular disorders include synchronised cardioversion, defibrillation and pacemaker insertion.

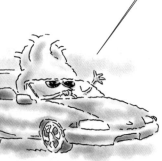

I think if I take the coronary artery bypass instead of the freeway, I can avoid anginal pain AND make good time.

Synchronised cardioversion
Synchronised cardioversion (synchronised countershock) is an elective or emergency procedure used to treat unstable tachyarrhythmias (such as atrial flutter, atrial fibrillation and supraventricular tachycardia and VT). It's also the treatment of choice for patients with arrhythmias that don't respond to drug therapy.

Electrifying experience

In synchronised cardioversion, an electric current is delivered to the heart to correct an arrhythmia. Compared with defibrillation, it uses much lower energy levels and is synchronised to deliver an electric charge to the myocardium at the peak R wave.

The procedure causes immediate depolarisation, interrupting reentry circuits (abnormal impulse conduction resulting when cardiac tissue is activated two or more times, causing reentry arrhythmias) and allowing the SA node to resume control.

Synchronising the electrical charge with the R wave ensures that the current won't be delivered on the vulnerable T wave and disrupt repolarisation. Thus, it reduces the risk that the current will strike during the relative refractory period of a cardiac cycle and induce VF.

Practice pointers

- Ensure that this elective procedure has been explained to the patient and that an informed consent is obtained
- Ensure a baseline 12-lead ECG is available
- Withhold food beginning as soon as possible (ideally at least for 4 hours)
- Give a sedative as ordered.

The practitioner conducting the procedure will:

- Attach defibrillation pads to the chest wall; positioning the pads so that one pad is to the right of the sternum, just below the clavicle, and the other is at the fifth or sixth ICS in the left anterior axillary line
- Turn on the defibrillator and select the ordered energy level, usually between 50 and 200 J. (See *Choosing the correct cardioversion energy level*)
- Activate the synchronised mode by depressing the synchroniser switch
- Check that the machine is sensing the R wave correctly
- Instruct other personnel to stand clear of the patient and the bed to avoid the risk of an electric shock by stating 'all clear'
- Discharge the current.

Stay on the ball

Choosing the correct cardioversion energy level

When choosing an energy level for cardioversion, the lowest energy level is first tried. If the arrhythmia isn't corrected, the procedure is repeated using the next energy level. This procedure is repeated until the arrhythmia is corrected or until the highest energy level is reached. The recommended (the final decision however will be that of the medical practitioner) energy doses used for cardioversion are as follows:

- 200 J for sustained VT
- 50 J for SVT
- 50 to 100 J for AF
- 50 J for unstable atrial flutter.

Repeat, repeat and repeat again

- If cardioversion is unsuccessful, the procedure is repeated two or three times, gradually increasing the energy with each additional countershock
- If normal rhythm is restored, the patient must be monitored continually, a 12-lead ECG performed and supplemental ventilation provided for as long as needed
- If the patient's cardiac rhythm changes to VF or pulseless VT, the mode is switched from *synchronised* to *defibrillate* and the patient defibrillated immediately after charging the machine
- If using handheld paddles, the paddles are held on the patient's chest until the energy is delivered.

In sync

- It is important that the *SYNC MODE* on the defibrillator is reset after each synchronised cardioversion. Resetting this switch is necessary, because most defibrillators automatically reset to an unsynchronised mode
- The use of synchronised cardioversion, the rhythm before and after cardioversion, the amperage used and how the patient tolerated the procedure must be documented.

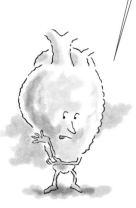

Resetting the SYNC MODE defibrillator switch after each cardioversion ensures that the machine stays synchronised.

Defibrillation

In defibrillation, electrode pads are used to direct an electric current through the patient's heart. The current causes the myocardium to depolarise, which in turn encourages the SA node to resume control of the heart's electrical activity.

The electrode pads delivering the current may be placed on the patient's chest or, during cardiac surgery, directly on the myocardium.

One or both

Defibrillators can be monophasic or biphasic. *Monophasic defibrillators* deliver a single current of electricity that travels in one direction between the two pads on the patient's chest. A large amount of electrical current is needed for effective monophasic defibrillation.

Positively speaking

A *biphasic defibrillator* delivers the electrical current in a positive direction for a specified duration and then reverses and flows in a negative direction for the remaining time of the electrical discharge. The biphasic defibrillator delivers two currents of electricity and lowers the defibrillation threshold of the heart muscle, making it possible to successfully defibrillate VF with smaller amounts of energy. For example, instead of using 200 J, an initial shock of 150 J is commonly effective.

Adjustable

Additionally, the biphasic defibrillator is able to adjust for differences in impedance or the resistance of the current through the chest, thereby reducing the number of shocks needed to terminate VF. Also, damage to the myocardial muscle is reduced because of the lower energy levels used and fewer shocks needed.

Act early and quickly

If not corrected, some arrhythmias such as VF can cause death. Therefore, the success of defibrillation depends on early recognition and quick treatment. In addition to treating VF, defibrillation may also be used to treat VT that doesn't produce a pulse.

Transcutaneous pacemaker

A transcutaneous pacemaker, also referred to as *external* or *noninvasive pacing*, is a temporary pacemaker that's used in an emergency. The device consists of an external, battery-powered pulse generator and a lead or electrode system.

Dire straits

In a life-threatening situation, a transcutaneous pacemaker works by sending an electrical impulse from the pulse generator to the patient's heart by way of two electrodes that are placed on the front and back of the patient's chest. Ideally patients will go to a cardiac catheterisation laboratory until a transvenous pacing wire can be inserted.

Transcutaneous pacing is quick and effective but can cause the patient pain and is only used until the practitioner can institute transvenous pacing. You should familiarise yourself with the transcutaneous pacing equipment and procedures used in your hospital. It is not a good idea to wait until you need to use it!

Practice pointers

• Attach monitoring electrodes to the patient in the lead I, II or III position. Do so even if the patient is already on telemetry monitoring, because you must connect the electrodes to the pacemaker. If you select the lead II position, adjust the LL electrode placement to accommodate the anterior pacing electrode and the patient's anatomy
• Plug the patient cable into the ECG input connection on the front of the pacing generator. Set the selector switch to the MONITOR ON position
• You should see the ECG waveform on the monitor. Adjust the R-wave beeper volume to a suitable level and activate the alarm by pressing the ALARM ON button. Set the alarm for 10 to 20 beats lower and 20 to 30 beats higher than the intrinsic rate
• Press the START/STOP button for a printout of the waveform
• Now the patient is ready for the application of the two pacing electrodes.

Proper placement

• First, make sure the patient's skin is clean and dry to ensure good skin contact

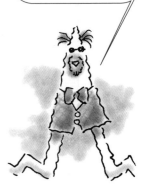

I'll never be dark or handsome, but as long as I'm tall you can turn on the transcutaneous pacemaker.

- The protective strip from the posterior electrode (marked BACK) is pulled off, and the electrode is applied on the left side of the back, just below the scapula and to the left of the spine
- The anterior pacing electrode (marked FRONT) has two protective strips – one covering the jellied area and one covering the outer ring. The jellied area is exposed and applied to the skin in the anterior position – to the left of the precordium in the usual V_2 to V_5 position. This electrode is moved around to get the best waveform. The electrode's outer rim is then exposed and pressed firmly onto the skin. (See *Proper electrode placement*.)

Proper electrode placement

The two pacing electrodes for a transcutaneous pacemaker at heart level on the patient's chest and back are placed (as shown). This placement ensures that the electrical stimulus must travel only a short distance to the heart.

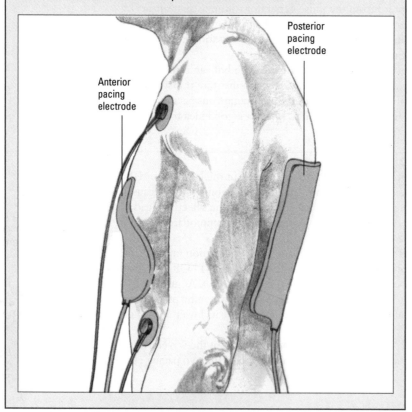

Now to pacing

- After making sure the energy output in milliamperes (mA) is on, the electrode cable is connected to the monitor output cable
- The waveform is checked looking for a tall QRS complex in lead II
- Next, the selector switch is turned to PACER ON. The patient will be told that he may feel a thumping or twitching sensation. The patient should be reassured that he will be given medication if he can't tolerate the discomfort.

Setting the beat

The doctor will set up the transcutaneous pacemaker. The following information is general guidance only as you will need to check with your local procedures and the specifics of the defibrillator being used:
- The rate dial is usually set to 10 to 20 beats higher than the patient's intrinsic rate. Pacer artifact or spikes, which will appear as you increase the rate, are looked for. If the patient doesn't have an intrinsic rhythm, the rate is usually set at 60
- The amount of energy delivered to the heart is increased slowly by adjusting the OUTPUT MA dial. This continues until capture is achieved; you'll see a pacer spike followed by a widened QRS complex (that resembles a permanent ventricular contraction). This setting is the pacing threshold. To ensure consistent capture, increase output by 10%. This should not go higher than required as this could cause the patient needless discomfort
- With full capture, the patient's heart rate should be approximately the same as the pacemaker rate set on the machine. The usual pacing threshold is between 40 and 60 mA.

Them bones, them bones

- The electrodes must not be placed over a bony area, because bone conducts current poorly. For female patients, the anterior electrode is placed under the patient's breast but not over her diaphragm.

Check back with the vitals

- After placement of a transcutaneous pacemaker, the patient's vital signs, such as skin colour, LOC and peripheral pulses to determine the effectiveness of the paced rhythm must be assessed. A 12-lead ECG is performed to serve as a baseline, and then additional ECGs are performed daily or with clinical changes. If possible, a rhythm strip is also obtained before, during and after pacemaker placement; any time that pacemaker settings are changed; and whenever the patient receives treatment because of a complication due to the pacemaker
- The ECG reading is monitored continuously noting capture, sensing, rate, intrinsic beats and competition of paced and intrinsic rhythms. If the pacemaker is sensing correctly, the sense indicator on the pulse generator should flash with each beat.

Common disorders

In the ED, you're likely to encounter patients with common cardiac emergencies, especially cardiac arrest, acute coronary syndrome, aortic aneurysm, cardiac contusion, cardiac tamponade, heart failure and hypertensive crisis. Regardless of the disorder, the priorities are always to ensure vital functioning – that is, airway, breathing and circulation.

Cardiac arrest

Cardiac arrest is the absence of mechanical functioning of the heart muscle. The heart stops beating or beats abnormally and doesn't pump effectively. If blood circulation isn't restored within minutes, cardiac arrest can lead to the loss of arterial BP, brain damage and death.

What causes it

Cardiac arrest can be caused by a wide variety of conditions, including acute MI, severe trauma, hypovolaemia, metabolic disorders, brain injury, respiratory arrest, drowning or drug overdose.

How it happens

In cardiac arrest, myocardial contractility stops, resulting in a lack of cardiac output. An imbalance in myocardial oxygen supply and demand follows, leading to myocardial ischaemia, tissue necrosis and death.

What to look for

The patient experiencing a cardiac arrest suddenly loses consciousness. Spontaneous respirations are absent, and the patient has no palpable pulse.

What tests tell you

No specific diagnostic tests are used to confirm a cardiac arrest. However, cardiac monitoring or ECG may reveal an underlying cardiac arrhythmia, such as VF, pulseless VT, pulseless electrical activity (PEA), or asystole. (See *Understanding cardiac arrhythmias*, pages 152–158.)

Treatment

In hospital resuscitation

• In hospital resuscitation (See *In-hospital resuscitation*) protocols are instigated immediately and Advanced Life Support (ALS) commenced as soon as possible. Resuscitative measures aim to maintain adequate ventilation and circulation until the cause of the arrest can be reversed.

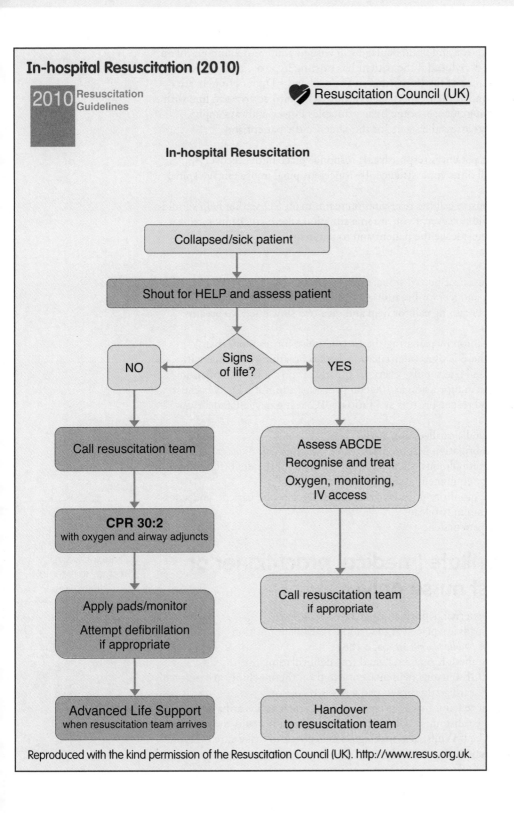

In-hospital Resuscitation (2010)

2010 Resuscitation Guidelines

Resuscitation Council (UK)

In-hospital Resuscitation

Collapsed/sick patient

Shout for HELP and assess patient

Signs of life?

NO

YES

Call resuscitation team

CPR 30:2
with oxygen and airway adjuncts

Apply pads/monitor

Attempt defibrillation
if appropriate

Advanced Life Support
when resuscitation team arrives

Assess ABCDE
Recognise and treat
Oxygen, monitoring,
IV access

Call resuscitation team
if appropriate

Handover
to resuscitation team

Reproduced with the kind permission of the Resuscitation Council (UK). http://www.resus.org.uk.

Cerebral hypoxia and brain damage will ensue within 3 to 4 minutes of an arrest-this time is reduced if the patient has existing hypoxia. In the UK we follow the guidance of the Resuscitation Council and ED practitioners are required to maintain their expertise in dealing with cardiac arrest in line with the most current guidance. Some basic principles however always apply:

• Scene Safety- assess the scene for the safety of the patient and yourself
• Check if the patient is responsive. If responds place in the recovery position and call or go for assistance. If suspected spinal injury engage spinal injury protocols

If not responsive call the resuscitation team. In an ED setting help should always be at hand however if you are in a situation where you cannot call for help then you must leave the patient and to get help.

• Assess Airway
• Open Airway
• Use jaw thrust if suspected spinal injuries
• Look, listen and feel for breathing – if breathing place in recovery position. If not breathing call for help and give two slow effective breaths (rescue breaths)
• Assess circulation by palpating the carotid pulse for no more than 10 seconds. If there is signs of circulation but no breathing continue with rescue breaths and check pulse every 10 breaths. If no signs of circulation commence chest compression at 100 compressions a minute. Deliver chest compression and rescue breaths at a ratio of 30:2 using oxygen and airway adjuncts
• Apply pads and a cardiac monitor
• Attempt defibrillation if appropriate. (See *Advanced Life Support*, page 189)
• Perform cardiopulmonary resuscitation (CPR) until the defibrillator and other emergency equipment arrive
• Connect the monitoring leads of the defibrillator to the patient, and assess his cardiac rhythm in two leads
• Expose the patient's chest

To defibrillate (medical practitioner or specialist nurse only)

• Automated external defibrillator (AED)
• Conductive pads are placed at the paddle placement positions. (See *Defibrillator paddle placement*, page 188)
• Most EDs in the UK now use 'hand free defibrillation
• The CHARGE buttons, which are located on the machine, are pressed
• The patient's cardiac rhythm in two leads is reassessed
• If the patient remains in VF or pulseless ventricular tachycardia (PVT), the doctor or specialist nurse will instruct all personnel to stand clear of the patient and the bed. Whilst also making a visual check to make sure everyone is clear of the patient and the bed.

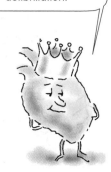

Having jewels would be nice, but I'd rather have 360 joules when it comes to external defibrillation.

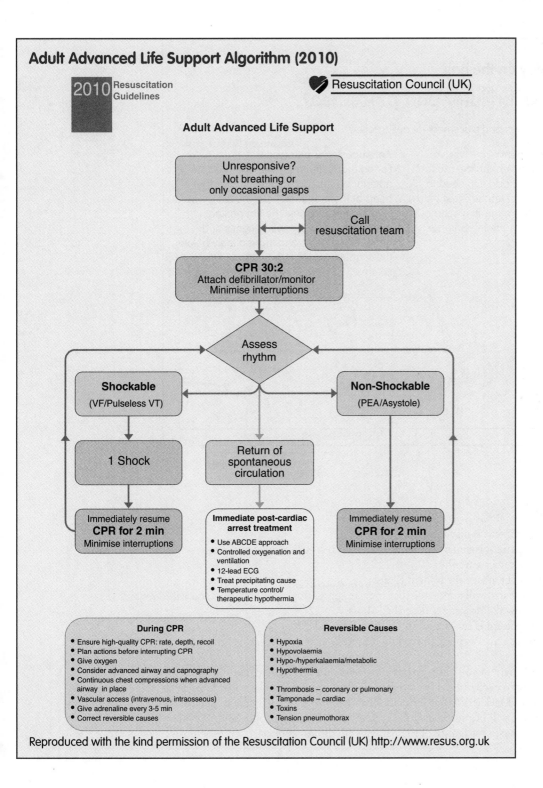

Adult Advanced Life Support Algorithm (2010)

2010 Resuscitation Guidelines

Resuscitation Council (UK)

Adult Advanced Life Support

Unresponsive?
Not breathing or
only occasional gasps

Call
resuscitation team

CPR 30:2
Attach defibrillator/monitor
Minimise interruptions

Assess
rhythm

Shockable
(VF/Pulseless VT)

Non-Shockable
(PEA/Asystole)

1 Shock

Return of
spontaneous
circulation

Immediately resume
CPR for 2 min
Minimise interruptions

**Immediate post-cardiac
arrest treatment**
• Use ABCDE approach
• Controlled oxygenation and
  ventilation
• 12-lead ECG
• Treat precipitating cause
• Temperature control/
  therapeutic hypothermia

Immediately resume
CPR for 2 min
Minimise interruptions

During CPR
• Ensure high-quality CPR: rate, depth, recoil
• Plan actions before interrupting CPR
• Give oxygen
• Consider advanced airway and capnography
• Continuous chest compressions when advanced
  airway in place
• Vascular access (intravenous, intraosseous)
• Give adrenaline every 3-5 min
• Correct reversible causes

Reversible Causes
• Hypoxia
• Hypovolaemia
• Hypo-/hyperkalaemia/metabolic
• Hypothermia

• Thrombosis – coronary or pulmonary
• Tamponade – cardiac
• Toxins
• Tension pneumothorax

Reproduced with the kind permission of the Resuscitation Council (UK) http://www.resus.org.uk

Stay on the ball

Defibrillator pad placement

Here's a guide to correct pad placement for defibrillation.

Anterolateral placement

For anterolateral placement (the most usual approach), one pad is placed to the right of the upper sternum, just below the right clavicle. The other is placed over the fifth or sixth ICS at the left anterior axillary line.

Anteroposterior placement

For anteroposterior placement, the anterior pad is placed directly over the heart at the precordium, to the left of the lower sternal border. The flat posterior pad is placed under the patient's body beneath the heart and immediately below the scapula (but not under the vertebral column).

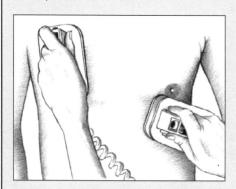

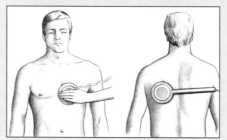

And discharge!

- The current is discharged
- The patient is given 2 minutes of CPR. His cardiac rhythm is reassessed using the cardiac monitor
- It may be necessary to defibrillate a second time at 200 J. The doctor or nurse specialist will announce that they are preparing to defibrillate, and will then follow the procedure described above
- The patient is reassessed and CPR continued
- A pulse check is performed only if there is a change in cardiac rhythm or patient status
- If the patient still has no heart rate visible on the cardiac monitor after the first two cycles of defibrillation and CPR, supplemental oxygen is give via Bag Valve Mask (BVM) or intubation, and appropriate medications such as adrenaline will begin to be administered. Also, consideration is given to other possible causes for failure of the patient's rhythm to convert, such as acidosis and hypoxia.

Rhythm restoration

- If defibrillation restores a normal rhythm, the patient is assessed. A baseline ABG levels and a 12-lead ECG are obtained. Supplemental oxygen, ventilation, and medications are provided as needed. The defibrillator is prepared for immediate reuse
- The procedure must be documented, including the patient's ECG rhythms before and after defibrillation; the number of times defibrillation was performed; the voltage used during each attempt; whether a pulse returned; the dosage, route, and time of drugs administered; whether CPR was used; how the airway was maintained; and the patient's outcome
- The patient may be assessed for possible insertion of an ICD.

Advanced Life Support

Practitioners working in emergency settings will have been prepared to offer advanced life support (ALS). It is essential to commence ALS as soon as possible. These measures include:
- Prompt defibrillation of shockable rhythms (VF and pulseless VT) with a single shock followed by resumption of CPR. After two minutes of CPR the cardiac rhythm is checked and another shock given if appropriate. (When using Biphasic defibrillators 150 to 200 J second and subsequent shocks at 150 to 360 J if using a monophasic defibrillator 360 J is used for the first and subsequent shocks)
- There is some evidence to suggest that a pre-cordial thump in cases where the arrest is witnessed and a defibrillator is not readily available can convert VT to sinus rhythm. This intervention is only delivered by health care professionals trained in its use
- Ventilation-Intubation-oropharyngeal or nasopharyngeal airway insertion to maintain a patent airway by securing the tongue position. Laryngeal mask airways (LMAs) or Combitubes improved ventilation, are relatively easy to insert and protect the lungs from pulmonary aspiration. ET intubation is the optimal method but only in the hands of an experienced (and quick) practitioner. Remember there should always be something on the patient's chest-hands or defibrillation!
- Intravenous assess- IV adrenaline 1 mg if VF/VT persists after a second shock and repeat every 3 to 5 minutes if VF/VT persists. (If PEA or asystole 1 mg adrenaline IV is given as soon as possible and repeated every 3 to 5 minutes)
- Other drugs include anti-arrhythmic drugs, such as amiodarone, magnesium, bicarbonate, atropine and calcium.

During resuscitation
- Remember the patient's family and friends. Ensure that they have been kept informed and their needs attended to. The family may wish to witness the resuscitation, so you will need to know what your hospital's policy is

- Ensure that a record of the duration of the arrest, drugs given and interventions provided are all recorded in a chronological order for the patient's notes. Someone can be given this task
- Be conscious of patient dignity and of the possibility of other patients and visitors hearing the resuscitation and remember just how alarming and distressing this can be.

Special cases

- Pregnant women present particular challenges due to the body changes that pregnancy causes. To successfully provide chest compressions and to provide defibrillation, the patient needs to be back angled at 15 to 30 degrees from a left lateral position to ensure lateral displacement of the uterus
- Children and babies – refer to current Resuscitation Council Guidelines found at http://www.resus.org.uk. At time of printing recommendations suggest five rescue breaths. Chest compression is achieved by approximately one-third of its depth. Use two fingers for an infant under 1 year; use one or two hands for a child over 1 year as needed to achieve an adequate depth of compression. Regardless of the child's age, the ratio of compression to breaths is 15:2 with 100 compressions a minute.

After resuscitation

- Airway, breathing, circulation, disability and exposure
- Check the patient. Are there any broken ribs? Is a nasogastric tube required?
- Maintain ECG and pulse oximetry recording
- Bloods-ABG, U & Es and blood sugars
- Treat seizures
- Obtain a Chest X-ray. Is the ET tube correctly positioned? Are there signs of a pneumothorax?
- Monitor level of consciousness (where appropriate)
- Monitor and treat hypo- or hyperthermia
- Consider use of therapeutic hypothermia (cooling a person after cardiac arrest with return of spontaneous circulation but without return of consciousness) shown to improve outcomes post VF arrest
- Help ascertain if possible what lead to the arrest
- Ensure the patient's notes are completed correctly
- If resuscitation not successful, when appropriate, consider discussing organ or tissue donation with the family especially if the patient carried a donor card.

Acute coronary syndrome

Patients with acute coronary syndrome have some degree of coronary artery occlusion. The degree of occlusion defines whether the acute coronary syndrome is:

- unstable angina
- non-ST-segment elevation MI (non-STEMI)
- ST-segment elevation MI (STEMI).

Plaque's place

The development of acute coronary syndrome begins with a rupture or erosion of plaque, an unstable and lipid-rich substance. The rupture results in platelet adhesions, fibrin clot formation and thrombin activation.

What causes it

Patients with certain risk factors appear to face a greater likelihood of developing acute coronary syndrome. These factors include:

- Diabetes
- Family history of heart disease
- Hypertension
- Obesity
- High-fat, high-carbohydrate diet
- Sedentary lifestyle
- Menopause
- Hyperlipoproteinaemia
- Smoking
- Stress.

How it happens

Acute coronary syndrome most commonly results when a thrombus progresses and occludes blood flow. (An early thrombus doesn't necessarily block blood flow.) The effect is an imbalance in myocardial oxygen supply and demand.

Degree and duration

The degree and duration of blockage dictate the type of infarct:

- If the patient has *unstable angina*, a thrombus partially occludes a coronary vessel. This thrombus is full of platelets. The partially occluded vessel may have distal microthrombi that cause necrosis in some myocytes
- If smaller vessels infarct, the patient is at higher risk for MI, which may then progress to a *non-STEMI*. Usually, only the innermost layer of the heart is damaged
- *STEMI* results when reduced blood flow through one of the coronary arteries causes myocardial ischaemia, injury and necrosis. The damage extends through all myocardial layers.

Angina – It hurts when I do this

Angina most commonly follows physical exertion but may also follow emotional excitement, cold exposure or a large meal. Angina is commonly relieved by GTN. It's less severe and shorter-lived than the pain of acute MI.

Angina has four major forms:

Stable – predictable pain, in frequency and duration, which can be relieved with nitrates and rest

Ages and stages

Identifying symptoms of MI

The cardinal symptom of an MI is persistent, intense substernal pain that may radiate to the left arm, jaw, neck or shoulder blades. This pain is unrelieved by rest or GTN and may last for several hours. Some patients with an MI, such as older adults and those with diabetes, may not experience pain at all. Other patients experience only mild pain; for example, female patients who experience atypical chest pain with an MI may present with complaints of indigestion and fatigue. Any patient may experience atypical chest pain, but it's more common in women.

Unstable – increased pain, which is easily induced

Prinzmetal's or a variant – pain from unpredictable coronary artery spasm

Microvascular – angina-like chest pain due to impairment of vasodilator reserve in a patient with normal coronary arteries.

Other signs and symptoms of MI include:
- Anxiety
- Pallor
- Feeling of impending doom
- Nausea and vomiting
- Perspiration
- Shortness of breath
- Cool extremities
- Fatigue
- Hypotension or hypertension
- Muffled heart sounds
- Palpable precordial pulse.

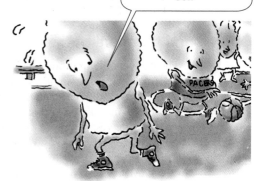

Patients with angina often experience a burning or squeezing sensation after physical exertion. I think I'll sit this one out!

What tests tell you
The following tests are used to diagnose acute coronary syndrome:
- ECG during an anginal episode shows ischaemia
- Serial 12-lead ECGs may be normal or inconclusive during the first few hours after an MI. Abnormalities include non-STEMI and STEMI. (See *Pinpointing infarction*)
- Coronary angiography reveals coronary artery stenosis or obstruction and collateral circulation and shows the condition of the arteries beyond the narrowing
- Myocardial perfusion imaging with thallium-201 during treadmill exercise discloses ischaemic areas of the myocardium, visualised as 'cold spots'

Pinpointing infarction

The site of MI depends on the vessels involved:
- Occlusion of the circumflex branch of the left coronary artery causes a lateral wall infarction.
- Occlusion of the anterior descending branch of the left coronary artery leads to an anterior wall infarction.
- True posterior or inferior wall infarctions generally result from occlusion of the right coronary artery or one of its branches.
- Right ventricular infarctions can also result from right coronary artery occlusion, can accompany inferior infarctions and may cause right-sided heart failure.
- In an STEMI, tissue damage extends through all myocardial layers; in a non-STEMI, damage occurs only in the innermost layer.

- With MI, serial serum cardiac marker measurements show elevated CK, especially the CK-MB isoenzyme (the cardiac muscle fraction of CK), troponin T and I and myoglobin
- With a Q-wave MI, echocardiography shows ventricular wall dyskinesia.

Cardiac marker studies

Analysis of cardiac markers (proteins) aids diagnosis of acute MI.

Release those enzymes!

After infarction, damaged cardiac tissue releases significant amounts of enzymes into the blood. Serial measurement of enzyme levels reveals the extent of damage and helps monitor the progress of healing. The risk of morbidity following an acute coronary syndrome event correlates directly to cardiac troponins T and I levels. These enzymes are highly specific for cardiac damage. Patients with no detectable troponins have a good short-term prognosis. Troponin levels increase within 3 to 6 hours after myocardial damage. Troponin I peaks in 14 to 20 hours, with a return to baseline in 5 to 7 days. Troponin T peaks in 12 to 24 hours, with a return to baseline in 10 to 15 days. Because troponin levels stay elevated for a long time, they can be used to detect an infarction that occurred several days earlier. Myocardial muscle creatine kinase CK-MB levels increase 4 to 8 hours after the onset of acute MI, peak after 20 hours and may remain elevated for up to 72 hours. (See *Release of cardiac enzymes and proteins*, page 194.)

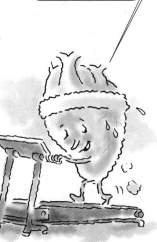

Myocardial perfusion imaging during treadmill exercise reveals the myocardium's ischaemic areas.

Practice pointers
- Before CK measurement, make certain that the patient hasn't ingested alcohol, aminocaproic acid or Lithium. If the patient has recently taken these substances, note this on the laboratory request
- Avoid administering intramuscular injections, because they can cause muscle damage and elevate some cardiac markers

Release of cardiac enzymes and proteins

Because they're released by damaged tissue, serum proteins and isoenzymes (catalytic proteins that vary in concentration in specific organs) can help identify the compromised organ and assess the extent of damage. After an acute MI, cardiac enzymes and proteins rise and fall in characteristic patterns, as shown in the graph.

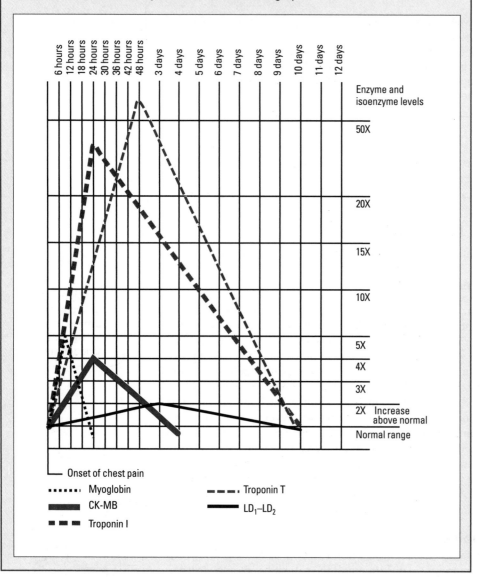

• After any cardiac enzyme test, handle the collection tube gently to prevent haemolysis and send the sample to the laboratory immediately. A delay can affect test results.

How angina is treated

For patients with angina, the goal of treatment is to reduce myocardial oxygen demand or increase oxygen supply. These treatments are used to manage angina:

• Oxygen saturation monitored by pulse oximetry. Oxygen given to maintain saturation within target saturation range usually between 94% and 98% (and 88%–92% for those at risk of hypercapnic respiratory failure)
• Nitrates and rest to reduce myocardial oxygen consumption
• Beta-adrenergic blockers may be administered to reduce the workload and oxygen demands of the heart
• If angina is caused by coronary artery spasm, calcium channel blockers may be given
• Antiplatelet drugs minimise platelet aggregation and the danger of coronary occlusion
• Antilipemic drugs can reduce elevated serum cholesterol or triglyceride levels
• Obstructive lesions may necessitate longer term interventions such as CABG or primary percutaneous coronary intervention (PCI). Other alternatives include laser angioplasty, minimally invasive surgery, rotational atherectomy or stent placement.

This mnemonic does *not* indicate the order in which these treatments are to be given. Unless there is a complication of hypotension give in this order: (1) oxygen (following British Thoracic Society (BTS) Guidelines), (2) aspirin, (3) GTN and (4) morphine.

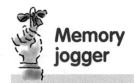

Memory jogger

To institute treatment of a patient's ischaemic chest pain or suspected acute coronary syndrome, use the mnemonic *MONA*:

Morphine
Oxygen
Nitroglycerin
Aspirin

MI relief-save the muscle!

The goals of treatment for MI are to relieve pain, stabilise heart rhythm, revascularise the coronary artery, preserve myocardial tissue and reduce cardiac workload. Here are some guidelines for treatment:

• 300 mg of aspirin is administered to inhibit platelet aggregation. Check that the patient does not have an aspirin allergy or gastrointestinal bleeding
• High-flow oxygen (12 to 15 L/minute) likely to be administered to increase oxygenation of the blood and may help to limit ischaemic myocardial injury and reduce amount of S-T elevation in line with BTS Guidelines
• GTN is administered sublingually to relieve chest pain, unless systolic BP is less than 90 mm Hg or heart rate is less than 50 or >100 beats/minute
• Morphine is administered as analgesia because pain stimulates the sympathetic nervous system, leading to an increase in heart rate and vasoconstriction
• So urgent referral for PCI if the unit has access increasingly paramedics will take patients to these expert centres directly
• PCI is the preferred treatment to thrombolytic therapy.

See NICE Guidelines 95. *Chest Pain of Recent Onset* at http://www.nice. org.uk/

What to do

• Monitor the patient's oxygen saturation levels, and notify the doctor or nurse practitioner if oxygen saturation falls below target range
• Monitor and record the patient's pulse, ECG, BP, temperature, ABG, respirations, LOC and physical appearance. Also, assess and record the severity, location, type and duration of pain
• Monitor the patient's haemodynamic status closely. Be alert for indicators suggesting decreased cardiac output, such as decreased BP, increased heart rate and increased confusion or disorientation
• Offer support and explanations to the patient and his family. Attempt to lessen patient anxiety. Physiological responses to anxiety may compound pathological physical status
• Obtain a 12-lead ECG and assess heart rate and BP when the patient experiences acute chest pain
• CXR to exclude cardiomegaly
• Assess urine output hourly
• Check the patient's BP before and after giving GTN, especially the first dose
• Serial measurements of cardiac enzyme levels will be ordered
• Watch for crackles, cough and tachypnoea (signs of acute pulmonary oedema) that may indicate impending left-sided heart failure. Carefully monitor weight, urinary intake and output, respiratory rate, serum enzyme levels, ECG waveforms and BP
• Prepare the patient for reperfusion therapy as indicated
• Administer and titrate medications as ordered. Avoid giving I.M. injections; I.V. administration provides more rapid symptom relief.

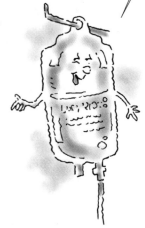

I.V. heparin, nitroglycerin and beta-adrenergic blocker can help patients with MI.

Aortic dissection

Aortic dissection is a medical and/or surgical emergency. If untreated it has a mortality rate of over 90% over a 1-year period. This condition is caused following a tear in the intima (lining layer) of the aorta and the blood in the aortic, which is at high pressure, forces itself into the media (muscle layers) of the aorta. Blood then travels in two channels, one where the blood is travelling normally and one where blood cannot move onwards and so pools and builds up at pressure.

High-risk groups are patients with arteriosclerosis and/or hypertension.

Presenting signs and symptoms

• Usually severe sudden onset of chest pain – commonly anterior chest pain – radiates to the interscapular region. Patients may terms such as 'tearing' 'ripping' or 'stabbing' to describe the pain. However, it can be painless

- Sudden death or shock due to aortic rupture or cardiac tamponade. (See *Understanding cardiac tamponade*, page 204)
- Congestive cardiac failure due to aortic incompetence and/or MI
- Signs and symptoms indicating occlusion of one of the branches of the aorta.

Practice pointers
- Assess ABCDE
- Stabilise the patient
- If the ascending aorta is involved – emergency surgery and BP control
- If the descending aorta is involved – medical management initially and BP control.

Aortic aneurysm

An aortic dissection may also involve abnormal widening or ballooning of the aorta that is called an aneurysm. An aortic aneurysm is a localised outpouching or an abnormal dilation in a weakened arterial wall. Aortic aneurysm is typically found in the aorta between the renal arteries and the iliac branches, but the abdominal, thoracic or ascending arch of the aorta may be affected.

What causes it
The exact cause of an aortic aneurysm is unclear, but several factors place a person at risk, including:
- Pregnancy
- Marfan syndrome (a genetic disorder of connective tissue)
- Long-standing history of systemic hypertension and a pre-existing aneurysm (in advanced age)
- Trauma.

How it happens
Aneurysms arise from a defect in the middle layer of the arterial wall (*tunica media* or medial layer). When the elastic fibres and collagen in the middle layer are damaged, stretching and segmental dilation occur. As a result, the medial layer loses some of its elasticity. This results in its it fragmentation. Smooth-muscle cells are lost and the wall thins.

Thin and thinner

The thinned wall may contain calcium deposits and atherosclerotic plaque, making the wall brittle. As a person ages, elastin in the wall decreases, thus further weakening the vessel. If hypertension is present, blood flow slows, resulting in ischaemia and additional weakening.

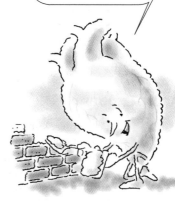

I wish my arterial walls were made of stuff this sturdy. I'd never have to worry about aneurysms again!

Wide vessel, slow flow

When an aneurysm begins to develop, lateral pressure increases, causing the vessel lumen to widen and blood flow to slow. Over time, mechanical stressors contribute to elongation of the aneurysm.

Blood forces

Haemodynamic forces may also play a role, causing pulsatile stresses on the weakened wall and pressing on the small vessels that supply nutrients to the arterial wall. In aortic aneurysms, this stress and pressure causes the aorta to become bowed and tortuous.

What to look for

Most patients with aortic aneurysms are asymptomatic until the aneurysms enlarge and compress surrounding tissue. A large aneurysm may produce signs and symptoms that mimic those of an MI, renal calculi, lumbar disc disease or duodenal compression.

When symptoms arise

Usually, the patient exhibits symptoms if rupture, expansion, embolisation, thrombosis or pressure from the mass on surrounding structures exists. Rupture is more common if the patient also has hypertension or if the aneurysm is larger than 6 cm. If the patient has a suspected thoracic aortic aneurysm, assess for the following:
• Pallor
• Difficulty breathing
• Complaints of sudden, excruciating, tearing pain that moves from the anterior to the posterior
• Hoarseness or coughing
• Nausea and vomiting
• Sweating
• Haematemesis
• Dysphagia
• Aortic insufficiency murmur
• Haemoptysis
• Palpable pulsations at the left sternoclavicular joint
• Tachycardia
• Unequal BP and pulse when measured in both arms.

Acute expansion

When there's an acute expansion of a thoracic aortic aneurysm, assess for the followings:
• Severe hypertension
• Neurologic changes
• Jugular vein distention
• New murmur of aortic sufficiency

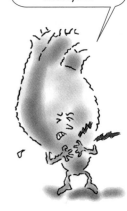

A sudden, tearing pain that moves from the anterior to the posterior is a sure sign of aortic aneurysm.

- Right sternoclavicular lift
- Tracheal deviation.

What tests tell you

No specific laboratory test diagnoses an aortic aneurysm; however, several other tests may be helpful:
- If blood is leaking from the aneurysm, leucocytosis and a decrease in haemoglobin and haematocrit may be noted
- Computed tomography (CT) scan and magnetic resonance imaging (MRI) can disclose the aneurysm's size and effect on nearby organs. The gold standard for diagnosing an aortic aneurysm is the use of MRI
- Transthoracic Echo (TOE) allows visualisation of the thoracic aorta. It's commonly combined with Doppler flow studies to provide information about blood flow
- Abdominal ultrasonography or echocardiography can be used to determine the size, shape, length and location of the aneurysm
- Anteroposterior and lateral X-rays of the chest or abdomen can be used to detect aortic calcification and widened areas of the aorta
- Angiography can be used to determine the aneurysm's approximate size and the patency of visceral vessels. This has however been largely been superseded by CT and MRI scans.

How it's treated

Aneurysm treatment usually involves surgery and appropriate drug therapy. Aortic aneurysms usually require resection and replacement of the aortic section using a vascular or Dacron graft. However, keep the following points in mind:
- If the aneurysm is small and produces no symptoms, surgery may be delayed, with regular physical examination and ultrasonography performed to monitor its progression
- Large or symptomatic aneurysms are at risk for rupture and need immediate repair if the aneurysm is dissecting
- Endovascular grafting may be an option for a patient with an abdominal aortic aneurysm. This procedure, which can be done using local or regional anaesthesia, is a minimally invasive procedure whereby the walls of the aorta are reinforced to prevent expansion and rupture of the aneurysm
- Medications to control BP, relieve anxiety and control pain are also prescribed.

Emergency measures: ABCDE

Rupture of an aortic aneurysm is a medical emergency requiring prompt treatment and resuscitation:
- Assess and record respiratory and cardiovascular status frequently (including respirations, heart rate and rhythm and pulse in extremities). Set up continuous cardiac monitoring. Monitor BP and compare findings

bilaterally. If the difference in systolic BP exceeds 10 mm Hg, notify the doctor immediately. The frequencies of these observations depend on the severity of the patient's condition
• Set up pulse oximetry. Give oxygen to maintain oxygen saturations within target saturation range as in accordance with BTS Guidelines. Usually 94%–98% for most acutely ill patients or 88%–92% for those at risk of hypercapnic respiratory failure
• Observe the patient for signs of rupture, which may be immediately fatal. Watch closely for signs of acute blood loss, such as increasing confusion and/or decreased level of consciousness, restlessness, cool clammy skin, increasing pulse and respiratory rates, decreasing BP (a later response)
• Ensure that the family has been seen, and they have a realistic understanding of the patient's prognosis
• An arterial line insertion may be undertaken to allow for continuous BP monitoring
• Cardiac enzyme levels may be taken. An MI can appear if an aneurysm ruptures along the coronary arteries
• Venous access with large-bore cannula is required
• Blood to be taken for full blood count (FBC), for evidence of blood loss, including decreased haemoglobin, haematocrit and red blood cell (RBC) count, U & Es (to evaluate kidney function) and cross match – it is recommended that at least 10 units of blood be ordered
• Resuscitation by the delivery of rapid intravenous volume using colloids and blood replacement will be needed
• Measure urinary intake and output, hourly if necessary, depending on the patient's condition. A urethral catheter may be ordered
• Analgesics to relieve pain (for example diamorphine plus metoclopramide)
• Beta-blockers to decrease BP, heart rate and left ventricular contractility
• Assist with insertion of PA wedge catheter (Swan-Ganz)
• Arrange transfer to ICU or to theatre.

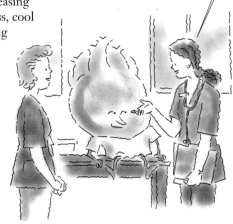

Pay close attention to blood pressure in an aortic aneurysm patient. Check it every 2 to 4 hours or more.

What tests tell you
• ECG will reveal rhythm disturbances, such as PVCs, premature atrial contractions, VT, atrial tachycardia and VF, along with nonspecific ST segment or T-wave changes occurring within 24 to 48 hours after the injury
• Echocardiogram will show evidence of abnormal ventricular wall movement and decreased ejection fraction
• Multiple-gated acquisition scan will show decreased ability of effective heart pumping
• Cardiac enzyme levels will show elevations of CK-MB to >8% of total CK within 3 to 4 hours after the injury
• Cardiac troponin I levels may be elevated 24 hours after the injury.

Cardiac contusion

Cardiac contusion refers to the bruising of the myocardium. It's the most common type of injury sustained from blunt trauma to the chest such as following car accidents due to seat belt bruising.

What causes it

A cardiac contusion typically results from blunt trauma. This trauma can be related to vehicular collisions or falls. The right ventricle is the most common site of injury, because it's located directly behind the sternum.

How it happens

During deceleration injuries, the myocardium strikes the sternum when the heart and aorta move forward; shearing forces may lacerate the aorta. Direct force may also be applied to the sternum, causing injury. Crushing and compressive forces may result in contusion as the heart is compressed between the sternum and vertebral column.

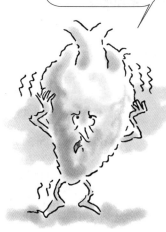

Ventricular irritability is a sure sign of cardiac contusion.

What to look for

Cardiac contusion should be suspected after any blow to the chest and/or sternal fractures, especially after head on impacts in road traffic accidents. Be alert for the following signs and symptoms of trauma:
- Shortness of breath
- Bruising on the chest
- Murmurs
- Bradycardia or tachycardia
- Precordial chest pain.

And also...

Keep these signals in mind as well:
- Arrhythmias due to ventricular irritability
- Cardiac tamponade
- Haemodynamic instability.

How it's treated

Maintaining haemodynamic stability and adequate cardiac output are key concerns. I.V. fluid therapy may be necessary. Continuous ECG monitoring is used to detect arrhythmias. Lidocaine may be administered to treat ventricular arrhythmias, and Digoxin may be given to treat pump failure. Inotropic agents may be used to assist with improving cardiac output and ejection fraction.

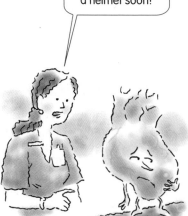

Another contusion? We're going to have to buy you a helmet soon!

Close watch

The patient with a cardiac contusion must be monitored closely for signs and symptoms of cardiopulmonary compromise because trauma leading to cardiac contusion is commonly associated with pulmonary trauma. Supplemental oxygen therapy may be necessary. If the extent of pulmonary trauma is great, ET intubation and mechanical ventilation may be necessary.

No if hypo

I.V. morphine may be used to treat severe pain, unless the patient is hypotensive. In the latter case, other less potent analgesics may be used.

What to do: ABCDE
• Assess ABCDE
• Auscultate breath sounds at least hourly, reporting signs of congestion or fluid accumulation. Evaluate peripheral pulses and capillary refill to detect decreased peripheral tissue perfusion. Give oxygen as ordered to maintain blood oxygenation within target range
• Assess the patient's cardiopulmonary status at least hourly, or more frequently if indicated, to detect signs and symptoms of possible injury
• Monitor heart rate and rhythm, heart sounds and BP every hour for changes; institute haemodynamic monitoring, including CVP, PAWP and cardiac output as indicated, at least every 1 to 2 hours
• Intravenous access and administer fluid replacement therapy, including blood component therapy as prescribed, typically to maintain systolic BP above 90 mm Hg
• Monitor urine output every hour, notifying the doctor if output is less than 0.5 ml/kg/hour
• Institute continuous cardiac monitoring to detect arrhythmias or conduction defects. If arrhythmias appear, administer antiarrhythmic agents as ordered
• Assess the patient's degree of pain and administer analgesic therapy as ordered, monitoring him for effectiveness. Position the patient comfortably, usually with the head of the bed elevated 30 to 45 degrees
• Prepare the patient and his family for surgery, if indicated
• Anticipate transfer of the patient to a critical care unit when appropriate.

Understanding cardiac tamponade

Cardiac tamponade is a rapid, unchecked increase in pressure in the pericardial sac. This increased pressure compresses the heart, impairs diastolic filling and reduces cardiac output. Cardiac tamponade should be suspected in any patient with the followings:
• Increased heart rate
• Increased respiratory rate (in a clear chest)
• Pulsus paradoxous (inspiratory drop in systemic BP >15 mm Hg)
• Falling BP.

Pericardial pressure

The increase in pressure usually results from blood or fluid accumulation in the pericardial sac. Even a small amount of fluid (50 to 100 ml) can cause a serious tamponade if it accumulates rapidly. If fluid accumulates rapidly, cardiac tamponade requires emergency lifesaving measures to prevent death. A slow accumulation and increase in pressure may not produce immediate symptoms because the fibrous wall of the pericardial sac can gradually stretch to accommodate as much as 1 to 2 L of fluid. (See *Understanding cardiac tamponade*, page 204.)

What causes it
Cardiac tamponade may result from acute or subacute causes. These include:
- Viral or post-irradiation pericarditis
- Acute MI
- Chronic renal failure requiring dialysis
- Connective tissue disorders (such as rheumatoid arthritis, systemic lupus erythematosus, rheumatic fever, vasculitis and scleroderma)
- Effusion (from cancer, bacterial infections, tuberculosis and rarely acute rheumatic fever)
- Haemorrhage due to nontraumatic causes (such as anticoagulant therapy in patients with pericarditis or rupture of the heart or great vessels)
- Haemorrhage due to trauma (such as gunshot or stab wounds of the chest)
- Idiopathic causes (such as Dressler's syndrome – a postmyocardial infarction syndrome characterised by pericarditis This is believed to be an immunological reaction. Found also after other forms of cardiac damage such as heart surgery)
- Drug reaction from Procainamide, Hydralazine, Minoxidil, Isoniazid, Penicillin or Daunorubicin.

> Good thing they aren't in a pericardial sac – too much blood accumulation there can lead to cardiac tamponade.

How it happens
In cardiac tamponade, accumulation of fluid in the pericardial sac causes compression of the heart chambers. This compression obstructs blood flow into the ventricles and reduces the amount of blood that can be pumped out of the heart with each contraction.

What to look for
Cardiac tamponade has the following three classic features (be careful only seen in 30% of patients diagnosed with cardiac tamponade) known as *Beck's triad:*

 Elevated CVP with jugular vein distension

 Muffled heart sounds

 Hypotension.

Understanding cardiac tamponade

The pericardial sac, which surrounds and protects the heart, is composed of several layers:
- The fibrous pericardium is the tough, outermost membrane.
- The inner membrane, called the *serous membrane*, consists of the visceral and parietal layers.
- The visceral layer of the heart, also known as the *epicardial layer*, clings to the heart.
- The parietal layer lies between the visceral layer and the fibrous pericardium.

- The pericardial space – between the visceral and parietal layers – contains 10 to 30 ml of pericardial fluid. This fluid lubricates the layers and minimises friction when the heart contracts.

In cardiac tamponade (shown below right), blood or fluid fills the pericardial space, compressing the heart chambers, increasing intracardiac pressure and obstructing venous return. As blood flow into the ventricles decreases, so does cardiac output. Without prompt treatment, low cardiac output can be fatal.

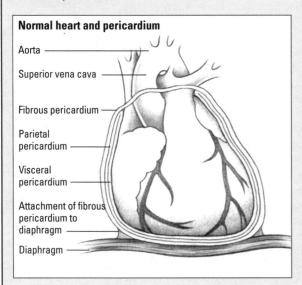

Normal heart and pericardium

Aorta

Superior vena cava

Fibrous pericardium

Parietal pericardium

Visceral pericardium

Attachment of fibrous pericardium to diaphragm

Diaphragm

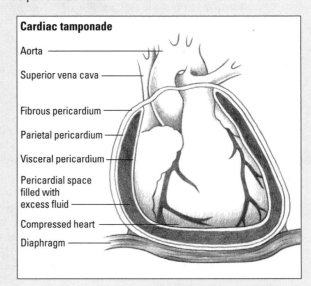

Cardiac tamponade

Aorta

Superior vena cava

Fibrous pericardium

Parietal pericardium

Visceral pericardium

Pericardial space filled with excess fluid

Compressed heart

Diaphragm

That's not all

Other signs include:
- Restlessness
- Anxiety
- Cold, clammy skin
- Cyanosis
- Sweating
- Dyspnoea/orthopnoea
- Decreased arterial pressure, decreased systolic BP and narrow pulse pressure
- Tachycardia and a weak, thready pulse.

What tests tell you
• Chest X-ray shows a slightly widened mediastinum and an enlarged cardiac silhouette
• ECG may show a low-amplitude QRS complex and electrical alternans, or an alternating beat-to-beat change in amplitude of the P wave, QRS complex and T wave. Generalised ST-segment elevation is noted in all leads. An ECG is used to rule out other cardiac disorders; it may reveal changes produced by acute pericarditis
• Other tests such as PA catheterisation, echocardiography, CT or MRI scan may be done if the situation isn't a medical emergency.

How it's treated
• Ensure adequate oxygenation
• Establish intravenous access and give IV fluids.
The goal of treatment is to relieve intrapericardial pressure and cardiac compression by removing accumulated blood or fluid, which can be done by the following three different ways:

 Pericardiocentesis (needle aspiration of the pericardial cavity)

 Insertion of a drain into the pericardial sac to drain the effusion

 Surgical creation of an opening, called a *pericardial window*.

When pressure is low

If the patient is hypotensive, trial volume loading with crystalloids, such as I.V. normal saline solution, may be used to maintain systolic BP. An inotropic drug, such as dopamine, may be necessary to improve myocardial contractility until fluid in the pericardial sac can be removed. Anticipated cardiac arrest is usually PEA in this case.

Additional treatments

Depending on the cause, additional treatment may be necessary. Examples of such causes and treatments are:
• Heparin-induced tamponade – administration of the heparin antagonist protamine sulphate
• Traumatic injury – blood transfusion or a thoracotomy to drain reaccumulating fluid or repair bleeding sites
• Warfarin-induced tamponade – vitamin K administration.

What to do
• Monitor the patient's cardiovascular status frequently, at least every hour, noting the extent of jugular vein distension, quality of heart sounds, and BP
• Assess haemodynamic status, including CVP, right atrial pressure, and PAP, and determine cardiac output

- Monitor for pulsus paradoxus
- Be alert for ST-segment and T-wave changes on the ECG. Note rate and rhythm, and report evidence of arrhythmias.

Keep an eye on the increase

- Watch closely for signs of increasing tamponade, increasing dyspnoea and arrhythmias; report them immediately
- Infuse I.V. solutions and inotropic drugs, such as dopamine, as ordered to maintain the patient's BP
- Administer 100% oxygen therapy and assess oxygen saturation levels to maintain within prescribed target levels in accordance with BTS Guidelines. Monitor the patient's respiratory status for signs of respiratory distress, such as severe tachypnoea and changes in the patient's LOC. Anticipate the need for ET intubation and mechanical ventilation if the patient's respiratory status deteriorates
- Prepare the patient for pericardiocentesis or thoracotomy
- If the patient has trauma-induced tamponade, assess for other signs of trauma and institute appropriate care, including the use of colloids, crystalloids and blood component therapy under pressure or by rapid volume infuser if massive fluid replacement is needed; administration of protamine sulphate for heparin-induced tamponade; and vitamin K administration for warfarin-induced tamponade
- Assess renal function status closely; monitoring urine output every hour and notifying the practitioner if output is less than 0.5 ml/kg/hour (adult)
- Monitor CRT, LOC, peripheral pulses and skin temperature for evidence of diminished tissue perfusion
- Anticipate transfer of the patient to a critical care unit when appropriate.

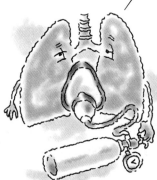

Oxygen therapy is just one aspect of cardiac tamponade treatment.

Heart failure

Heart failure results when the heart can't pump enough blood to meet the metabolic needs of the body. It results in intravascular and interstitial volume overload and poor tissue perfusion. An individual with heart failure experiences reduced exercise tolerance, a reduced quality of life and a shortened life span.

What causes it

The most common cause of heart failure is CAD, but it also occurs in infants, children and adults with congenital and acquired heart defects.

How it happens

Heart failure may be classified into the following four general categories:

 Left-sided heart failure

 Right-sided heart failure

Systolic dysfunction

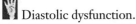 Diastolic dysfunction.

When the left loses its faculties

Left-sided heart failure is a result of ineffective left ventricular contractile function. As the pumping ability of the left ventricle fails, cardiac output drops. Blood is no longer effectively pumped out into the body; it backs up into the left atrium and then into the lungs, causing pulmonary congestion, dyspnoea and activity intolerance. If the condition persists, pulmonary oedema and right-sided heart failure may result. Common causes include:
- Hypertension
- Aortic and mitral valve stenosis
- Left ventricular infarction.

When right goes wrong

Right-sided heart failure results from ineffective right ventricular contractile function. When blood isn't pumped effectively through the right ventricle to the lungs, blood backs up into the right atrium and into the peripheral circulation. The patient gains weight and develops peripheral oedema and engorgement of the kidney and other organs.

Blame it on the left

Right-sided heart failure may be due to an acute right ventricular infarction or a pulmonary embolus. However, the most common cause is profound backward flow due to left-sided heart failure.

Just can't pump enough

Systolic dysfunction results when the left ventricle can't pump enough blood out to the systemic circulation during systole and the ejection fraction falls. Consequently, blood backs up into the pulmonary circulation and pressure increases in the pulmonary venous system. Cardiac output decreases; weakness, fatigue and shortness of breath may occur. Causes of systolic dysfunction include MI and dilated cardiomyopathy.

It all goes to swell from here

Diastolic dysfunction results when the ability of the left ventricle to relax and fill during diastole is reduced and the stroke volume falls. Therefore, higher volumes are needed in the ventricles to maintain cardiac output. Consequently, pulmonary congestion and peripheral oedema develop. Diastolic dysfunction may occur as a result of left ventricular hypertrophy, hypertension or restrictive cardiomyopathy. This type of heart failure is less common than heart failure resulting from systolic dysfunction, and treatment isn't as clear.

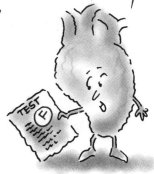

I can't believe failure was an option. I'm in real trouble!

Compensatory mechanisms

All types of heart failure eventually lead to reduced cardiac output, which triggers compensatory mechanisms that improve cardiac output at the expense of increased ventricular work. These compensatory mechanisms include:

- Increased sympathetic activity
- Activation of the renin–angiotensin–aldosterone system
- Ventricular dilation
- Ventricular hypertrophy.

Increased sympathetic activity

Increased sympathetic activity – a response to decreased cardiac output and BP – enhances peripheral vascular resistance, contractility, heart rate and venous return. Signs of increased sympathetic activity, such as cool extremities and clamminess, may indicate impending heart failure.

Renin–angiotensin–aldosterone system

Increased sympathetic activity also restricts blood flow to the kidneys, causing them to secrete renin, which in turn converts angiotensinogen to angiotensin I. Angiotensin I then becomes angiotensin II – a potent vasoconstrictor. Angiotensin causes the adrenal cortex to release aldosterone, leading to sodium and water retention and an increase in circulating blood volume.

This renal mechanism is helpful; however, if it persists unchecked, it can aggravate heart failure as the heart struggles to pump against the increased volume.

Ventricular dilation

In ventricular dilation, an increase in end-diastolic ventricular volume (preload) causes increased stroke work and stroke volume during contraction. This increased volume stretches cardiac muscle fibres so that the ventricle can accept the increased volume. Eventually, the muscle becomes stretched beyond optimal limits and contractility declines.

Ventricular hypertrophy

In ventricular hypertrophy, an increase in ventricular muscle mass allows the heart to pump against increased resistance to the outflow of blood, improving cardiac output. However, this increased muscle mass also increases the myocardial oxygen requirements.

Compromising situation

An increase in the ventricular diastolic pressure necessary to fill the enlarged ventricle may compromise diastolic coronary blood flow, limiting the oxygen supply to the ventricle and causing ischaemia and impaired muscle contractility.

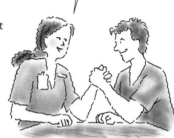

Check extremities for signs of sympathetic activity. Cold hands could mean impending heart failure.

Counterregulatory substances

In heart failure, counterregulatory substances – prostaglandins and atrial natriuretic factor – are produced in an attempt to reduce the negative effects of volume overload and vasoconstriction caused by the compensatory mechanisms.

Kidneys' contributions

The kidneys release the prostaglandins prostacyclin and prostaglandin E_2, which are potent vasodilators. These vasodilators also act to reduce volume overload produced by the renin–angiotensin–aldosterone system by inhibiting sodium and water reabsorption by the kidneys.

Counteracting hormone

Atrial natriuretic factor is a hormone that's secreted mainly by the atria in response to stimulation of the stretch receptors in the atria caused by excess fluid volume. Atrial natriuretic factor works to counteract the negative effects of sympathetic nervous system stimulation and the renin–angiotensin–aldosterone system by producing vasodilation and diuresis.

What to look for

Early signs and symptoms of left-sided heart failure include:
- Fatigue
- Nonproductive cough
- Orthopnoea
- Dyspnoea
- Paroxysmal nocturnal dyspnoea.

Later, on the left

Later clinical manifestations of left-sided heart failure can be an acute emergency:
- Acute dyspnoea
- Cool, pale skin
- Distress, restlessness and confusion
- Displacement of the PMI towards the left anterior axillary line
- Haemoptysis and/or frothy expectoration
- Crackles on auscultation
- S_3 heart sound
- S_4 heart sound
- Tachycardia.

On the right side

Clinical manifestations of right-sided heart failure include:
- Usually slower onset
- Weight gain

- Anorexia, fullness and nausea
- Oedema
- Ascites or anasarca (extreme generalised oedema)
- Hepatojugular reflux and hepatomegaly
- Jugular vein distension
- Nocturia
- Right upper quadrant pain.

What tests tell you
- Chest X-ray shows increased pulmonary vascular markings, interstitial oedema or pleural effusion and cardiomegaly
- ECG may indicate hypertrophy, ischaemic changes or infarction and may also reveal tachycardia and extrasystoles
- Laboratory testing may reveal abnormal liver function tests (LFTs) U & Es and creatinine levels
- ABG analysis may reveal hypoxaemia from impaired gas exchange and respiratory alkalosis because the patient blows off more carbon dioxide as the respiratory rate increases in compensation
- Echocardiography may reveal left ventricular hypertrophy, dilation and abnormal contractility
- PA monitoring typically demonstrates elevated PAP and PAWP, left ventricular end-diastolic pressure in left-sided heart failure and elevated right atrial pressure or CVP in right-sided heart failure
- Radionuclide ventriculography may reveal an ejection fraction less than 40%; in diastolic dysfunction, the ejection fraction may be normal.

How it's treated
The goal of therapy is to improve pump function. Correction of heart failure may involve:
- ACE inhibitors for patients with left ventricular dysfunction to reduce production of angiotensin II, resulting in preload and afterload reduction
- Beta-adrenergic blockers to prevent remodelling in patients with mild to moderate heart failure caused by left ventricular systolic dysfunction
- CABG surgery or angioplasty for patients with heart failure due to CAD
- Digoxin for patients with heart failure due to left ventricular systolic dysfunction to increase myocardial contractility, improve cardiac output, reduce the volume of the ventricle and decrease ventricular stretch
- Diuretics to reduce fluid volume overload, venous return and preload
- Diuretics, nitrates, morphine, and oxygen to treat pulmonary oedema
- Continuous Positive Airway Pressure (CPAP)
- Treatment of the underlying cause, if known.

Longer term
- Heart transplantation in patients receiving aggressive medical treatment but still experiencing limitations or repeated hospitalisations

- Other surgery or invasive procedures, such as cardiomyoplasty, insertion of an intra-aortic balloon pump (IABP), partial left ventriculectomy, use of a mechanical VAD and implantation of an ICD or a biventricular pacemaker
- Lifestyle modifications, such as weight loss (if obese), limited sodium (to 2 g/day) and alcohol intake, reduced fat intake, smoking cessation, stress reduction and development of an exercise program to reduce symptoms.

What to do

- Place the patient in supported sitting position with the bed raised under the knees slightly (Fowler's position) to maximise chest expansion. Give supplemental oxygen as prescribed. Monitor oxygen saturation levels and ABGs as indicated. If respiratory status deteriorates, anticipate the need for ET intubation and mechanical ventilation
- Institute continuous cardiac monitoring and notify the doctor of changes in rhythm and rate. If the patient develops tachycardia, administer beta-adrenergic blockers as ordered; if atrial fibrillation is present, administer anticoagulants or antiplatelet agents, as ordered, to prevent thrombus formation
- If the patient develops a new arrhythmia, obtain a 12-lead ECG immediately
- Monitor haemodynamic status, including cardiac output, cardiac index and pulmonary and systemic vascular pressures, at least hourly, noting trends
- Administer medications as ordered. Check the apical heart rate before administering Digoxin.

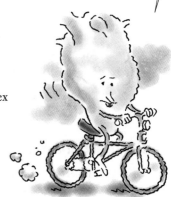

Developing an exercise program is just one lifestyle modification that can reduce symptoms of heart failure.

Pump up the potassium

- Expect to administer electrolyte replacement therapy (especially potassium) after the administration of diuretics to prevent such imbalances as hypokalaemia and the resultant cardiac arrhythmias that may arise from potassium imbalance
- Assess respiratory status frequently – at least every hour. Auscultate lungs for abnormal breath sounds, such as crackles and wheezes. Encourage coughing and deep breathing
- Obtain a baseline weight and observe for peripheral oedema
- Assess hourly urine output. Also, monitor fluid intake, including I.V. fluids
- Organise all activities to provide maximum rest periods. Assess for signs of activity intolerance, such as increased shortness of breath, chest pain, increased arrhythmias, heart rate >120 beats/minute and ST-segment changes and have the patient stop activity
- Prepare the patient for surgical intervention or insertion of an IABP or ICD or transfer to the ITU or specialist unit as indicated.

Hypertensive crisis

A hypertensive emergency, commonly called *hypertensive crisis*, refers to the abrupt, acute, marked increase in BP from the patient's baseline that ultimately leads to acute and rapidly progressing end-organ damage.

Rapid rise

Typically, in a hypertensive crisis, the patient's diastolic BP is >120 mm Hg. The increased BP value, although important, is probably less important than how rapidly the BP increases.

What causes it

Most patients who develop hypertensive crisis have long histories of chronic, poorly controlled or untreated primary hypertension. Conditions that cause secondary hypertension, such as pheochromocytoma or Cushing's syndrome, may also be responsible.

How it happens

Arterial BP is a product of total peripheral resistance and cardiac output:
• Cardiac output is increased by conditions that increase heart rate, stroke volume or both
• Peripheral resistance is increased by factors that increase blood viscosity or reduce the lumen size of vessels, especially the arterioles.

Faulty mechanisms

Hypertension may result from a disturbance in one of the body's intrinsic mechanisms, including:
• Sympathetic nervous system
• Antidiuretic hormone
• Autoregulation
• Renin–angiotensin system.

Up with pressure

The renin–angiotensin system increases BP in several ways:
• Sodium depletion, reduced BP and dehydration stimulate renin release
• Renin reacts with angiotensinogen, a liver enzyme, and converts it to angiotensin I, which increases preload and afterload
• Angiotensin I converts to angiotensin II in the lungs; angiotensin II is a potent vasoconstrictor that targets the arterioles
• Circulating angiotensin II increases preload and afterload by stimulating the adrenal cortex to secrete aldosterone. This secretion increases blood volume by conserving sodium and water.

Maintaining flow

In autoregulation, several intrinsic mechanisms together change an artery's diameter to maintain tissue and organ perfusion despite fluctuations in systemic BP. These mechanisms include:
- Stress relaxation, in which blood vessels gradually dilate when BP increases, reducing peripheral resistance
- Capillary fluid shift, in which plasma moves between vessels and extravascular spaces to maintain intravascular volume.

Taking control

Sympathetic nervous system mechanisms control BP. When BP decreases, baroreceptors in the aortic arch and carotid sinuses decrease their inhibition of the medulla's vasomotor centre.

Consequent increases in sympathetic stimulation of the heart by noradrenaline increases cardiac output by:
- Strengthening the contractile force
- Raising the heart rate
- Augmenting peripheral resistance by vasoconstriction.

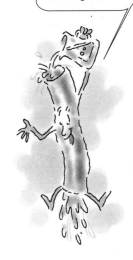

Capillary fluid shift is part of autoregulation.

Regulating reabsorption

Stress can also stimulate the sympathetic nervous system to increase cardiac output and peripheral vascular resistance. The release of antidiuretic hormone can regulate hypotension by increasing reabsorption of water by the kidney. In reabsorption, blood plasma volume increases, thus raising BP. In hypertensive crisis, one or more of these regulating mechanisms is disrupted. (See *What happens in hypertensive crisis*, page 214.)

Strain for the brain

In hypertensive crisis, the BP-regulating mechanism is disturbed, causing cerebral vasodilation. Blood flow increases, causing an increase in pressure and subsequent cerebral oedema. This increase in pressure damages the intimal and medial lining of the arterioles.

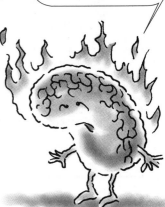

Bad for the heart, bad for the head. Hypertensive crisis can lead to cerebral edema.

What to look for

Your assessment of a patient in hypertensive crisis almost always reveals a history of hypertension that's poorly controlled or hasn't been treated. Signs and symptoms may include:
- Dizziness
- Confusion, somnolence or stupor
- Irritability
- Nausea
- Vomiting
- Anorexia
- Oedema
- Acute retinopathy and haemorrhage, retinal exudates and papilloedema

What happens in hypertensive crisis

Hypertensive crisis is a severe rise in arterial BP caused by a disturbance in one or more of the regulating mechanisms. If untreated, hypertensive crisis may result in renal, cardiac or cerebral complications and, possibly, death. This flowchart outlines the process.

Causes of hypertensive crisis

- Abnormal renal function
- Eclampsia
- Hypertensive encephalopathy
- Intracerebral haemorrhage
- Monoamine oxidase inhibitor interactions
- Myocardial ischaemia
- Phaeochromocytoma
- Withdrawal of antihypertensive drugs (abrupt)

▼

Prolonged hypertension

▼

Inflammation and necrosis of arterioles

▼

Narrowing of blood vessels

▼

Restriction of blood flow to major organs

▼

Organ damage

▼

Renal
- Decreased renal perfusion
- Progressive deterioration of nephrons
- Decreased ability to concentrate urine
- Increased serum creatinine and blood urea nitrogen
- Increased renal tubule permeability with protein leakage into tubules
- Renal insufficiency
- Uraemia
- Renal failure

Cardiac
- Decreased cardiac perfusion
- Coronary artery disease
- Angina or myocardial infarction
- Increased cardiac workload
- Left ventricular hypertrophy
- Heart failure

Cerebral
- Decreased cerebral perfusion
- Increased stress on vessel wall
- Arterial spasm
- Ischaemia
- Transient ischaemic attacks
- Weakening of vessel intima
- Aneurysm formation
- Intracranial haemorrhage

- Angina
- Dyspnoea on exertion, orthopnoea or paroxysmal nocturnal dyspnoea
- Possible left ventricular heave palpated at the mitral valve area
- Severe, throbbing headache in the back of the head
- S_4 heart sound
- Vision loss, blurred vision or diplopia.

Check the head

If the patient has hypertensive encephalopathy, you may note:
- Headache, nausea and vomiting, hypertensive retinopathy
- Decreased GCS
- Late features – neurological signs, fits and coma.

Kidney-related consequences

If the hypertensive emergency has affected the kidneys, you may note reduced urine output as well as abnormal U & Es results.

What tests tell you
- BP measurement, when obtained several times at an interval of at least 2 minutes, revealing an elevated diastolic pressure >120 mm Hg – confirms the diagnosis of hypertensive crisis
- FBC count may be decreased secondary to haematuria if the kidneys are involved
- U & Es may demonstrate renal impairment. Special attention to serum potassium (K+) levels-risk of low levels
- ECG may reveal ischaemic changes or left ventricular hypertrophy. ST-segment depression and T-wave inversion suggest repolarisation problems from endocardial fibrosis associated with left ventricular hypertrophy
- Echocardiography may reveal increased wall thickness with or without an increase in left ventricle size
- Chest X-ray may reveal enlargement of the cardiac silhouette with left ventricular dilation, or pulmonary congestion and pleural effusions with heart failure
- Urinalysis results may be normal unless renal impairment occurs; then specific gravity is low (<1.010), and haematuria, casts and proteinuria may also be found. If the patient's condition is due to a disease condition such as pheochromocytoma, a 24-hour urine test reveals increases in vanillylmandelic acid (VMA) and urinary catecholamines
- Drug screen – rule out cocaine, amphetamine and others.

How it's treated
Treatment of hypertensive crisis immediately focuses on reducing the patient's BP with I.V. antihypertensive therapy. However, a rapid reduction in BP can be dangerous – two situations that may require BP rapid reduction are aortic dissection and MI.

Slow pressure cuts

The aim is for an initial BP reduction of up to 25% over 1 to 4 hours with a less rapid reduction over 24 hours to a diastolic of 100 mm Hg. The next several days should bring further reductions.

Here are some additional guidelines:
- If patient is conscious and otherwise well then oral therapy can be used to lower BP gradually
- First line treatment should be with a beta blocker (unless contraindicated) with a thiazide diuretic or a low- dose calcium antagonist
- Sodium nitroprusside, may be given as an I.V. infusion and titrated according to the patient's response (first line therapy for LVF and hypertensive encephalopathy). It has a rapid onset of action, and its effects cease within 1 to 5 minutes of stopping the drug. Thus, if the patient's BP drops too low, stopping the drug enables the BP to increase almost immediately
- Other agents that may be used include labetalol GTN the drug of choice for treating hypertensive crisis when myocardial ischaemia, acute MI, or pulmonary oedema and hydralazine specifically indicated for treating hypertension in pregnant women with pre-eclampsia
- Lifestyle changes may include weight reduction, smoking cessation, exercise and dietary changes
- After the acute episode is controlled, maintenance pharmacotherapy to control BP plays a key role.

What to do
- Immediately obtain the patient's BP
- Institute continuous cardiac and arterial pressure monitoring to assess BP directly; determine the patient's MAP
- Assess ABG. Monitor the patient's blood oxygen saturation level using pulse oximetry; if you're monitoring the patient haemodynamically assess mixed venous oxygen saturation. Administer supplemental oxygen, as ordered to maintain target levels
- Administer I.V. antihypertensive therapy as ordered
- Titrate I.V. antihypertensive medications according to the desired response and parameters set by the doctor.

Much monitoring

- Monitor BP every 1 to 5 minutes while titrating drug therapy, then every 15 minutes to 1 hour as the patient's condition stabilises
- Continuously monitor ECG and institute treatment as indicated if you find arrhythmias. Auscultate the patient's heart, noting signs of heart failure such as S_3 or S_4 heart sounds
- Assess the patient's neurologic status frequently – every 15 to 30 minutes initially and then every hour, based on the patient's response to therapy. Patient is at risk of hypertensive encephalopathy.

Education edge

Teaching about hypertensive crisis

Hypertensive crisis is an emergency situation that most commonly results from inadequately controlled hypertension or untreated hypertension. As a result, the patient will need to be educated about measures to control his hypertension to reduce the risk of complications and a recurrence of the crisis once his condition has stabilised.

Check in on output

- Monitor urine output every hour, and notify the practitioner if output is less than 0.5 ml/kg/hour. Evaluate U & Es and serum creatinine levels for changes. Try and get a baseline weight
- Administer other antihypertensives as ordered. If the patient is experiencing fluid overload, administer diuretics as ordered
- Assess the patient's vision and report changes, such as increased blurred vision, diplopia or loss of vision may indicate retinopathy, indicating accelerated and malignant hypertension
- Administer analgesics as ordered for headache; keep your patient's environment quiet, with low lighting
- Anticipate transfer of the patient to the CCU/ICU as indicated
- Provide support to the patient and his family; begin patient teaching related to the condition and measures to reduce the risk of complications as the patient's condition begins to stabilise. (See *Teaching about hypertensive crisis*.)

> Stay in the know about your patient's urine flow! For adults less than 0.5 ml/kg/hour means there's a problem.

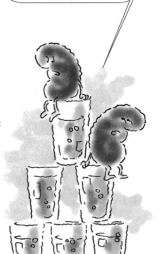

Quick quiz

1. Which sign or symptom would the nurse expect to assess in a patient who's admitted to the ED with a diagnosis of cardiac tamponade?
   A. Shortness of breath.
   B. Pulsus paradoxus.
   C. Holosystolic murmur.
   D. Bounding peripheral pulse.

Answer: B. Pulsus paradoxus (inspiratory drop in systemic BP >15 mm Hg) is one of the three classic signs of cardiac tamponade. The other classic signs are elevated CVP with jugular vein distension and muffled heart sounds.

2. Which assessment finding would the nurse expect to find elevated in a client admitted with right-sided heart failure?
   A. CVP.
   B. Left-ventricular end-diastolic pressure.
   C. PAWP.
   D. Cardiac output.

Answer: A. CVP is elevated in right-sided heart failure.

3. When performing synchronised cardioversion, the nurse understands that the electrical charge is delivered at which point?
    A.   Initiation of the QRS complex.
    B.   During the ST segment.
    C.   At the peak of the R wave.
    D.   Just before the onset of the P wave.

Answer: *C.* Synchronised cardioversion delivers an electrical charge to the myocardium at the peak of the R wave.

4. Defibrillation is a key treatment for dealing with cardiac arrest due to certain arrhythmias. Which of these are shockable rhythms?
    A.   VF
    B.   Pulseless VT
    C.   Asystole

Answer: *A* and *B* only. Defibrillation is not used for asystole.

Scoring

☆☆☆   If you answered all four questions correctly, let your heart swell with pride. You're tops when it comes to cardiac emergencies!

☆☆   If you answered three questions correctly, congratulations on all your 'heart' work. You're a member of the cardiac emergency team!

☆   If you answered fewer than three questions correctly, don't be heartbroken. Just go back and review the chapter!

7 Respiratory emergencies

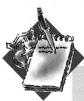

Just the facts

In this chapter, you'll learn:

♦ Assessment of the respiratory system
♦ Respiratory disorders and treatments
♦ Diagnostic tests and procedures used in respiratory emergencies.

Understanding respiratory emergencies

Respiratory emergencies can be caused by obstructions, infections or injury of the respiratory system. Any trauma that alters the integrity of the respiratory system can alter gas exchange. Respiratory emergencies can be life-threatening and require your expert assessment techniques and prompt interventions.

Assessment

Respiratory assessment is a critical nursing responsibility in the emergency department. Conduct a thorough assessment to detect subtle and obvious respiratory changes.

History

Build your patient's health history by asking short, open-ended questions. Conduct the interview in several short sessions if you have to, depending on the severity of your patient's condition. Ask his family or friends to provide information if he can't.

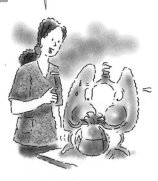

I know respiratory emergencies can be life-threatening, but don't panic! This chapter helps you deal with them.

Cover all the bases

Respiratory disorders may be caused or exacerbated by obesity, smoking and workplace conditions, so be sure to ask about these factors.

Current health status

Begin by asking why your patient is seeking care. Because many respiratory disorders are chronic, ask how his latest acute episode compares with the previous episode and which relief measures are helpful and not helpful. Patients with respiratory disorders commonly report such complaints as:
- Chest pain
- Cough
- Shortness of breath
- Sleep disturbance
- Sputum production
- Wheezing.

Chest pain

If the patient has chest pain, ask: Where's the pain? What does it feel like? Is it sharp, stabbing, burning or aching? Does it move to another area? How long does it last? What causes it? What makes it better?

Pain provocations

Chest pain due to a respiratory problem is usually the result of pleural inflammation, inflammation of the costochondral junctions, soreness of chest muscles because of coughing or indigestion. Less common causes of pain include rib or vertebral fractures caused by coughing or osteoporosis.

Cough

Ask the patient with a cough: At what time of day do you cough most often? Is the cough productive? If the cough is a chronic problem, has it changed recently? If so, how? What makes the cough better? What makes it worse?

Shortness of breath

Assess your patient's shortness of breath by asking him to rate his usual level of dyspnoea on a scale of 1 to 10, in which 1 means no dyspnoea and 10 means the worst he has experienced. Then ask him to rate the level that day. Other scales grade dyspnoea as it relates to activity, such as climbing a set of stairs or walking 50 yards. (See *Grading dyspnoea*.)

Pillow talk

A patient with orthopnoea (shortness of breath when lying down) tends to sleep with his upper body elevated. Ask the patient how many pillows he uses; the answer reflects the severity of the orthopnoea. For instance, a patient who uses three pillows can be said to have *three-pillow orthopnoea*.

Grading dyspnoea

To assess dyspnoea as objectively as possible, ask your patient to briefly describe how various activities affect his breathing. Then document his response using this grading system:
- *Grade 0* – not troubled by breathlessness except with strenuous exercise
- *Grade 1* – troubled by shortness of breath when hurrying on a level path or walking up a slight hill
- *Grade 2* – walks more slowly than people of the same age on a level path because of breathlessness or has to stop to breathe when walking on a level path at own pace
- *Grade 3* – stops to breathe after walking about 100 yards (91 m) on a level path
- *Grade 4* – too breathless to leave the house or becomes breathless when dressing or undressing.

Don't forget to ask

In addition to using a severity scale, ask: What do you do to relieve the shortness of breath? How well does it usually work?

Sleep disturbance
Sleep disturbances may be related to obstructive sleep apnoea or another sleep disorder requiring additional evaluation.

Daytime drowsiness

If the patient complains of being drowsy or irritable in the daytime, ask: How many hours of continuous sleep do you get at night? Do you wake up often during the night? Does your family complain about your snoring or restlessness?

Sputum production
If a patient produces sputum, ask how much in numbers of teaspoons or some other common measurement. Also ask: What's the colour and consistency of the sputum? If sputum is a chronic problem, has it changed recently? If so, how? Do you cough up blood? If so, how much and how often?

Wheezing
If a patient wheezes, ask: When do you wheeze? What makes you wheeze? Do you wheeze loudly enough for others to hear it? What helps stop your wheezing?

Previous health status
Look at the patient's health history, being especially watchful for:
• Allergies
• Respiratory diseases, such as pneumonia and tuberculosis (TB)
• Smoking habit
• Exposure to second-hand smoke
• Previous operations.
    Ask about current immunisations, such as an influenza or pneumococcal vaccine. Also determine whether the patient uses respiratory equipment, such as oxygen nebulisers or other respiratory support at home.

Family history
Ask the patient whether he has a family history of cancer, sickle cell anaemia, heart disease or chronic illness, such as asthma and emphysema. Determine whether the patient lives with anyone who has an infectious disease, such as TB or influenza.

Lifestyle patterns
Ask about the patient's workplace, because some jobs, such as coal mining and construction work, expose workers to substances that can cause lung disease.

Also ask about the patient's home, community and other environmental factors that may influence how he deals with his respiratory problems. For example, you may ask questions about interpersonal relationships, stress management and coping methods. Ask about any at risk behaviours, such as drug use, which may be connected with acquired immunodeficiency syndrome-related pulmonary disorders.

Physical examination

In most cases, the physical examination will take place after taking the patient's history. However, a complete history may have to wait if the patient develops an ominous sign such as acute respiratory distress. If your patient is in respiratory distress, establish the priorities of your nursing assessment, progressing from the most critical factors to less critical factors. (See *Emergency respiratory assessment.*)

You will need to be guided by your level of practice or local policies as to the level of investigative assessment you will undertake. These assessments may be conducted solely by the doctor or the emergency nurse practitioner, however increasingly these assessments are being undertaken by all emergency nurses. It is of course essential that the

---

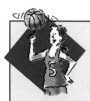

Stay on the ball

Emergency respiratory assessment

If your patient is in acute respiratory distress, immediately assess ABCDE. Be ready to start cardiopulmonary resuscitation.

Next, quickly check for these signs of impending crisis:

- Is the patient having trouble breathing?
- Is the patient using accessory muscles to breathe? If chest excursion is less than the normal (3 to 6 cm), look for evidence that the patient is using accessory muscles when he breathes, including shoulder elevation, intercostal muscle retraction and use of the scalene muscles (lateral muscles in the neck) and sternocleidomastoid muscles
- Has the patient's level of consciousness diminished?
- Is he confused, anxious or agitated?

- Does he change his body position to ease breathing?
- Does his skin look pale? Is there excessive sweating? Is the patient cyanotic?

Setting priorities

If your patient is in respiratory distress, establish priorities for your nursing assessment. Don't assume the obvious. Note positive and negative factors, starting with the most clinically critical factors and progressing to less critical factors.

If you don't have time to go through each step of the nursing process, make sure you gather enough data to answer vital questions. A single sign or symptom has many possible meanings, so gather a group of findings to assess the patient and develop interventions.

nurse and the student nurse understand the rationale for and the correct conduct of respiratory assessment even if they are not actually undertaking them.

Four steps

A systematic approach is used to detect subtle and obvious respiratory changes. The four steps for conducting a physical examination of the respiratory system are:

 Inspection

 Palpation

 Percussion

 Auscultation.

Back, then front

The back of the chest is examined first, using inspection, palpation, percussion and auscultation. One side is always compared with the other. Then the front of the chest is examined using the same sequence. The patient can lie back when the front of the chest is being examined if that's more comfortable for him.

Inspection

Make a few key observations about the patient as soon as you enter the patient care area and include these observations in your assessment. Note the patient's position on the stretcher. Does the patient appear comfortable? Is he sitting up, lying quietly or shifting about? Is he anxious? Is the patient having trouble breathing? Is oxygen required?

Muscles in motion

When the patient inhales, his diaphragm should descend and the intercostal muscles should contract. This dual motion causes the abdomen to push out and the lower ribs to expand laterally.

When the patient exhales, his abdomen and ribs return to their resting positions. The upper chest shouldn't move much. Accessory muscles may hypertrophy, indicating frequent use. This may be normal in some athletes, but for most patients it indicates a respiratory problem, especially when the patient purses his lips and flares his nostrils when breathing.

Chest inspection

Inspect the patient's chest configuration, tracheal position, chest symmetry, skin condition, nostrils (for flaring) and accessory muscle use.

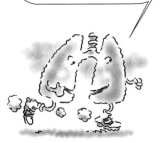

Hypertrophy in accessory muscles can be normal in some athletes, but in most patients it signals respiratory problems.

Beauty in symmetry

Look for chest wall symmetry. Both sides of the chest should be equal at rest and expand equally as the patient inhales. The diameter of the chest, from front to back, should be about one-half of the width of the chest.

A new angle

Also, look at the costal angle (the angle between the ribs and the sternum at the point immediately above the xiphoid process). This angle should be less than 90 degrees in an adult. The angle is larger if the chest wall is chronically expanded because of an enlargement of the intercostal muscles, as can happen with chronic obstructive pulmonary disease (COPD).

Chest wall abnormalities

Inspect for chest wall abnormalities, keeping in mind that a patient with a deformity of the chest wall might have completely normal lungs that could be cramped in the chest. The patient may have a smaller-than-normal lung capacity and limited exercise tolerance.

Raising a red flag

Watch for paradoxical (uneven) movement of the patient's chest wall. Paradoxical movement may appear as an abnormal collapse of part of the chest wall when the patient inhales or an abnormal expansion when the patient exhales. In either case, such uneven movement indicates a loss of normal chest wall function.

Breathing rate and pattern

Assess and record your patient's respiratory function by determining the rate, rhythm and quality of respirations. One respiration is a breath in and out.

Count on it

The counting and recording of the patient's respiratory rate is very important and must not be ignored. The respiratory pattern should be even, coordinated and regular, with occasional sighs. Normal rate for adults is between 10 and 18 breaths per minute. Eupnoea is the term used to describe normal breathing at rest.

Abnormal respiratory patterns

Cheyne-Stokes respirations are initially shallow but gradually become deeper and deeper; then a period of apnoea follows, lasting up to 20 seconds, and the cycle starts again. This respiratory pattern is seen in patients with heart failure, kidney failure or central nervous system (CNS) damage. Cheyne-Stokes respirations can be a normal breathing pattern during sleep in the older person.

Biot's (cluster) respirations

Biot's respirations involve rapid, deep breaths that alternate with abrupt periods of apnoea. It's an ominous sign of severe CNS damage or can be found in opiate overdose.

Inspecting related structures

Inspect the patient's skin for cyanosis and fingers and toes for clubbing. Clubbing is a sign of long-standing respiratory or cardiac disease and indicates chronic tissue hypoxia. Look for abnormal enlargement and for nail thinning and alterations in the normal angle of the finger and toe bases. The fingernail normally enters the skin at an angle of less than 180 degrees. In clubbed fingers, the angle is greater than or equal to 180 degrees.

Don't be blue

Skin colour varies considerably among patients, but a patient with a bluish tint to his skin, nail beds and mucous membranes is considered cyanotic. Cyanosis, which results when oxygenation to the tissues is poor, is a late sign of hypoxaemia.

Palpation

Palpation of the chest provides some important information about the respiratory system and the processes involved in breathing.

Leaky lungs

The chest wall should feel smooth, warm and dry. Crepitus, which feels like puffed-rice cereal crackling under the skin, indicates that air is leaking from the airways or lungs.

Probing palpation pain

Gentle palpation shouldn't cause the patient pain. If the patient complains of chest pain, try to find a painful area on the chest wall. Here's a guide to assessing some types of chest pain:
• Painful costochondral joints are typically located at the mid-clavicular line or next to the sternum
• A rib or vertebral fracture is quite painful over the fracture
• Protracted coughing may cause sore muscles
• A collapsed lung can cause pain in addition to dyspnoea.

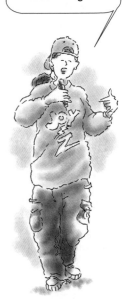

Don't hate me cuz I palpate; I'm only tryin' to get the pain in your chest straight!

Evaluating symmetry

The patient's chest wall symmetry and expansion can be evaluated by the placing of hands on the front of the chest wall with the thumbs touching each other at the second intercostal space. As the patient inhales deeply, watch the thumbs. They should separate simultaneously and equally to a distance several centimetres away from the sternum. The measurement is repeated at the fifth intercostal space. The same measurement can be made on the back of the chest near the 10th rib. (See *Feeling for Fremitus*.)

Warning signs

The patient's chest may expand asymmetrically if he has:
• Pneumonia
• Atelectasis
• Pleural effusion
• Pneumothorax.
   Chest expansion may be decreased at the level of the diaphragm if the patient has:
• Respiratory depression
• Emphysema

Feeling for fremitus

Tactile fremitus (palpable vibrations caused by the transmission of air through the bronchopulmonary system) is palpated for. Fremitus decreases over areas where pleural fluid collects, when the patient speaks softly and with pneumothorax, atelectasis and emphysema.

Fremitus is increased normally over the large bronchial tubes and abnormally over areas in which alveoli are filled with fluid or exudates, as happens in pneumonia.

What to do

When checking the back of the thorax for tactile fremitus, the patient is asked to fold his arms across his chest. This movement shifts the scapulae out of the way. Open palms are placed lightly on both sides of the patient's back without touching his back with fingers, as shown here. The patient is asked to repeat the phrase 'ninety-nine' loudly enough to produce palpable vibrations. The front of the chest is then palpated using the same hand positions.

What the results mean

Vibrations that feel more intense on one side than on the other indicate tissue consolidation on that side. Less intense vibrations may indicate emphysema, pneumothorax or pleural effusion. Faint or no vibrations in the upper posterior thorax may indicate bronchial obstruction or a fluid-filled pleural space.

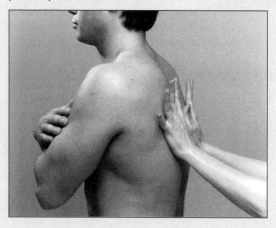

- Obesity
- Ascites
- Atelectasis
- Diaphragm paralysis.

Percussion

The chest is percussed to:
- Find the boundaries of the lungs
- Determine whether the lungs are filled with air, fluid or solid material
- Evaluate the distance the diaphragm travels between the patient's inhalation and exhalation.

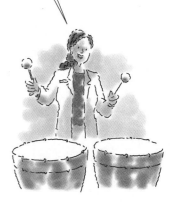

Percuss the chest to determine whether lungs are filled with air, fluid or solid material.

Sites and sounds

Normal, resonant sounds are listened for over most of the chest. In the left front chest wall from the third or fourth intercostal space at the sternum to the third or fourth intercostal space at the mid-clavicular line, there is a dull sound over the space occupied by the heart. Careful percussion aids the identification of the borders of the heart when lung tissue is normal. Resonance resumes at the sixth intercostal space. The sequence of sounds in the back is slightly different. (See *Percussion sequences*, page 228.)

Warning sounds

Hyperresonance heard during percussion means that an area of increased air in the lung or pleural space has been found. We expect to hear hyperresonance in patients with:
- Acute asthma
- Pneumothorax
- Bullous emphysema (large cavities left by septal rupture).

When abnormal dullness is heard it means that areas of decreased air in the lungs have been found. Abnormal dullness is expected in the presence of pleural fluid, consolidation, atelectasis and tumour.

Detecting diaphragm movement

Percussion also allows the assessment of how much the diaphragm moves during inspiration and expiration. The normal diaphragm descends 3 to 5 cm when the patient inhales. The diaphragm doesn't move as far in patients with emphysema, respiratory depression, diaphragm paralysis, atelectasis, obesity or ascites.

Auscultation

As air moves through the bronchi, it creates sound waves that travel to the chest wall. The sound produced by breathing changes as air moves from larger to smaller airways. Sounds also change if they pass through fluid, mucus or narrowed airways. You can hear breath sounds at Web sites such as: http://www.nlm.nih.gov/medlineplus/ency/article/003323.htm

Percussion sequences

These percussion sequences aid the distinguishing between normal and abnormal sounds in the patient's lungs. Sound variations are compared from one side with the other. Abnormal sounds are described and their locations noted. (The same sequence for auscultation is followed.)

Anterior

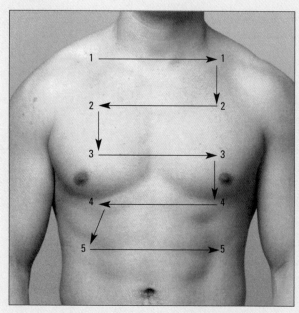

Posterior

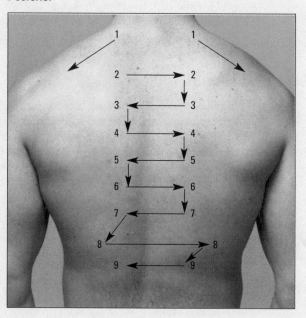

Auscultation preparation

Auscultation sites are the same as percussion sites. Using the diaphragm of the stethoscope, a full cycle of inspiration and expiration at each site is listened to. The patient will be asked to breathe through his mouth if it doesn't cause discomfort; nose breathing alters the pitch of breath sounds.

Be firm

To auscultate for breath sounds, the diaphragm side of the stethoscope is pressed firmly against the skin. If listened for through clothing or chest hair, breath sounds won't be heard clearly and unusual and deceptive sounds may be heard.

Interpreting breath sounds

Each breath sound is classified during auscultation by its intensity, pitch, duration, characteristic and location. Note is made whether it occurs during inspiration, expiration or both.

Normal breath sounds

During auscultation, four types of breath sounds over normal lungs are listened for. (See *Locations of normal breath sounds.*) Here's a rundown of the normal breath sounds and their characteristics:

• Tracheal breath sounds, heard over the trachea, are harsh and discontinuous. They're present when the patient inhales or exhales
• Bronchial breath sounds, usually heard next to the trachea just above or below the clavicle, are loud, high-pitched and discontinuous. They're loudest when the patient exhales
• Bronchovesicular sounds are medium-pitched and continuous. They're best heard over the upper third of the sternum and between the scapulae when the patient inhales or exhales
• Vesicular sounds, heard over the rest of the lungs, are soft and low-pitched. They're prolonged during inhalation and shortened during exhalation. (See *Qualities of normal breath sounds.*)

Abnormal breath sounds

Because solid tissue transmits sound better than air or fluid, breath sounds (as well as spoken or whispered words) are louder than normal over areas of consolidation. If pus, fluid or air fills the pleural space, breath sounds are quieter than normal. If a foreign body or secretions obstruct a bronchus, breath sounds are diminished or absent over lung tissue distal to the obstruction.

Detect the unexpected

Breath sounds heard in an unexpected area are also abnormal. For instance, if bronchial sounds are heard where vesicular sounds are expected, the area being auscultated might be filled with fluid or exudates, as in pneumonia. The vesicular sounds expected in those areas are absent because no air is moving through the small airways. Some common abnormal breath sounds are vocal fremitus and adventitious breath sounds.

Locations of normal breath sounds

These photographs show the normal locations of different types of breath sounds.

Anterior thorax

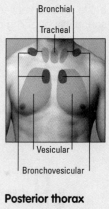

Posterior thorax

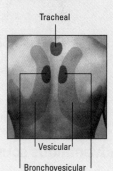

Qualities of normal breath sounds

Use this chart as a quick reference for the qualities of normal breath sounds.

Breath sound	Quality	Inspiration-expiration ratio	Location
Tracheal	Harsh, high-pitched	I < E	Over trachea
Bronchial	Loud, high-pitched	I > E	Next to trachea
Bronchovesicular	Medium in loudness and pitch	I = E	Next to sternum, between scapula
Vesicular	Soft, low-pitched	I > E	Remainder of lungs

Abnormal breath sounds

Here's a quick guide to assessing abnormal breath sounds.

Crackles

Crackles are intermittent, nonmusical, crackling sounds heard during inspiration. They're classified as *fine* or *coarse* and are common in older adults when small sections of the alveoli don't fully aerate and secretions accumulate during sleep. Alveoli re-expand or pop open when the patient takes deep breaths upon awakening. Fine crackles sound like strands of hair being rubbed between the fingers. Coarse crackles sound like bubbling or gurgling as air moves through secretions in larger airways.

Wheezes

Wheezes are high-pitched sounds caused by blocked airflow and are heard on exhalation or also on inspection as the block increases. Patients may wheeze as a result of asthma, infection or airway obstruction from a tumour or foreign body.

Stridor

Stridor is a loud, high-pitched sound heard during inspiration.

Pleural friction rub

Pleural friction rub is a low-pitched, grating sound heard during inspiration and expiration and is accompanied by pain.

Vocal fremitus

Vocal fremitus is the sound produced by chest vibrations as the patient speaks. Voice sounds can transmit abnormally over consolidated areas because sound travels well through fluid. There are three common abnormal voice sounds:

 Bronchophony – The patient is asked to say 'ninety-nine' or 'blue moon'. Over normal tissue, the words sound muffled, but over consolidated areas, the words sound unusually loud

Egophony – The patient is asked to say 'E'. Over normal lung tissue, the sound is muffled, but over consolidated areas, it sounds like the letter A

Whispered pectoriloquy – The patient is asked to whisper '1, 2, 3'. Over normal lung tissue, the numbers are almost indistinguishable. Over consolidated tissue, the numbers sound loud and clear.

Adventitious sounds

Adventitious sounds are abnormal no matter where you hear them in the lungs. (See *Abnormal breath sounds*.) There are four types of adventitious breath sounds:

 Crackles

 Wheezes

 Stridor

 Pleural friction rub.

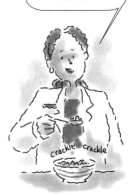

Crackles aren't just for breakfast – they also signal problems with alveoli.

Diagnostic tests

If your patient's history and the physical examination findings reveal evidence of pulmonary dysfunction, diagnostic tests can identify and evaluate the dysfunction. These tests include:
- Peak flow meter readings
- Blood and sputum studies
- Endoscopy and imaging
- Pulmonary angiography.

Peak flows

Peak flow meters measure the peak flow of air on forced expiration. This gives a base line reading and is a useful reading to be taken pre and post use of bronchodilators. The patient sits upright and is asked to ensure his lips are sealed tightly around the mouthpiece. The patient exhales with force. This is done three times and the highest reading is recorded.

Pulse oximetry

Pulse oximetry is a relatively simple procedure used to monitor arterial oxygen saturation noninvasively. It's performed intermittently or continuously.

Shedding light on the subject

In this procedure, two diodes send red and infrared light through a pulsating arterial vascular bed such as the one in the fingertip. A photodetector (also called a *sensor* or *transducer*) slipped over the finger measures the transmitted light as it passes through the vascular bed, detects the relative amount of colour absorbed by arterial blood and calculates the saturation without interference from the venous blood, skin or connective tissue. The percentage expressed is the ratio of oxygen to haemoglobin. (See *Interfering factors*, page 232.)

Note denotation

In pulse oximetry, arterial oxygen saturation values are usually denoted with the symbol SpO_2. Arterial oxygen saturation values that are measured invasively using arterial blood gas (ABG) analysis are denoted by the symbol SaO_2.

Practice pointers
- Place the sensor over the finger or other site – such as the toe, bridge of the nose or earlobe – so that the light beams and sensors are opposite each other.

Interfering factors

Certain factors can interfere with the accuracy of oximetry readings. For example, an elevated bilirubin level may falsely lower oxygen saturation readings, whereas elevated carboxyhaemoglobin or methaemoglobin levels can falsely elevate oxygen saturation readings.

Certain intravascular substances, such as lipid emulsions and dyes, can also prevent accurate readings. Other interfering factors include excessive light (such as from phototherapy or direct sunlight), excessive patient movement, excessive ear pigment, hypothermia, hypotension and vasoconstriction.

Some acrylic nails and certain colours of nail polish (blue, green, black and brown-red) may also interfere with readings.

* Protect the sensor from exposure to strong light, such as fluorescent lighting, because it interferes with results. Check the sensor site frequently to make sure the device is in place and examine the skin for abrasion and circulatory impairment
* The pulse oximeter displays the patient's pulse rate and oxygen saturation reading. The pulse rate on the oximeter must correspond to the patient's actual pulse. If the rates don't correspond, the saturation reading can't be considered accurate. You may need to reposition the sensor to obtain an accurate reading
* Rotate the sensor site at least every 4 hours, following the manufacturer's instructions and your local policy for site rotation, to avoid skin irritation and circulatory impairment
* If oximetry is done properly, the oxygen saturation readings are usually within 2% of ABG values. A normal reading is 95% to 100%. Remember to note on your records if oxygen is being used and at what rate.

Poisoning precludes pulse oximetry

* Pulse oximetry isn't used when carbon monoxide poisoning is suspected because the oximeter doesn't differentiate between oxygen and carbon monoxide bound to haemoglobin. An ABG analysis should be performed in such cases.

End-tidal carbon dioxide monitoring

End-tidal carbon dioxide monitoring ($ETco_2$) is used to measure the carbon dioxide concentration at end expiration. An $ETco_2$ monitor may be a separate monitor or part of the patient's bedside haemodynamic monitoring system.

Indications for $ETco_2$ monitoring include:
* Monitoring apnoea, respiratory function and patency of the airway in acute airway obstruction

- Early detection of hypercapnia, hyperthermia and changes in carbon dioxide production and elimination with hyperventilation therapy
- Assessing effectiveness of such interventions as mechanical ventilation, neuromuscular blockade used with mechanical ventilation and prone positioning.

In-lightened

In $ETco_2$ monitoring, a photodetector measures the amount of infrared light absorbed by the airway during inspiration and expiration. (Light absorption increases along with carbon dioxide concentration.) The monitor converts these data to a carbon dioxide value and a corresponding waveform or capnogram, if capnography is used.

Crunching the numbers

Values are obtained by monitoring samples of expired gas from an endotracheal (ET) tube or an oral or nasopharyngeal airway. Although the values are similar, the $ETco_2$ values are usually 2 to 5 mm Hg lower than the partial pressure of arterial carbon dioxide ($Paco_2$) value. End exhalation contains the highest carbon dioxide concentration. Normal $ETco_2$ is 35 to 45 mm Hg.

Capnograms and $ETco_2$ monitoring reduce the need for frequent ABG sampling.

Practice pointers

- Explain the procedure to the patient and his family
- Assess the patient's respiratory status, vital signs, oxygen saturation and $ETco_2$ readings
- Observe waveform quality and trends of $ETco_2$ readings and observe for sudden increases (which may indicate hypoventilation, partial airway obstruction or respiratory depressant effects from drugs) or decreases (due to complete airway obstruction, a dislodged ET tube or ventilator malfunction). Notify the doctor of a 10% increase or decrease in readings.

ABG analysis

ABG analysis enables evaluation of gas exchange in the lungs by measuring the partial pressures of gases dissolved in arterial blood.

ABCs of ABGs

Arterial blood is measured because it reflects how much oxygen is available to peripheral tissues. Together, ABG values tell the story of how well a patient is oxygenated and whether he's developing acidosis or alkalosis.

Here's a summary of commonly assessed ABG values and what the findings indicate:

- pH measurement of the hydrogen ion (H^+) concentration is an indication of the blood's acidity or alkalinity
- $Paco_2$ reflects the adequacy of ventilation of the lungs
- Partial pressure of arterial oxygen (Pao_2) reflects the body's ability to pick up oxygen from the lungs
- Bicarbonate (HCO_3^-) level reflects the activity of the kidneys in retaining or excreting bicarbonate
- Sao_2 is the ratio of actual haemoglobin oxygen content to potential maximum oxygen carrying capacity of the haemoglobin. (See *Normal ABG values*.)

Valuable values

Here's an interpretation of possible ABG values:

- A Pao_2 value greater than 100 mm Hg reflects more-than-adequate supplemental oxygen administration. A value less than 80 mm Hg indicates hypoxaemia
- A Sao_2 value less than 95% represents decreased saturation and may contribute to a low Pao_2 value
- A pH value above 7.45 (alkalosis) reflects an H^+ deficit; a value below 7.35 (acidosis) reflects an H^+ excess.

A sample scenario

If a patient has a pH value greater than 7.45, indicating alkalosis then this will be investigated further by checking the $PaCO_2$ value, which is known as the *respiratory parameter*. This value reflects how efficiently the lungs eliminate carbon dioxide. A $PaCO_2$ value below 35 mm Hg indicates respiratory alkalosis and hyperventilation.

Next, check the HCO_3^- value, called the *metabolic parameter*. An HCO_3^- value greater than 28 mEq/L indicates metabolic alkalosis.

Likewise, a pH value below 7.35 indicates acidosis. A $PaCO_2$ value above 45 mm Hg indicates respiratory acidosis; an HCO_3^- value below 22 mEq/L indicates metabolic acidosis.

See-saw systems

The respiratory and metabolic systems work together to keep the body's acid-base balance within normal limits. If respiratory acidosis develops, for example, the kidneys compensate by conserving HCO_3^-. That's why you expect to see an above-normal HCO_3^- value.

Similarly, if metabolic acidosis develops, the lungs compensate by increasing the respiratory rate and depth to eliminate carbon dioxide. (See *Understanding acid-base disorders*.)

Normal ABG values

Arterial blood gas (ABG) values provide information about the blood's acid-base balance and oxygenation. Normal values are:

- pH: 7.36 to 7.44
- $Paco_2$: 35 to 45 mm Hg (4.5 to 6.1 kPa)
- PaO_2: 80 to 100 mm Hg (12 to 14 kPa)
- HCO_3^-: 23 to 28 mEq/L (23 to 28 mmol/L)
- SaO_2: 95% to 100%.

Understanding acid-base disorders

This chart provides an overview of selected acid-base disorders.

Disorder and arterial blood gas findings	Possible causes	Signs and symptoms
Respiratory acidosis (excess carbon dioxide retention) pH < 7.35 Bicarbonate (HCO_3^-) > 26 mEq/L (if compensating) Partial pressure of arterial carbon dioxide ($Paco_2$) > 45 mm Hg	• Asphyxia • Central nervous system depression from drugs, injury or disease • Hypoventilation from pulmonary, cardiac, musculoskeletal or neuromuscular disease	Diaphoresis; headache; tachycardia; confusion; restlessness; apprehension; flushed face
Respiratory alkalosis (excess carbon dioxide excretion) pH > 7.45 HCO_3^- < 22 mEq/L (if compensating) $Paco_2$ < 35 mm Hg	• Gram-negative bacteraemia • Hyperventilation from anxiety, pain or improper ventilator settings • Respiratory stimulation by drugs, disease, hypoxia, fever or high room temperature	Rapid, deep respirations; paraesthesia; light-headedness; twitching; anxiety; fear
Metabolic acidosis (bicarbonate loss, acid retention) pH < 7.35 HCO_3^- < 22 mEq/L $Paco_2$ < 35 mm Hg (if compensating)	• Bicarbonate depletion from diarrhoea • Excessive production of organic acids from hepatic disease, endocrine disorders, shock or drug intoxication • Inadequate excretion of acids from renal disease	Rapid, deep breathing; fruity breath; fatigue; headache; lethargy; drowsiness; nausea; vomiting; coma (if severe); abdominal pain
Metabolic alkalosis (bicarbonate retention, acid loss) pH > 7.45 HCO_3^- > 26 mEq/L $Paco_2$ > 45 mm Hg (if compensating)	• Excessive alkali ingestion • Loss of hydrochloric acid from prolonged vomiting or gastric suctioning • Loss of potassium from increased renal excretion (as in diuretic therapy) or steroids	Slow, shallow breathing; hypertonic muscles; restlessness; twitching; confusion; irritability; apathy; tetany; seizures; coma (if severe)

Practice pointers

• ABG samples are drawn usually from an arterial line if the patient has one. If a percutaneous puncture must be done, the site is chosen carefully. The most common site is the radial artery, but the brachial or femoral arteries can be used

• After obtaining the sample, pressure is applied to the puncture site for 5 minutes and a gauze pad taped firmly in place. The site is monitored regularly for bleeding and the arm checked for signs of complications, such as swelling, discolouration, pain, numbness and tingling. (See *Obtaining an ABG sample*, page 236)

• Whether the patient is breathing room air or oxygen is noted. If the patient is on oxygen, document the number of litres. If the patient is receiving mechanical ventilation, document the fraction of inspired oxygen

• Any air bubbles in the sample syringe must be removed because air bubbles also alter results

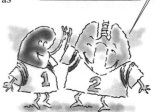

Here's the game plan: If you develop respiratory acidosis, I'll cover you and conserve HCO_3^-. Ready? Break!

Obtaining an ABG sample

These steps are followed to obtain a sample for arterial blood gas (ABG) analysis:
- The procedure is explained to the patient and consent gained (where possible)
- After performing a test for the patency of the radial or ulnar artery (Allen's test), a cutaneous arterial puncture is performed. Or, if an arterial line is in place, blood is drawn from the arterial line
- A heparinised blood gas syringe is used to draw the sample
- All air is eliminated from the sample and it is placed on ice immediately and transported rapidly for analysis
- Pressure is applied to the puncture site for 5 minutes. If the patient is receiving anticoagulants or has a coagulopathy, hold the puncture site longer than 5 minutes, if necessary
- A gauze pad is tapped firmly over the puncture site. If the puncture site is on the arm, don't tape the entire circumference because this may restrict circulation.

- The sample of arterial blood is kept cold, preferably on ice and delivered as soon as possible to the laboratory for analysis.

Sputum analysis

Sputum analysis assesses sputum specimens to diagnose respiratory disease, identify the cause of pulmonary infection (including viral and bacterial causes), identify abnormal lung cells and manage lung disease.

Practice pointers
- When he's ready to expectorate, instruct the patient to take three deep breaths and force a deep cough
- Before sending the specimen to the laboratory, make sure it's sputum, not saliva. Saliva has a thinner consistency and more bubbles (froth) than sputum.

Chest X-ray

During chest radiography (commonly known as chest X-ray), X-ray beams penetrate the chest and form an image on specially sensitised film. Because normal pulmonary tissue is radiolucent, such abnormalities as infiltrates, foreign bodies, fluid and tumours appear dense on the film.

More is better

A chest X-ray is most useful when compared with the patient's previous films, allowing the radiologist to detect changes. By themselves, chest X-rays may not provide definitive diagnostic information. For example, they may not reveal mild to moderate obstructive pulmonary disease. However, they can show the location and size of lesions and can also be used to identify structural abnormalities that influence ventilation.

Comparing two chest X-rays can paint a better picture of respiratory change than looking at just one.

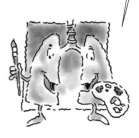

X-ray vision

Examples of abnormalities visible on X-ray include:
- Fibrosis
- Infiltrates
- Atelectasis
- Pneumothorax
- Haemothorax
- Bowel perforation (may show evidence).

Practice pointers
- When a patient in the ED can't be moved, a chest X-ray maybe performed at the bedside
- Make sure that female patients of childbearing age wear a lead apron. Males should have protection for the testes.

Magnetic resonance imaging

Magnetic resonance imaging (MRI) is a noninvasive test that employs a powerful magnet, radio waves and a computer. It's used to diagnose respiratory disorders by providing high-resolution, cross-sectional images of mediastinal structures and by tracing blood flow.

View that's see-through

The greatest advantage of MRI is that it enables the distinguishing of bone and delineates fluid-filled soft tissue in great detail without using ionising radiation or contrast media. It's used to discriminate tumours from other structures such as blood vessels.

Practice pointers
- Provide information and reassurance. Check that consent, where possible, has been gained
- Ensure that a prescan checklist has been completed
- All metal objects must be removed from the patient before entering the scanning room. (See *MRI and technology don't mix*)
- If the patient is claustrophobic, he may be sedated before the test
- Tell the patient that the test usually takes 15 to 30 minutes. Some facilities can perform open MRIs, which are more tolerable for patients who are claustrophobic.

Thoracic computed tomography scan

Thoracic computed tomography (CT) scan provides cross-sectional views of the chest by passing an X-ray beam from a computerised scanner through the body at different angles and depths. A contrast agent is sometimes used to highlight blood vessels and allow greater visual discrimination.

MRI and technology don't mix

Before your patient undergoes a MRI, make sure he doesn't have a pacemaker or surgically implanted joints, pins, clips, valves or pump containing metal. Such objects could be attracted to the strong MRI magnet.

Ask your patient whether he's ever worked with metals or has metal in his eyes. If he has such a device, the test can't be done. Some facilities have a checklist that covers all pertinent questions regarding metals, clips, pins, pacemakers and other devices.

CT in 3-D

Thoracic CT scan provides a three-dimensional image of the lung, allowing the practitioner to assess abnormalities in the configuration of the trachea or major bronchi and evaluate masses or lesions, such as tumours and abscesses and abnormal lung shadows.

Practice pointers
• Confirm that the patient isn't allergic to iodine or shellfish. A patient with these allergies may have an adverse reaction to the contrast medium
• If a contrast medium is used, explain that it's injected into the existing I.V. line or that a new line may be inserted
• Explain to the patient that he may feel flushed or notice a metallic or salty taste in his mouth when the contrast medium is injected
• Explain that the CT scanner involves an X-ray beam which rotates around the patient during the procedure which lasts for 10 minutes in total
• Instruct the patient to lie still during the test
• Encourage oral fluid intake to flush the contrast medium out of the patient's system unless it's contraindicated or the patient is on nothing-by-mouth status. The practitioner may write an order to increase the rate of I.V. fluid infusion
• Monitor for adverse reactions to the contrast medium, which may include restlessness, tachypnoea and respiratory distress, tachycardia, urticaria and nausea and vomiting. Keep emergency equipment nearby in case of a reaction.

Bronchoscopy

Bronchoscopy allows direct visualisation of the larynx, trachea and bronchi through a fibre-optic bronchoscope (a slender, flexible tube with mirrors and a light at its distal end). The flexible fibre-optic bronchoscope is preferred to metal because it's smaller, allows a better view of the bronchi and carries less risk of trauma. This procedure usually requires the patient to go to an endoscopy unit or to theatre.

Treatments

Respiratory disorders interfere with airway clearance, breathing patterns and gas exchange. If not corrected, they can adversely affect many other body systems and can be life threatening. Treatments for patients with respiratory disorders include drug therapy, inhalation therapy and surgery.

Drug therapy

Drugs are used for airway management in patients with such disorders as acute respiratory failure, acute respiratory distress syndrome (ARDS), asthma, emphysema and chronic bronchitis. Some types of drugs commonly seen in the ED include anti-inflammatory agents, bronchodilators, neuromuscular blocking agents and sedatives.

Anti-inflammatory agents

Anti-inflammatory agents (corticosteroids) are used to reduce bronchial inflammation.

Reversing obstruction

Corticosteroids are the most effective anti-inflammatory agents used to treat patients with reversible airflow obstruction. They work by suppressing immune responses and reducing inflammation.

Systemic drugs, such as Dexamethasone, Methylprednisolone and Prednisone are given to manage an acute respiratory event, such as acute respiratory failure or exacerbation of COPD. These drugs are initially given I.V.; when the patient stabilises, the dosage is tapered and oral dosing may be substituted.

Patients with asthma commonly use inhaled steroids. These agents also work by suppressing immune response and reducing airway inflammation. (See *Understanding corticosteroids*.)

Bronchodilators

Bronchodilators relax bronchial smooth muscles and are used to treat patients with bronchospasms. Here's how some types of bronchodilators are used:
- Short-acting inhaled beta$_2$-adrenergic agonists, such as Salbutamol, are used to relieve acute symptoms in asthma and bronchospasm

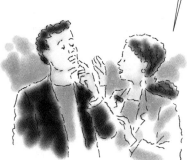

Spontaneous conversations need quick wit; spontaneous breathing efforts need neuromuscular blocking agents if they hamper ventilator function.

Understanding corticosteroids

Use this table to learn about the indications, adverse reactions and practice pointers associated with corticosteroids.

Drug	Indications	Adverse reactions	Practice pointers
Systemic steroids dexamethasone methylprednisolone prednisone	• Anti-inflammatory for acute respiratory failure, acute respiratory distress syndrome and chronic obstructive pulmonary disease • Anti-inflammatory and immunosuppressant for asthma	• Arrhythmias • Circulatory collapse • Heart failure • Pancreatitis • Peptic ulcer • Thromboembolism	• Use cautiously in patients with recent myocardial infarction, hypertension, renal disease and GI ulcer • Monitor blood pressure and blood glucose levels.
Inhaled steroids beclomethasone budesonide	• Long-term asthma control	• Bronchospasm • Dry mouth • Hoarseness • Oral candidiasis • Wheezing	• Don't use for treatment of acute asthma attack • Use a spacer to reduce adverse effects. • Rinse the patient's mouth after use to prevent oral fungal infection.

Understanding bronchodilators

Use this table to learn about the indications, adverse reactions and practice pointers associated with bronchodilators.

Drug	Indications	Adverse reactions	Practice pointers
Beta$_2$-adrenergic agonists			
Salbutamol	• Short-acting relief of acute symptoms with asthma and bronchospasm	• Hyperactivity • Palpitations • Paradoxical bronchospasm • Tachycardia • Tremor	• Warn the patient about the possibility of paradoxical bronchospasm. If it occurs, stop the drug and seek medical treatment • The older adult may require a lower dose • Monitor respiratory status, vital signs and heart rhythm.
Adrenaline	• Relaxation of bronchial smooth muscle through stimulation of beta$_2$-adrenergic receptors; used for bronchospasm, hypersensitivity reaction, anaphylaxis and asthma	• Cerebral hemorrhage • Palpitations • Tachycardia • Ventricular fibrillation	• Use cautiously in the older adult and those with long-standing asthma and emphysema with degenerative heart disease • Monitor respiratory status, vital signs and heart rhythm • This drug is contraindicated in patients with angle-closure glaucoma, coronary insufficiency and cerebral arteriosclerosis.
Anticholinergic agents			
ipratropium bromide	• Bronchospasm associated with chronic bronchitis and emphysema	• Bronchospasm • Chest pain • Nervousness • Palpitations	• Because of delayed onset of bronchodilation, this drug isn't recommended for acute respiratory distress • Use cautiously in patients with angle-closure glaucoma, bladder neck obstruction and prostatic hypertrophy • Monitor respiratory status, vital signs and heart rhythm.

• Adrenaline acts on alpha- and beta-adrenergic receptors. It's used to relieve anaphylactic, allergic and other hypersensitivity reactions. Its beta-adrenergic effects relax bronchial smooth muscle and relieve bronchospasm
• Anticholinergic agents, such as ipratropium bromide act by inhibiting the action of acetylcholine at bronchial smooth-muscle receptor sites and thus produce bronchodilation. (See *Understanding bronchodilators*.)

Inhalation therapy

Inhalation therapy employs carefully controlled ventilation techniques to help the patient maintain optimal ventilation in the event of respiratory failure. Techniques include aerosol treatments, non-invasive ventilation (NIV) known also as non-invasive positive pressure ventilation (NIPPV), ET intubation, mechanical ventilation and oxygen therapy.

Aerosol treatments

Aerosol therapy is a means of administering medication into the airways. The administration method can use handheld nebulisers or metered-dose inhalers. These devices deliver topical medications to the respiratory tract, producing local and systemic effects. The mucosal lining of the respiratory tract absorbs the inhalant almost immediately.

NIV/NIPPV

NIV/NIPPV delivers ventilator support via a non-invasive interface, such as a nasal mask. Use of this ventilatory support can be use for long term support at home and also used in acute respiratory episodes, for instance acute exacerbation of COPD with respiratory failure.

Use of a laryngeal mask airway (LMA)

The laryngeal mask airway (LMA) is used in an emergency setting when endotracheal intubation or use of multilumen airways (such as Combitube) is not possible. The LMA provides better oxygenation than a bag-valve-mask airway but is not a primary airway device for the emergency patient. The LMA is placed so it surrounds the opening of the larynx with an inflatable silicone cuff; this enables ventilation from the glottic opening. It does not, however, protect against aspiration.

Endotracheal (ET) Intubation

ET intubation involves insertion of a tube into the lungs through the mouth or nose to establish a patent airway. It protects patients from aspiration by sealing off the trachea from the digestive tract and permits removal of tracheobronchial secretions in patients who can't cough effectively. ET intubation also provides a route for mechanical ventilation.

Conversation stopper

Drawbacks of ET intubation are that it bypasses normal respiratory defenses against infection, reduces cough effectiveness, may be uncomfortable and prevents verbal communication.

Potential complications of ET intubation include:

- Aspiration of blood, secretions or gastric contents
- Bronchospasm or laryngospasm
- Cardiac arrhythmias
- Hypoxaemia (if attempts at intubation are prolonged or oxygen delivery interrupted)
- Injury to the lips, mouth, pharynx or vocal cords
- Tooth damage or loss
- Tracheal stenosis, erosion and necrosis.

Open up

In orotracheal intubation, the oral cavity is used as the route of insertion. It's preferred in emergency situations because it's easier and faster. However, maintaining exact tube placement is more difficult because the tube must be well secured to avoid kinking and prevent bronchial obstruction or accidental extubation. It's also uncomfortable for conscious patients because it stimulates salivation, coughing and retching.

Be quick about it

Rapid sequence intubation (RSI) is the standard of care for ET intubation. RSI minimises the complications of endotracheal intubation, such as airway trauma and aspiration and is more comfortable for the patient. (See *The seven Ps of RSI*.)

The six Ps of RSI

Rapid sequence intubation (RSI) is used to rapidly produce optimal conditions for intubation in emergency situations, especially for patients who are conscious or combative but who need intubation.

Prepare patient and equipment

- Explain procedure to the patient. Reassure the patient that he will be asleep during the procedure as he will likely be very anxious
- Cardiac monitor and pulse oximeter to be attached to the patient
- Ensure equipment to be used is to hand and in good working order including suction.

Pre-oxygenate

- For instance, following the doctor's prescription, you may administer 100% O_2 for 3 minutes using a tight-fitting face mask with reservoir.

Pre-treatment

- A sedating agent will be prescribed
- Additional drugs maybe prescribed to minimise the effects of intubation.

Medication

- If there is time the doctor will prescribe a small dose of a non-depolarising paralytic (a defasciculating dose)
- Atropine sulphate maybe ordered to reduce the potential for bradycardia when using suxamethonium
- Sedation is given if the patient is haemodynamically stable (systolic BP greater than 90 Hg mm)

- A neuro-muscular block is undertaken using suxamethonium (usually takes 30 seconds and will be complete within 2 minutes).

Placement

- The larynx is compressed against the oesophagus (Sellick manoeuvre or posterior cricoid pressure) to prevent aspiration
- The patient is intubated rapidly. If not achieved within 30 seconds stop and ventilate slowly using a bag-valve mask whilst maintaining cricoid pressure to prevent regurgitation
- The cuff is inflated, stylet removed, position verified and cricoid pressure removed
- Endotracheal (ET) tube placement is verified by observation, auscultation, end-tidal carbon dioxide ($ETCO_2$) detector and chest X-ray.

Post-intubation management

- Secure the ET tube using tape or a commercial device. Ensure not too tight
- Maintain continuous $ETCO_2$ monitoring
- Continue sedation or paralysis as indicated
- Monitor the patient's response, including vital signs, arterial blood gas values, cardiac monitor and arterial oxygen saturation.

Not for everyone

Orotracheal intubation is contraindicated in patients with orofacial injuries, acute cervical spinal injury and degenerative spinal disorders.

Through the nose

Oral ET intubation is the preferred method of airway management in patients who are apnoeic. However, nasal intubation may be an alternative if the oral route is contraindicated. In nasal intubation, a nasal passage is used as the route of insertion. Nasal intubation is preferred for elective insertion when the patient is capable of spontaneous ventilation for a short period.

A conscious choice

Nasal intubation is more comfortable than oral intubation and is typically used in conscious patients who are at risk for imminent respiratory arrest or who have cervical spinal injuries. It's contraindicated in patients with facial or basilar skull fractures.

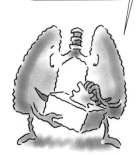

This tissue I can replace. I have less luck with the tissue damaged by nasal intubation.

Difficult and damaging

Although it's more comfortable than oral intubation, nasal intubation is more difficult to perform. Because the tube passes blindly through the nasal cavity, it causes more tissue damage, increases the risk of infection by nasal bacteria introduced into the trachea and increases the risk of pressure necrosis of the nasal mucosa.

Practice pointers
- If possible, explain the procedure to the patient and family
- Obtain the correct size of ET tube. The typical size for an oral ET tube is 7.5 mm (the size of the lumen) for women and 8 mm for men
- Administer medication, as ordered, to decrease respiratory secretions, induce amnesia and/or analgesia and help calm and relax the conscious patient. Remove dentures and bridgework, if present.

Note breath sounds
- After securing the ET tube, reconfirm tube placement by noting bilateral breath sounds and $ETCO_2$ readings
- Auscultate breath sounds and watch for chest movement to ensure correct tube placement and full lung ventilation
- A chest X-ray may be ordered to confirm tube placement
- Disposable $ETCO_2$ detectors are commonly used to confirm tube placement in EDs, postanesthesia care units and critical care units (CCUs) that don't use continual $ETCO_2$ monitoring. Follow the manufacturer's instructions for proper use of the device. Don't use the detector with a heated

humidifier or nebuliser because humidity, heat and moisture can interfere with the device
• Follow standard precautions and suction through the ET tube as the patient's condition indicates to clear secretions and prevent mucus plugs from obstructing the tube
• After suctioning, use a handheld resuscitation bag to hyperoxygenate the patient who's being maintained on a ventilator. (See *Understanding manual ventilation*)
• If available, use a closed tracheal suctioning system, which permits the ventilated patient to remain on the ventilator during suctioning.

Understanding manual ventilation

A handheld resuscitation bag is an inflatable device that can be attached to a face mask or directly to a tracheostomy or endotracheal (ET) tube to allow manual delivery of oxygen or room air to the lungs of a patient who can't breathe independently.

Although usually used in an emergency, manual ventilation can also be performed while the patient is disconnected temporarily from a mechanical ventilator (such as during a tubing change), during transport or before suctioning. In such instances, use of the handheld resuscitation bag maintains ventilation. Oxygen administration with a resuscitation bag can help improve a compromised cardiorespiratory system.

Ventilation guidelines

To manually ventilate a patient with an ET or tracheostomy tube, follow these guidelines:
• If oxygen is readily available, connect the handheld resuscitation bag to the oxygen. Attach one end of the tubing to the bottom of the bag and the other end to the nipple adapter on the flowmeter of the oxygen source
• Turn on the oxygen and adjust the flow rate according to the patient's condition

• Before attaching the handheld resuscitation bag, suction the ET or tracheostomy tube to remove any secretions that may obstruct the airway
• Remove the mask from the ventilation bag and attach the handheld resuscitation bag directly to the tube
• Keeping your nondominant hand on the connection of the bag to the tube, exert downward pressure to seal the mask against his face. For an adult patient, use your dominant hand to compress the bag every 5 seconds to deliver approximately 1 L of air

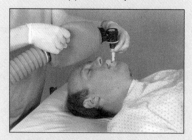

• Deliver breaths with the patient's own inspiratory effort if any is present. Don't attempt to deliver a breath as the patient exhales
• Observe the patient's chest to ensure that it rises and falls with each compression. If ventilation fails to occur, check the connection

and the patency of the patient's airway; if necessary, reposition his head and suction
• Be alert for possible underventilation, which commonly occurs because the handheld resuscitation bag is difficult to keep positioned while ensuring an open airway. In addition, the volume of air delivered to the patient varies with the type of bag used and the hand size of the person compressing the bag. An adult with a small- or medium-sized hand may not consistently deliver 1 L of air. For these reasons, have someone assist with the procedure, if possible
• Keep in mind that air is forced into the patient's stomach with manual ventilation, placing the patient at risk for aspiration of vomitus (possibly resulting in pneumonia) and gastric distention
• Record the date and time of the procedure, reason and length of time the patient was disconnected from mechanical ventilation and received manual ventilation, any complications and the nursing action taken and the patient's tolerance of the procedure.

Mechanical ventilation

Mechanical ventilation involves the use of a machine to move air into a patient's lungs. Mechanical ventilators use positive or negative pressure to ventilate patients.

When to ventilate

Indications for mechanical ventilation include:
- Acute respiratory failure due to ARDS, pneumonia, acute exacerbations of COPD, pulmonary embolus, heart failure, trauma, tumours or drug overdose
- Respiratory centre depression due to stroke, brain injury or trauma
- Neuromuscular disturbances caused by neuromuscular diseases, such as: Guillain-Barré syndrome, multiple sclerosis and myasthenia gravis; trauma, including spinal cord injury; or CNS depression.

Accentuate the positive

Positive pressure ventilators exert positive pressure on the airway, which causes inspiration while increasing tidal volume (V_T). A high-frequency ventilator uses high respiratory rates and low V_T to maintain alveolar ventilation.

The inspiratory cycles of these ventilators may be adjusted for volume, pressure or time:
- A volume-cycled ventilator (the type used most commonly) delivers a preset volume of air each time, regardless of the amount of lung resistance
- A pressure-cycled ventilator generates flow until the machine reaches a preset pressure, regardless of the volume delivered or the time required to achieve the pressure
- A time-cycled ventilator generates flow for a preset amount of time.
   Several different modes of ventilatory control are found on the ventilator. The choice of mode depends on the patient's respiratory condition.

Be alarmed

- Make sure the ventilator alarms are on at all times to alert you to potentially hazardous conditions and changes in the patient's status. If an alarm sounds and the problem can't be easily identified, disconnect the patient from the ventilator and use a handheld resuscitation bag to ventilate him
- Assess and record cardiopulmonary status as ordered. Assess vital signs and auscultate breath sounds. Monitor pulse oximetry or $ETCO_2$ levels and haemodynamic parameters as ordered. Monitor intake and output and assess for fluid volume excess or dehydration
- Administer a sedative or neuromuscular blocking agent, as ordered, to relax the patient or eliminate spontaneous breathing efforts that can interfere with the ventilator's action.

Be extra vigilant

- Remember that the patient receiving a neuromuscular blocking agent requires close observation because he can't breathe or communicate. In addition, if the patient is receiving a neuromuscular blocking agent, make sure he also receives a sedative. Neuromuscular blocking agents cause paralysis without altering the patient's level of consciousness. Reassure the patient and his family that the paralysis is temporary
- Provide emotional support to the patient during all phases of mechanical ventilation to reduce anxiety and promote successful treatment. Even if the patient is unresponsive, continue to explain all procedures and treatments.

Oxygen therapy

In oxygen therapy, oxygen is delivered by mask or nasal prongs to prevent or reverse hypoxaemia and reduce the workload of breathing. Oxygen is given by medical prescription or in critical situation immediately to maintain blood oxygenation within a prescribed target range in line with British Thoracic Society Guidelines. These guidelines are found at: http://www.brit-thoracic.org.uk/clinical-information/emergency-oxygen/emergency-oxygen-use-in-adult-patients.aspx.

Fully equipped

Therapy equipment depends on the patient's condition and the required fraction of inspired oxygen. High-flow systems, such as Venturi masks and ventilators, deliver a precisely controlled air oxygen mixture. Low-flow systems, such as nasal prongs or masks, allow variation in the oxygen percentage delivery based on the patient's respiratory pattern.

Concentrate on concentration

Nasal cannula provide a flow rate of 1-6L minute (oxygen concentration of 24%–44%). A Venturi mask delivers oxygen concentrations dependent on the adapter used and will be used for patients with Chronic Obstruction Pulmonary Disease (COPD) and other chronic respiratory diseases.

Practice pointers

- Be sure to humidify oxygen flow exceeding 3 L/minute to help prevent drying of mucous membranes. However, humidity isn't added with Venturi masks because water can block the Venturi jets
- Assess for signs of hypoxia, including decreased LOC, tachycardia, arrhythmias, diaphoresis, restlessness, altered blood pressure or respiratory rate, clammy skin and cyanosis. If these occur, notify the practitioner, obtain pulse oximetry readings and check the oxygen equipment to see if it's malfunctioning
- Use a low flow rate if your patient has COPD. However, don't use a simple face mask, because low flow rates won't flush carbon dioxide from the mask and the patient will rebreathe carbon dioxide. Watch for alterations in LOC, heart rate and respiratory rate, which may signal carbon dioxide narcosis or worsening hypoxaemia.

Surgery

If drugs or other therapeutic modes fail to maintain the patient's airway patency and protect healthy tissues from disease, surgery may be necessary. Some types of respiratory surgeries are chest-tube insertion and tracheotomy.

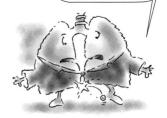

Chest-tube insertion gives me the chance to reinflate – maybe a little TOO much this time!

Chest-tube insertion

Chest-tube insertion may be needed when treating patients with pneumothorax, haemothorax, empyema or pleural effusion. The tube, which is inserted into the pleural space, allows blood, fluid, pus or air to drain and allows the lung to reinflate. Most chest tubes are placed at the fourth intercostal space in the anterior axillary line.

Gotta have some negative pressure

The tube restores negative pressure to the pleural space through an underwater-seal drainage system. The water in the system prevents air from being sucked back into the pleural space during inspiration. If a leak through the bronchi can't be sealed, suction applied to the underwater-seal system removes air from the pleural space faster than it can collect. The draining system may have one drainage bottle of increasingly multi-function chest drainage systems have been designed. These are used primarily for post-cardiothoracic surgery and chest trauma management. The multifunction systems allow single or multi-catheter drainage and are suitable for both gravity and suction-assisted drainage. The following gives general considerations. The nurse must be familiar with the equipment used in the department in which he or she works.

Practice pointers

• Assess respiratory function and obtain vital signs and oxygen saturation levels immediately after insertion. Routinely assess and record chest-tube function. Describe and record the amount of drainage. Notify the doctor immediately if the amount of drainage is greater than 200 ml in 1 hour (indicates bleeding)
• The fluid in the water-seal chamber typically rises on inspiration and decreases on expiration. However, if the patient is receiving positive-pressure ventilation, the opposite is normal
• Avoid creating dependent loops, kinks or pressure in the tubing. Don't lift the drainage system above the patient's chest because fluid may flow back into the pleural space. Keep two rubber-tipped clamps at the bedside to clamp the chest tube if the system cracks or to locate an air leak in the system. (See *Checking for chest-tube leaks*, page 248)
• If the drainage collection chamber fills, replace it according to your hospital's policy. To do so, double-clamp the chest tube close to the insertion site (using two clamps facing in opposite directions), exchange the system, remove the clamps and retape the connection

---

Checking for chest-tube leaks

When trying to locate a leak in your patient's chest-tube system, try:
- Briefly clamping the tube at various points along its length, beginning at the tube's proximal end and working down toward the drainage system
- Paying special attention to the seal around the connections
- Pushing any loose connections back together and taping them securely.

Bubble may mean trouble

The bubbling of the system stops when a clamp is placed between an air leak and the water seal. If you clamp along the tube's entire length and the bubbling doesn't stop, you probably need to replace the drainage unit because it may be cracked. Bubbling can indicate a bronchopleural leak.

- To prevent a tension pneumothorax (which can result when clamping stops air and fluid from escaping), never leave the chest tube clamped for more than 1 minute
- Notify the doctor immediately if the patient develops cyanosis, rapid or shallow breathing, subcutaneous emphysema, chest pain or excessive bleeding.

Tracheotomy

A tracheotomy is a surgical procedure that creates an opening into the trachea, called a *tracheostomy*. This opening allows insertion of an indwelling tube to keep the patient's airway open. The tracheostomy tube may be made of plastic, polyvinyl chloride or metal and comes in various sizes, lengths and styles, depending on the patient's needs. A patient receiving mechanical ventilation needs a cuffed tube to prevent backflow of air around the tube. A cuffed tracheostomy tube also prevents an unconscious or a paralyzed patient from aspirating food or secretions.

Emergency or planned procedure

In emergency situations, such as foreign body obstruction and laryngeal with anaphylactic shock, tracheotomy should be done as soon as possible.

Practice pointers
- Quickly obtain equipment and a tracheotomy tray
- Before an emergency tracheotomy, explain briefly the procedure to the patient if time permits and ensure that the patient has signed a consent form (provided they have mental capacity otherwise the doctor will carry out the procedure without consent as the treatment would be in the patient's best interest)
- Ensure that samples for ABG analysis and other diagnostic tests have been collected.

Afterward ward

- After the procedure, assess the patient's respiratory status, breath sounds, oxygen saturation levels, vital signs and heart rhythm. Note any crackles, wheezes or diminished breath sounds
- Assess the patient for such complications as haemorrhage, into tracheal tissue causing airway obstruction, aspiration of secretions, hypoxaemia and introduction of air into surrounding tissue causing subcutaneous emphysema
- Document the procedure: the amount, colour and consistency of secretions, stoma and skin conditions; the patient's respiratory status; the duration of any cuff deflation; and cuff pressure readings with inflation.

Common disorders

Some common respiratory disorders seen in the ED include airway obstruction, inhalation injuries, near drowning, pneumothorax and acute severe asthma.

Airway obstruction

The body uses coughing as its main mechanism to clear the airway. Yet coughing may not clear the airway during some disease states or even under normal, healthy conditions if an obstruction is present.

Upper airway obstruction is an interruption in the flow of air through the nose, mouth, pharynx or larynx. Obstruction of the upper airway is considered a life-threatening situation; if not recognised early, it will progress to respiratory arrest. Respiratory arrest will lead to cardiac arrest, which requires cardiopulmonary resuscitation (CPR).

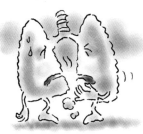

If coughing doesn't clear a patient's airway, he may have an obstruction.

What causes it

A patient's airway can become obstructed or compromised by vomitus, food or his tongue, teeth or saliva. Although there are several causes of upper airway obstruction, the most common cause is the tongue. Because muscle tone decreases when a person is unconscious or unresponsive, the potential for the tongue and epiglottis to obstruct the airway increases. Partial airway obstruction is commonly caused by oedema or a small foreign object that doesn't completely obstruct the airway.

It's anatomical

The presence of oedema – oedema of tongue (caused by trauma), laryngeal oedema and smoke inhalation oedema – in anatomical structures of the upper airway can lead to an upper airway obstruction. Other potential causes include:
- Anaphylaxis
- Aspiration of a foreign object
- Burns to the head, face or neck area
- Cerebral disorders (stroke)
- Croup

- Epiglottitis
- Laryngospasms
- Peritonsillar or pharyngeal abscesses
- Tenacious secretions in the airway
- Trauma of the face, trachea or larynx
- Tumours of the head or neck.

How it happens

In airway obstructions, the patient is partially able or not able to take in oxygen through inhalation. Hypoxaemia results the longer the obstruction remains.

What to look for

Prompt detection and intervention can prevent a partial airway obstruction from progressing to a complete airway obstruction. Signs of a partial airway obstruction include diaphoresis, tachycardia, coughing and elevated blood pressure. Patients with a partial obstruction may also experience no symptoms. With a complete airway obstruction, the following symptoms may be observed:
- Sudden onset of choking or gagging
- Stridor
- Cyanosis
- Wheezing, whistling or any other unusual breath sound that indicates breathing difficulty
- Diminished breath sounds (bilateral or unilateral)
- Sense of impending doom.

What tests tell you

Physical examination may indicate decreased breath sounds. Tests aren't usually necessary to diagnose an upper airway obstruction but may include X-rays (particularly a chest X-ray), bronchoscopy and laryngoscopy. If there are persistent symptoms of an upper airway obstruction, a chest X-ray, neck X-rays, laryngoscopy or CT scan may be ordered to rule out the presence of a tumour, foreign body or infection.

How it's treated

- Rapid assessment of airway patency, breathing and circulation are foremost. (See *Opening an obstructed airway*.)
- Promptly assess the obstruction's cause. When an obstruction relates to the tongue or an accumulation of tenacious secretions, place the head in a slightly extended position and insert an oral airway
- Promptly remove objects visible in the mouth with suction, fingers or Magill forceps
- If the patient can breathe (partial obstruction) encourage him to sit forward and cough to relieve the obstruction. However, be aware that this might worsen the obstruction and may totally occlude the airway
- ET intubation and removal of the foreign object during insertion of the laryngoscope enables visualisation of the obstruction
- If an oral or ET airway doesn't provide ventilation, emergency cricothyroidotomy is indicated.

Opening an obstructed airway

To open an obstructed airway, use the head-tilt, chin-lift manoeuvre or the jaw-thrust manoeuvre as described here.

Head-tilt, chin-lift manoeuvre

In many cases of airway obstruction, the muscles controlling the patient's tongue have relaxed, causing the tongue to obstruct the airway. If the patient doesn't appear to have a neck injury, use the head-tilt, chin-lift manoeuvre to open his airway. Use these four steps to carry out this manoeuvre:

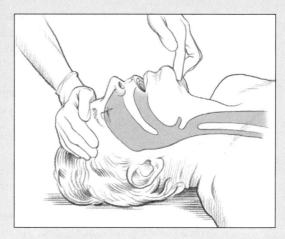

Place your hand that's closest to the patient's head on his forehead

Apply firm pressure – firm enough to tilt the patient's head back

Place the fingertips of your other hand under the bony portion of the patient's lower jaw, near the chin

Lift the patient's chin. Be sure to keep his mouth partially open. Avoid placing your fingertips on the soft tissue under the patient's chin because this may inadvertently obstruct the airway you're trying to open.

Using the jaw-thrust manoeuvre

If you suspect a neck or spinal injury, use the jaw-thrust manoeuvre to open the patient's airway. Use these four steps to carry out this manoeuvre:

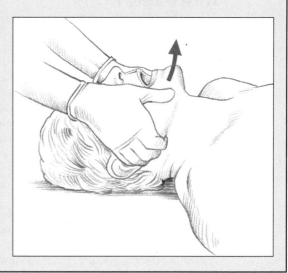

Kneel at the patient's head with your elbows on the ground (if the patient is on the floor)

Rest your thumbs on the patient's lower jaw near the corners of his mouth, pointing your thumbs toward his feet

Place your fingertips around the lower jaw

To open the airway, lift the lower jaw with your fingertips (as shown).

What to do
- Assess for the cause of the obstruction
- Assess the patient's breath sounds bilaterally
- Monitor oxygen saturation (using pulse oximetry) and cardiac rhythm continuously
- Continually assess for stridor, cyanosis and changes in LOC and notify the practitioner immediately if any of these changes occur
- Prepare for ET intubation if an airway can't be established
- Prepare for a cricothyroidotomy if the patient's ventilation isn't established by oral or ET intubation
- Anticipate cardiac arrest if the obstruction isn't cleared promptly
- Monitor chest X-ray and ABG results after the obstruction is relieved.

Inhalation injuries

Inhalation injuries result from trauma to the pulmonary system after inhalation of toxic substances or inhalation of gases that are nontoxic but interfere with cellular respiration. Inhaled exposure forms include fog, mist, fume, dust, gas, vapour or smoke. Inhalation injuries commonly accompany burns.

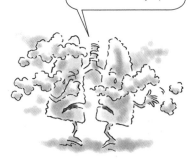

Fog, fumes, dust, gas – you name it! If it floats, it can probably cause inhalation injury.

What causes it?
There are many causes of inhalation injuries, including carbon monoxide poisoning and chemical and thermal inhalation.

Carbon monoxide poisoning
Carbon monoxide is a colourless, odourless, tasteless gas produced as a result of combustion and oxidation. Inhaling small amounts of this gas over a long period of time (or inhaling large amounts in a short period of time) can lead to poisoning. Carbon monoxide is considered a chemical asphyxiant. Accidental poisoning can result from exposure to heaters, smoke from a fire or use of a gas lamp, gas stove or charcoal grill in a small, poorly ventilated area.

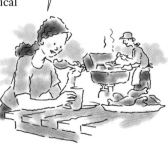

Accidental carbon monoxide poisoning can make any barbeque blue, so make sure to grill in a well-ventilated area.

Chemical inhalation
A wide variety of gases may be generated when materials burn. The acids and alkalis produced in the burning process can produce chemical burns when inhaled. The inhaled substances can reach the respiratory tract as insoluble gases and lead to permanent damage. Synthetic materials also produce gases that can be toxic. Plastic material has the ability to produce toxic vapours when heated or burned.

Inhaling unburned chemicals in a powder or liquid form can also cause pulmonary damage. Such substances as ammonia, cyanide, chlorine, sulphur dioxide and hydrogen chloride are considered pulmonary irritants.

Thermal inhalation

Pulmonary complications remain the leading cause of death following thermal inhalation trauma. This type of trauma is commonly caused by the inhalation of hot air or steam. The mortality rate exceeds 50% when inhalation injury accompanies burns of the skin. This type of injury should be suspected when the circumstances associated with the patient's injuries involves flames in a confined area, even if burns on the surface of the patient's skin aren't visible.

Other complications

Pulmonary complications can arise from tight eschar formation on the chest from circumferential chest burns. The eschar can restrict chest movement or can impair ventilation from compression of the anatomical structures of the throat and neck. Visual assessment of the chest will reveal the ease of respirations, depth of chest movement, rate of respirations and respiratory effort.

How it happens
Carbon monoxide poisoning

There are several gases (such as carbon monoxide and hydrogen cyanide) that are nontoxic to the respiratory system directly yet interfere with cellular respiration. Carbon monoxide has a greater attraction to haemoglobin than oxygen. When carbon monoxide enters the blood, it binds with the haemoglobin to form carboxyhaemoglobin. Carboxyhaemoglobin reduces the oxygen-carrying capacity of haemoglobin. This reduction results in decreased oxygenation to the cells and tissues.

Chemical inhalation

Irritating gases (chlorine, hydrogen chloride, nitrogen dioxide, phosgene and sulphur dioxide) commonly combine with water in the lungs to form corrosive acids. These acids cause denaturation of proteins, cellular damage and oedema of the pulmonary tissues. Smoke inhalation injuries generally fall into this category. Chemical burns to the airway are similar to burns on the skin, except that they're painless. The tracheobronchial tree is insensitive to pain. The inhalation of small quantities of noxious chemicals can also damage the alveoli and bronchi.

Thermal inhalation

Inhaled hot air or steam is rapidly cooled by the upper airway. Because the hot air or steam is confined to this area, the upper airway suffers the greatest damage. Inhaled hot air or steam can also injure the lower respiratory tract because water holds heat better than dry air. Even so, this injury is rare because reflexive closure of the vocal cords and laryngeal spasm commonly prevent full inhalation of the hot air or steam.

What to look for

Physical findings with an inhalation injury vary depending on the gas or substance inhaled and the duration of the exposure.

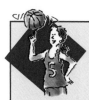

Stay on the ball

Oxygen saturation in CO poisoning

When assessing for carbon monoxide (CO) poisoning, be aware that pulse oximetry devices measure oxygenated and deoxygenated haemoglobin but don't measure dysfunctional haemoglobin such as carboxyhaemoglobin. Therefore, the oxygen saturation levels in the presence of carbon monoxide poisoning will be within normal ranges, as the carboxyhaemoglobin levels aren't measured.

Carbon monoxide poisoning

Carboxyhaemoglobin reduces the oxygen-carrying capacity of haemoglobin. This reduction commonly causes the patient's face to turn bright red and the lips cherry red. The symptoms of carbon monoxide (CO) poisoning vary with the concentration of carboxyhaemoglobin. (See *Oxygen saturation in CO poisoning*.)

When it's a little ...

Mild poisoning generally indicates a CO level from 11% to 20%. Symptoms at this concentration commonly include:
- Slight shortness of breath
- Headache
- Decreased visual acuity
- Decreased cerebral function.

When it's a lot ...

Moderate poisoning indicates a CO level from 21% to 41%. Symptoms at this concentration include:
- Altered mental status
- Confusion
- Headache
- Tinnitus
- Dizziness
- Drowsiness
- Irritability
- Nausea
- Changes in skin colour
- Electrocardiograph (ECG) changes
- Tachycardia
- Hypotension
- Stupor.

And when it's way too much ...

Severe poisoning is defined as a level of CO from 42% to 60%. Symptoms include:
- Convulsions
- Coma
- Generalised instability.

In the final stage (fatal poisoning), the CO level reaches 61% to 80% and results in death.

Chemical inhalation

The most common effects of smoke or chemical inhalation include atelectasis, pulmonary oedema and tissue anoxia. Respiratory distress usually occurs early in the course of smoke inhalation secondary to hypoxia. Patients also exhibiting no respiratory difficulties may suddenly develop respiratory distress. Intubation and mechanical ventilation equipment should be available for immediate use.

Thermal inhalation

The entire respiratory tract has the potential to be damaged by thermal inhalation injury; however, injury rarely progresses to the lungs. Ulcerations, erythema and oedema of the mouth and epiglottis are the initial symptoms of this type of injury. Oedema may rapidly progress to upper airway obstruction. You may also note stridor, wheezing, rales, increased secretions, hoarseness and shortness of breath. Direct thermal injury to the upper airway yields burns of the face and lips, burned nasal hairs and laryngeal oedema.

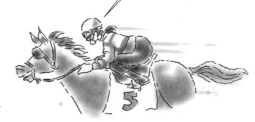

'Hoarse'-ness is a common symptom of thermal inhalation ... just like the silence I'm hearing now is a common symptom of bad puns.

What tests tell you

Initial laboratory studies commonly include urea and electrolytes, liver function studies and a full blood count (FBC). Obtaining these studies will provide baseline data for analysis. ABG analysis will provide valuable information on the acid-base status, ventilation and oxygenation status of the patient. In patients with suspected CO poisoning, a carboxyhaemoglobin level will be obtained. Cardiac monitoring will monitor ischaemic changes and ECG and chest X-ray will also be evaluated. A depressed ST segment on ECG is a common finding in the moderate stage of CO poisoning.

How it's treated

- Assessment (ABCDE) and resuscitative interventions are your first priority
- Obtain a history of the exposure and attempt to identify the toxic agent of exposure
- Immediately provide oxygen to the patient. Intubation and mechanical ventilation may be required if the patient demonstrates severe respiratory distress or an altered mental state
- Upper airway oedema requires urgent ET intubation
- Bronchodilators, antibiotics and I.V. fluids may be prescribed

- The preferred treatment for CO poisoning is administering 100% humidified oxygen and continuing until carboxyhaemoglobin levels fall to the nontoxic range of 10%
- Chest physical therapy may assist in the removal of necrotic tissue
- The use of hyperbaric oxygen for CO poisoning remains controversial, although it's known to lower carboxyhaemoglobin levels faster than humidified oxygen
- Fluid resuscitation is an important component of managing inhalation injury; however, careful monitoring of fluid status is essential because of the risk of pulmonary oedema.

What to do
- Remove the patient's clothing, but take care to prevent self-contamination from the toxic substance if the clothing has possibly been exposed to it
- Establish I.V. access for medication, blood products and fluid administration
- Obtain laboratory specimens to evaluate ventilation, oxygenation and baseline values
- Obtain chest X-ray, ECG and pulmonary function studies
- Implement cardiac monitoring to assess for ischaemic changes or arrhythmias
- Monitor for signs of pulmonary oedema that may accompany fluid resuscitation
- In the event of bronchospasms, provide oxygen, bronchodilators via a nebuliser and, possibly, aminophylline
- Monitor fluid balance and intake and output closely
- Administer antibiotics as prescribed
- Assess lung sounds frequently and notify the practitioner immediately of changes in those sounds or oxygenation
- Provide a supportive and educative environment for the patient, his family and significant others. (See *Inhalation injury in children*)
- Monitor laboratory studies for changes that may indicate multisystem complications.

Ages and stages
Inhalation injury in children

It's essential that your care of a child with inhalation injury address the emotional and psychological needs of the child and his family. Initially, care will focus on oxygenating and stabilising the child and managing the physical components of his injury. However, your care must eventually encompass the psychological needs of the frightened child and the emotional needs of his parents.

Parents may feel guilt if the injury could have been prevented or even if it couldn't. Be sure to provide information to the parents about their child's condition, prognosis, treatment plan and discharge needs. In addition to on going communication, psychological intervention may be needed to discuss feelings of guilt, emotional stress or fears of the parent and child.

Near drowning

Near drowning refers to surviving – at least temporarily – the physiologic effects of hypoxaemia and acidosis that result from submersion in fluid. Hypoxaemia and acidosis are the primary problems in victims of near drowning. Accidental drowning claimed 312 lives in 2006 in the UK. In 2007 27 children under 15 years of age died in the UK due to drowning and 170 were admitted to hospital following near drowning incidents.

What causes it

Near drowning results from an inability to swim or, in swimmers, from panic, a boating accident, a heart attack, a blow to the head while in the water, heavy drinking before swimming or a suicide attempt.

Near drowning takes three forms:
• *Dry*, in which the victim doesn't aspirate fluid but suffers respiratory obstruction or asphyxia (10% to 15% of patients)
• *Wet*, in which the victim aspirates fluid and suffers from asphyxia or secondary changes due to fluid aspiration (about 85% of patients)
• *Secondary*, in which the victim suffers a recurrence of respiratory distress (usually aspiration pneumonia or pulmonary oedema) within minutes or 1 to 2 days after a near-drowning incident.

How it happens

Regardless of the type of the fluid aspirated, hypoxaemia is the most serious consequence of near drowning, followed by metabolic acidosis. Other consequences depend on the kind of water aspirated.

After freshwater aspiration, changes in the character of lung surfactant result in exudation of protein-rich plasma into the alveoli. These changes, plus increased capillary permeability, lead to pulmonary oedema and hypoxaemia. (See *Physiologic changes in near drowning*, page 258.)

After saltwater aspiration, the hypertonicity of seawater exerts an osmotic force that pulls fluid from pulmonary capillaries into the alveoli. The resulting intrapulmonary shunt causes hypoxaemia. Also, the pulmonary capillary membrane may be injured and induce pulmonary oedema. In both kinds of near drowning, pulmonary oedema and hypoxaemia take place secondary to aspiration.

I like some aspirations: a good job, a happy home life. But freshwater and saltwater are aspirations I could do without.

What to look for

Near-drowning victims can display a host of clinical problems, including:
• Fever
• Confusion
• Unconsciousness
• Irritability
• Lethargy
• Restlessness
• Substernal chest pain
• Shallow or gasping respirations

Physiologic changes in near drowning

This flowchart shows the primary cellular alterations that occur during near drowning. Separate pathways are shown for saltwater and freshwater incidents. Hypothermia presents a separate pathway that may preserve neurologic function by decreasing the metabolic rate. All pathways lead to diffuse pulmonary oedema.

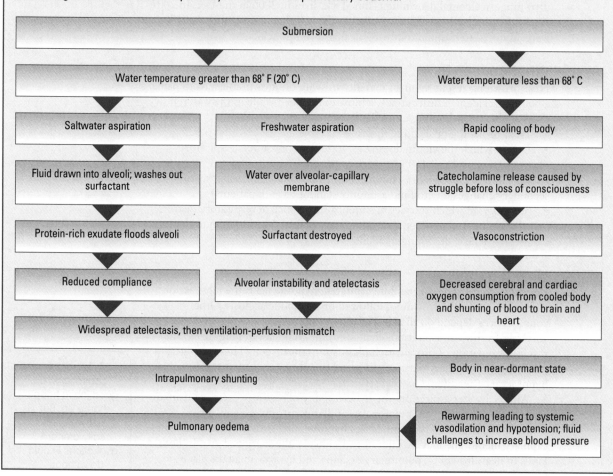

- Cough that produces a pink, frothy fluid
- Vomiting
- Abdominal distention
- Apnoea
- Asystole
- Bradycardia
- Tachycardia.

What tests tell you

Diagnosis requires a history of near drowning, including the type of water aspirated, along with characteristic features and auscultation of crackles and wheezing.

ABG analysis shows decreased oxygen content, low bicarbonate levels and low pH. Electrolyte levels may be elevated or decreased, depending on the type of water aspirated. Leukocytosis may occur. ECG shows arrhythmias and waveform changes.

How it's treated

- Assessment ABCDE
- Emergency treatment begins with CPR and administration of 100% oxygen
- If hypothermia is an issue, measures must be taken to warm the patient
- Ongoing support and monitoring of circulation and oxygenation should be maintained and haemodynamic monitoring should be instituted.

What to do

- Stabilise the patient's neck in case he has a cervical injury
- Assess for a patent airway and be prepared to administer high-flow oxygen and assist with ET intubation
- Assess the patient's core body temperature and be prepared to institute rewarming as necessary
- Continue CPR, intubation of the patient and provide respiratory assistance, such as mechanical ventilation with positive end-expiratory pressure (PEEP), if needed
- Assess ABG and pulse oximetry values
- If the patient's abdomen is distended, insert a nasogastric tube. (Intubate the patient first if he's unconscious)
- Start I.V. lines and insert an indwelling urinary catheter
- Give medications as ordered; drug treatment for near-drowning victims is controversial. Such treatment may include antibiotics to prevent infections and bronchodilators to ease bronchospasms
- Observe for pulmonary complications and signs of delayed drowning (confusion, substernal pain, adventitious breath sounds). Suction often. Pulmonary artery catheters may be useful in assessing cardiopulmonary status
- Monitor vital signs, intake and output and peripheral pulses.
- Check for skin perfusion and watch for signs of infection
- To facilitate breathing, raise the head of the bed slightly
- Prepare to administer prophylactic antibiotics as needed
- Correct acid-base imbalances
- Prepare the patient for transfer to an ICU or, if patient is a child, to a paediatric unit or facility.

> Make sure to check the near drowning patient's core body temperature to assess for hypothermia.

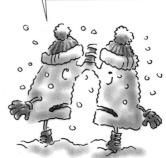

Pneumothorax

Pneumothorax is an accumulation of air in the pleural cavity that leads to partial or complete lung collapse. The amount of air trapped in the intrapleural space determines the degree of lung collapse. In some cases, venous return to the heart is impeded, causing a life-threatening condition called *tension pneumothorax*.

Pneumothorax can be classified as *traumatic* or *spontaneous*. Traumatic pneumothorax may be further classified as *open* or *closed*. (Note that an open, or penetrating, *wound* may cause *closed* pneumothorax.) Spontaneous pneumothorax, which is also considered *closed*, is most common the older adult with COPD but can appear in young, healthy patients as well. Spontaneous pneumothorax can occur with minimal signs and symptoms, classically in tall thin young men, this may be something that has happened before and the patient will tell you what is wrong or might only be detected on X-ray.

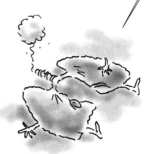

Air plus pleural cavity equals partial or complete lung collapse.

What causes it

The causes of pneumothorax vary according to classification.

Traumatic pneumothorax

Traumatic pneumothorax may be open or closed.

Open book

Causes of open pneumothorax include:
- Penetrating chest injury (stab or gunshot wound)
- Insertion of a central venous catheter
- Thoracentesis or closed pleural biopsy
- Transbronchial biopsy
- Chest surgery.

Closed call

Causes of closed pneumothorax include:
- Blunt chest trauma
- Interstitial lung disease such as eosinophilic granuloma
- Tubercular or cancerous lesions that erode into the pleural space
- Air leakage from ruptured blebs
- Rupture resulting from barotrauma caused by high intrathoracic pressures during mechanical ventilation.

Spontaneous pneumothorax

Spontaneous pneumothorax is usually caused by the rupture of a subpleural bleb (a small cystic space) at the surface of a lung.

Tension pneumothorax

Causes of tension pneumothorax include:
- Penetrating chest wound treated with an airtight dressing
- Fractured ribs
- Mechanical ventilation
- Chest tube occlusion or malfunction
- High-level PEEP that causes alveolar blebs to rupture.

How it happens

Traumatic pneumothorax

Open pneumothorax results from atmospheric air flowing directly into the pleural cavity (under negative pressure). As the air pressure in the pleural cavity becomes positive, the lung on the affected side collapses, causing decreased total lung capacity. As a result, the patient develops a V imbalance that leads to hypoxia.

Closed pneumothorax results when an opening is created between the intrapleural space and the parenchyma of the lung. Air enters the pleural space from within the lung, causing increased pleural pressure and preventing lung expansion during inspiration.

Spontaneous pneumothorax

In spontaneous pneumothorax, the rupture of a subpleural bleb causes air leakage into the pleural spaces, which causes the lung to collapse. Hypoxia results from decreased total lung capacity, vital capacity and lung compliance.

Tension pneumothorax

Tension pneumothorax results when air in the pleural space is under higher pressure than air in the adjacent lung. (See *Understanding tension pneumothorax*, page 262.) Here's what happens:
- Air enters the pleural space from the site of pleural rupture, which acts as a one-way valve. Thus, air enters the pleural space on inspiration but can't escape as the rupture site closes on expiration
- More air enters with each inspiration and air pressure begins to exceed barometric pressure
- The air pushes against the recoiled lung, causing compression atelectasis, and pushes against the mediastinum, compressing and displacing the heart and great vessels
- The mediastinum eventually shifts away from the affected side, affecting venous return and putting ever greater pressure on the heart, great vessels, trachea and contralateral lung. Without immediate treatment, this emergency can rapidly become fatal.

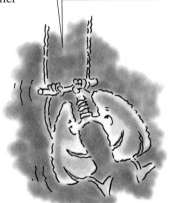

I try my best to hang loose – tension just isn't my thing, and neither is tension pneumothorax.

What to look for

Assessment findings depend on the severity of the pneumothorax. Spontaneous pneumothorax that releases a small amount of air into the pleural space may cause no signs or symptoms. Generally, tension pneumothorax causes the most severe respiratory signs and symptoms.

Understanding tension pneumothorax

In tension pneumothorax, air accumulates intrapleurally and can't escape. As intrapleural pressure increases, the lung on the affected side collapses.

On inspiration, the mediastinum shifts toward the unaffected lung, impairing ventilation.

On expiration, the mediastinal shift distorts the vena cava and reduces venous return.

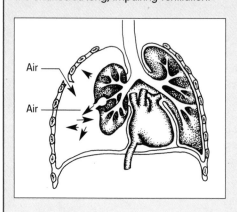

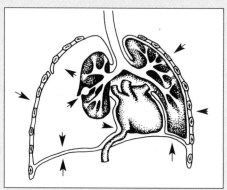

Every breath hurts

Your patient's history reveals sudden, sharp, pleuritic chest pain. The patient may report that chest movement, breathing and coughing exacerbate the pain. He may also report shortness of breath.

Further findings

Inspection reveals asymmetric chest wall movement with overexpansion and rigidity on the affected side. The skin may be cool, clammy and cyanotic. Palpation of the chest wall may reveal crackling beneath the skin (subcutaneous emphysema) and decreased vocal fremitus.

In addition, percussion may reveal hyperresonance on the affected side. Auscultation may disclose decreased or absent breath sounds on the affected side. Vital signs may follow the pattern of respiratory distress seen with respiratory failure.

Did we mention the tension?

Tension pneumothorax also causes:
• Distended jugular veins as a result of high intrapleural pressure, mediastinal shift and increased cardiovascular pressure
• Hypotension and tachycardia due to decreased cardiac output
• Tracheal deviation to the opposite side (a late sign).

What tests tell you
• Chest X-rays reveal air in the pleural space and a mediastinal shift, which confirm pneumothorax
• ABG analysis reveals hypoxaemia, usually with elevated $PaCO_2$ and normal bicarbonate ion levels in the early stages
• ECG may reveal decreased QRS amplitude, precordial T-wave inversion and rightward shift of the frontal QRS axis.

How it's treated
Treatment of pneumothorax depends on the cause and severity.

With trauma

Open or closed pneumothorax may necessitate surgical repair of affected tissues, followed by chest-tube placement with an underwater seal.

With less lung collapse

Spontaneous pneumothorax with less than 30% lung collapse, no signs of increased pleural pressure and no dyspnoea or indications of physiologic compromise may be corrected with:
• Aspiration of air from the intrapleural space with a large-bore needle attached to a syringe to restore negative pressure within the pleural space
• Oxygen administration to improve hypoxia
• Vital signs monitoring to detect physiologic compromise.

With more lung collapse

Lung collapse greater than 30% may necessitate other measures, such as:
• Placing a chest tube in the 5th or 6th intercostal space anterior mid-axillary line to re-expand the lung by restoring negative intrapleural pressure
• Connecting the chest tube to an underwater seal or a low-pressure suction to re-expand the lung.

With tension

Treatment for tension pneumothorax typically involves:
• Analgesics to promote comfort and encourage deep breathing and coughing
• Immediate large-bore needle insertion into the pleural space through the 2nd intercostal space mid-clavicular line to re-expand the lung, followed by insertion of a chest tube if large amounts of air escape through the needle after insertion.

What to do
• Assess the patient's respiratory status, including auscultation of bilateral breath sounds
• Monitor oxygen saturation levels closely for changes; obtain ABG analysis as ordered

- Monitor haemodynamic parameters frequently, as appropriate and indicated. Anticipate the need for cardiac monitoring because hypoxaemia can predispose the patient to arrhythmias
- Initiate and maintain vascular access
- Watch for complications, signalled by pallor, gasping respirations and sudden chest pain. Carefully monitor vital signs at least every hour for indications of shock, increasing respiratory distress or mediastinal shift. If your patient's respiratory status deteriorates, anticipate the need for ET intubation and mechanical ventilation and assist as necessary
- Assist with chest-tube insertion and connect to suction as ordered. Monitor your patient for possible complications associated with chest-tube insertion
- Maintain bed rest in high Fowler's position.

Acute severe asthma

Acute severe asthma is a potentially life-threatening situation. It begins with impaired gas exchange and – without rapid intervention – may lead to respiratory failure and, eventually, death. Patients present with:

- Wheeze
- Breathlessness
- Cough.

Asthma overview

Asthma is a chronic inflammatory airway disorder that causes episodic airway obstruction and hyperresponsiveness of the airway to multiple stimuli. It results from bronchospasms, increased mucus secretion and mucosal oedema.

Giving evidence-based care

You should ensure that you are delivering asthma care guided by the most recent guidelines from the British Thoracic Society. These can be found at – www.brit-thoracic.org.uk.

Making things worse

Asthma exacerbations are acute or subacute episodes of worsening shortness of breath, coughing and wheezing, with measurable decreases in expiratory airflow.

What causes it

Many asthmatics, especially children, have intrinsic and extrinsic asthma.

Outside factors

Extrinsic (or *atopic*) asthma begins in childhood. Patients are typically sensitive to specific external allergens. Extrinsic allergens that can trigger an asthma attack include pollen, animal dander, house dust or mold, kapok or feather pillows, food additives containing sulphites and other sensitising substances.

Extrinsic asthma in childhood is commonly accompanied by other hereditary allergies, such as eczema and allergic rhinitis.

Factors within

Patients with intrinsic (or *nonatopic*) asthma react to internal, nonallergenic factors. Intrinsic factors that can trigger an asthma attack include irritants, emotional stress, fatigue, endocrine changes, temperature variations, humidity variations, exposure to noxious fumes, anxiety, coughing or laughing and genetic factors. Most episodes take place after a severe respiratory tract infection, especially in adults.

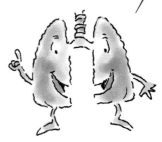

Irritants in the workplace – and no, the guy who hogs the copier doesn't count – can exacerbate existing asthma.

Irritants in the workplace

Many adults acquire an allergic form of asthma or exacerbation of existing asthma from exposure to agents in the workplace. Irritants include chemicals in flour, acid anhydrides and excreta of dust mites in carpet.

Genetic messes

Asthma is associated with two genetic influences:

 Ability to develop asthma because of an abnormal gene (atopy)

Tendency to develop hyperresponsive airways (without atopy).

A potent mix

Environmental factors interact with inherited factors to cause asthmatic reactions with associated bronchospasms.

How it happens

Acute severe asthma presentation may have a history of a worsening condition over minutes or days. The patient may then deteriorate suddenly and be even admitted as a respiratory or cardio-respiratory arrest. In asthma, bronchial linings overreact to various stimuli, causing episodic smooth-muscle spasms that severely constrict the airways. Here's how asthma develops into:

• Immunoglobulin (Ig) E antibodies attached to histamine-containing mast cells and receptors on cell membranes initiate intrinsic asthma attacks

• When exposed to an antigen, such as pollen, the IgE antibody combines with it

• On subsequent exposure to the antigen, mast cells degranulate and release mediators

• Mast cells in the lung are stimulated to release histamine and the slow-reacting substance of anaphylaxis.

Attachment disorder

- Histamine attaches to receptor sites in the larger bronchi, where it causes swelling in smooth muscles
- Mucous membranes become inflamed, irritated and swollen. The patient may experience dyspnoea, prolonged expiration and an increased respiratory rate
- Leukotrienes attach to receptor sites in the smaller bronchi and cause local swelling of the smooth muscle
- Leukotrienes also cause prostaglandins to travel by way of the bloodstream to the lungs, where they enhance the effect of histamine. A wheeze may be audible during coughing – the higher the pitch, the narrower the bronchial lumen
- Histamine stimulates the mucous membranes to secrete excessive mucus, further narrowing the bronchial lumen.

A not-so-good goblet

- Goblet cells secrete viscous mucus that's difficult to cough up, resulting in coughing, wheezing, higher-pitched wheezing and increased respiratory distress. Mucosal oedema and thickened secretions further block the airways
- On inhalation, the narrowed bronchial lumen can still expand slightly, allowing air to reach the alveoli. On exhalation, increased intrathoracic pressure closes the bronchial lumen completely. Air enters but can't escape
- If the acute asthma is not treated hypoxaemia worsens and the expiratory rate and volume decrease even further
- Obstructed airways impede gas exchange and increase airway resistance. The patient labours to breathe
- As breathing and hypoxaemia tire the patient, the respiratory rate drops to normal, $PaCO_2$ levels rise and the patient hypoventilates from exhaustion
- Respiratory acidosis develops as $PaCO_2$ increases
- The situation becomes life-threatening when no air is audible on auscultation (a silent chest) and $PaCO_2$ rises to over 70 mm Hg
- Without treatment, the patient experiences acute respiratory failure.

What to look for
A patient who comes to the ED during a severe asthma attack may demonstrate:
- Increased respiratory rate, breathlessness
- Wheezing
- Coughing
- Inability to speak more than a few words before pausing for breath
- Use of accessory muscles
- Fatigue
- Decreasing LOC
- Inability to lay flat
- Pulsus paradoxus greater than 20 mm Hg
- Long expiratory phase

- SpO_2 less than 90%
- Hypoxaemia
- Hypercarbia (elevated $PaCO_2$)
- Hypotension
- Metabolic acidosis
- Confusion or coma
- Cyanosis.

What tests tell you

- Pulmonary function tests reveal decreased vital capacity and increased total lung and residual capacities during an acute attack. Peak and expiratory flow rate measurements are less than 60% of baseline
- Pulse oximetry commonly shows that oxygen saturation is less than 90%
- Chest X-ray may show hyperinflation with areas of atelectasis and flat diaphragm due to increased intrathoracic volume
- ABG analysis reveals decreasing PaO_2 and increasing $PaCO_2$
- ECG shows sinus tachycardia during an attack
- Sputum analysis may indicate increased viscosity, mucus plugs, presence of Curschmann's spirals (casts of airways), Charcot-Leyden crystals (breakdown products of eosinophils) and eosinophils themselves. Culture may disclose causative organisms if infection is the trigger
- FBC shows an increased eosinophil count secondary to inflammation and an elevated white blood cell count and granulocyte count if an acute infection is present.

How it's treated

In acute severe asthma, the patient is monitored closely for respiratory failure. Oxygen, bronchodilators, adrenaline, corticosteroids and nebuliser therapies may be ordered. The patient may be intubated and placed on mechanical ventilation if $PaCO_2$ increases or if he experiences respiratory arrest.

Treatment may include the use of:
- Humidified oxygen to correct dyspnoea, cyanosis and hypoxaemia
- Mechanical ventilation, which is necessary if the patient doesn't respond to initial ventilatory support and drugs or develops respiratory failure.

Bucking bronchos

- Bronchodilators, such as oxygen driven nebulised salbutamol to decrease bronchoconstriction, reduce bronchial airway oedema and increase pulmonary ventilation. Consider adding nebulised ipratropium bromide
- Corticosteroids, such as prednisolone, oral or IV, or IV hydrocortisone, to decrease airway inflammation reduce bronchial airway oedema and increase pulmonary ventilation
- Anticholinergics to increase the effects of bronchodilators
- Single dose IV magnesium in cases that are not responding
- Relaxation exercises to increase circulation and aid recovery from an asthma attack.

Practice pointers

- Position the patient in a sitting up position and offer reassurance and explanation
- Monitor and record vital signs and ABGs as indicated
- Maintain continuous pulse oximetry
- Provide high-percentage oxygen as ordered to main oxygen saturation levels at prescribed levels often requiring 15 L/minute with a high-flow mask
- Administer nebulised bronchodilators such as salbutamol and undertake peak flow readings
- Establish and maintain vascular access
- Intravenous steroids (hydrocortisone) maybe ordered)
- Antibiotics if evidence of a chest infection
- Commence IV fluids as ordered to maintain adequate hydration
- Prepare for possible ET intubation
- Auscultate for breath sounds
- Assess the patient's mental status for confusion, agitation or lethargy
- Initiate cardiac monitoring and be alert for cardiac arrhythmias related to bronchodilator therapy or hypoxaemia
- Obtain ordered tests such as CXR, FBC, U&E, C-reactive protein (CRP) and report results promptly
- When the acute phase is over, position the patient for maximum comfort, usually in semi-recumbent position. Encourage coughing to clear secretions
- Provide emotional support and reassurance.

Quick quiz

1. When auscultating for breath sounds in a patient's lungs, what causes crackles?
   A.   Secretions blocking the bronchial airways.
   B.   Collapsed or fluid-filled alveoli snapping open.
   C.   Foreign body obstructing the trachea.
   D.   Consolidation.

Answer: *B*. Crackles are caused by alveoli opening and are usually associated with fluid in the alveolar space.

2. Which ABG analysis results would you expect to find in a patient with acute respiratory failure?
   A.   pH 7.25, PaO$_2$ 48, PaCO$_2$ 55.
   B.   pH 7.40, PaO$_2$ 82, PaCO$_2$ 45.
   C.   pH 7.50, PaO$_2$ 60, PaCO$_2$ 30.
   D.   pH 7.30, PaO$_2$ 85, PaCO$_2$ 48.

Answer: *A*. The patient with a PaO$_2$ less than 50, a decreased pH and an elevated PaCO$_2$ is hypoxemic and in respiratory acidosis.

3. ET tubes have inflatable cuffs to:
  A. Measure pressure on tracheal tissues.
  B. Drain gastric contents.
  C. Prevent backflow of oxygen.
  D. Treat laryngeal oedema.

Answer: C. ET tube cuffs prevent backflow of oxygen so that it's delivered fully to the lungs.

4. Which condition is a cause of spontaneous pneumothorax?
  A. Fractured ribs.
  B. Rupture of a small cystic area on the lung's surface.
  C. Interstitial lung disease.
  D. Mechanical ventilation.

Answer: B. In spontaneous pneumothorax, the rupture of a subpleural bleb results in air leakage into the pleural spaces, causing lung collapse. Hypoxia results from decreased total lung capacity, vital capacity and lung compliance.

5. Why are chemical burns to the airway from inhalation injury usually painless?
  A. The chemical alters the patient's sense of perception.
  B. The patient immediately becomes unconscious after the injury.
  C. The tracheobronchial tree is insensitive to pain.
  D. The burn damages the nerves and the patient can't sense the pain.

Answer: C. Chemical burns to the airway are similar to burns on the skin, except that they're painless. The tracheobronchial tree is insensitive to pain. The inhalation of small quantities of noxious chemicals can also damage the alveoli and bronchi.

6. The preferred treatment for carbon monoxide (CO) poisoning is:
  A. Administration of 100% humidified oxygen.
  B. Sedation.
  C. Hyperbaric oxygen therapy.
  D. Corticosteroid therapy.

Answer: A. The preferred treatment for CO poisoning is administering 100% humidified oxygen until carboxyhaemoglobin levels fall to the nontoxic range of 10%.

Scoring

☆☆☆ If you answered all six questions correctly, breathe a big sigh of relief. You're a respiratory mastermind!

☆☆ If you answered four or five questions correctly, don't wait to exhale. You're an inspiration!

☆ If you answered fewer than four questions correctly, you're on the verge of expiration. Take a deep breath and dive back into the chapter!

Neurological emergencies (8)

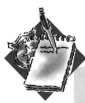

Just the facts

In this chapter, you'll learn:

♦ Key areas to assess when dealing with neurological emergencies

♦ Important diagnostic tests and procedures used for neurological emergencies

♦ Common neurological emergencies and their treatments.

Understanding neurological emergencies

The neurological system is a highly complex system that plays a major role in regulating many body functions. In the ED you're likely to encounter patients with common neurological emergencies, especially head trauma, increased intra cranial pressure (ICP), seizures, spinal cord injury, stroke, subarachnoid haemorrhage and extra and subdural haematomas. Regardless of the disorder, your priority is always to ensure assessment and prompt support of vital functioning – using the guide of airway, breathing, circulation, disability and exposure (ABCDE) as discussed in Chapter 3, *Initial assessment in emergency departments*.

When faced with an emergency, involving the neurological system, you must assess the patient thoroughly, always being alert for subtle neurological changes that might indicate a potential deterioration in the patient's condition. A focused assessment forms the basis for your interventions. These interventions must be instituted quickly to minimise the risks to the patient, which can be life-threatening. Often you will be involved in stabilising the patient's condition whilst he is waiting for neurosurgical intervention or whilst being transferred to a specialist (tertiary) neurosurgical unit, either by road or air ambulance.

Assessment

As patients with neurological conditions can deteriorate rapidly you must ensure that you conduct your initial assessment of ABCDE, including the Alert, Verbal, Painful, Unresponsive (AVPU) Scale and the Glasgow Coma Scale (GCS) assessment as soon as you receive the patient. (See *Using the Glasgow Coma Scale*, page 275). If the patient is drowsy or demonstrating any impairment in his level of consciousness (LOC), then ensure that you assess him for your baseline readings before the paramedic or the person who has brought the patient to the ED leaves the department. Ask yourself:

- Is the airway secure and ventilation adequate?
- Are the vital signs stable?
- Is there a non-neurological condition requiring immediate attention?
- Might there be an undiagnosed non-neurological medical reason such as diabetic ketoacidosis causing the symptoms?
- Have you undertaken a 'top to toe' examination to rule out other injuries?

Assessment of subtle and elusive changes in the complex nervous system can be difficult. When you assess a patient for possible neurological impairment, be sure to collect a thorough health history and investigate physical signs of impairment.

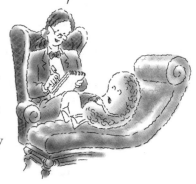

I know this is difficult, but a detailed history is the basis of neurologic emergency assessment.

Check the records

If you can't interview the patient because of his physical condition or mental impairment, you may gather history information from the patient's medical record. Family members and the paramedic team that transported the patient to the ED are important sources of information too. Patients or their families may have contacted a telephone advice service, such as NHS Direct, or community health services, such as general practitioners. Background information may be gained from these services also. Concerns regarding non-accidental injury must be referred to the appropriate bodies, such as the police or social services in line with hospital policies.

History

To collect a focused health history, gather details about the patient's current state of health, previous health status, lifestyle and family health.

Friends and family fill in

A patient with a neurological emergency may have trouble remembering or relating information. If the patient's family or close friends are available, include them in the assessment process. They may be able to corroborate or correct the details of the patient's health history.

Current health

Discover the patient's chief complaint by asking such questions as, 'Why did you come to the hospital?' or 'What has been bothering you lately?' Use the patient's words when you document these complaints.

Common complaints

If your patient is suffering from a neurological emergency, you may hear reports of headaches, motor disturbances (such as weakness, paresis, and paralysis), seizures, sensory deviations and altered LOC.

Details, please

Encourage the patient to describe details of the current condition by asking such questions as:
- Can you describe your headache?
- When did you start feeling dizzy?
- What were you doing when the numbness started?
- Have you ever had seizures or tremors? Have you ever had weakness or paralysis in your arms or legs?
- Do you have trouble urinating, walking, speaking, understanding others, reading or writing?
- How is your memory and ability to concentrate?

Previous health

Many chronic diseases affect the neurological system, so ask questions about the patient's past health and what medications he's taking. Specifically, ask whether the patient has had any:
- Major illnesses
- Recurrent minor illnesses
- Injuries
- History of hypertension
- Surgical procedures
- Allergies.

Lifestyle

Ask questions about the patient's cultural and social background because these affect care decisions. Note the patient's education level, occupation and hobbies. As you gather this information, also assess the patient's self-image. Also ask about smoking, alcohol consumption and recreational drug use. Be wary of ascribing a depressed LOC to drug or alcohol intoxication before brain injury has been excluded.

Physical examination

A complete neurological examination is long, detailed and unnecessary initially. The emergency nurse, the admitting doctor and/or the emergency nurse practitioner (ENP) will all contribute to this assessment. Because of the nature of the patient's condition, the examination will be limited to specific problem

A patient's hobbies can really 'play' into his neurologic assessment, so ask about them!

areas and the examination will be halted to intervene should the patient exhibit signs and symptoms of deterioration. If the initial screening indicates a neurological problem, the doctor may need to conduct a more detailed assessment.

You must be guided by your local practice and protocols. Work towards effective team work and communication to prevent the patient having assessments repeated unnecessarily. Ask your mentor and note the record keeping used in the ED where you are working.

Top-to-bottom examination

Examine the patient's neurological system in an orderly way. Beginning with the highest levels of neurological function and working down to the lowest, assess these five areas:

 Mental status

 Cranial nerve function

 Sensory function

 Motor function

 Reflexes.

Mental status
Mental status assessment begins when you talk to the patient. Responses to your questions reveal clues about the patient's orientation and memory. Use such clues as a guide during the physical assessment.

No easy answers

Be sure to ask questions that require more than yes-or-no answers, otherwise confusion or disorientation might not reveal themselves. If you have doubts about a patient's mental status, perform a screening examination. (See *Quick check of mental status*, page 274.)

Three-part exam

Use the mental status examination to check these three parameters:

 LOC

 Speech

 Cognitive function.

Level of consciousness
Watch for any change in the patient's LOC. It's the earliest and most sensitive indicator that his neurological status has changed.

Quick check of mental status

To quickly screen your patient for disordered thought processes, ask the questions below. An incorrect answer to any question may indicate the need for a complete mental status examination. Make sure that you (and the patient) know the correct answers before asking the questions. You may have to tell the patient the answers and then reassess. For instance, patients on spinal boards may not know where they are as they can only look upwards.

Question	Function screened
What's your name?	Orientation to person
What's your mother's name?	Orientation to other people
What year is it?	Orientation to time
What is the place that we're in?	Orientation to place
How old are you?	Memory
Where were you born?	Remote memory
What did you have for breakfast?	Recent memory
Who's the Prime Minister?	General knowledge
Can you count backwards from 20 to 1?	Attention span and calculation skills

Descriptions and definitions

Many terms are used to describe LOC, and definitions differ widely among practitioners. To avoid confusion, clearly describe the patient's response to various stimuli and *avoid* using words such as:

- Lethargic
- Stuporous
- Comatose.

Always start with a minimal stimulus, increasing intensity as necessary. The GCS offers an objective way to assess the patient's LOC. (See *Using the Glasgow Coma Scale*.)

Looking at LOC

Start by quietly observing the patient's behaviour. If the patient appears to be sleeping or unconscious, try to rouse him by providing an appropriate stimulus, in this order:

 Auditory

 Tactile

 Painful.

Using the Glasgow Coma Scale

You can use the GCS to describe the patient's baseline mental status and detect and interpret changes in his LOC.

To use the scale, test the patient's ability to respond to verbal, motor and sensory stimulation and score your findings based on the scale. A patient who's alert, can follow simple commands, and is oriented to time, place and person, will receive a score of 15 points. A lower score in one or more category may signal an impending neurological crisis. A GCS score of 8 or less means the airway is vulnerable and the patient is at risk of aspiration. A total score of 7 or less indicates severe neurological damage.

Test	Score	Patient's response
Eye-opening response		
Spontaneously	4	Opens eyes spontaneously
To speech	3	Opens eyes in response to verbal stimulus. (Child responds to shout or voice.)
To pain	2	Opens eyes only on painful stimulus
None	1	Doesn't open eyes in response to stimulus
Verbal response		
Oriented	5	Is oriented to person, place and time. (Child responds correct for age.)
Confused	4	Disorientated but can converse. (Child cries and/or uses inappropriate words for age.)
Inappropriate words	3	Replies randomly with incorrect word. (Child screams or cries inappropriately.)
Incomprehensible	2	Moans, screams or makes incomprehensible sounds. (Child grunts.)
None	1	Doesn't respond
Motor response		
Obeys commands	6	Responds to simple commands
Localises pain	5	Reaches towards painful stimulus and tries to remove it
Withdraws from pain	4	Moves away from painful stimulus
Abnormal flexion	3	Abnormal flexion to pain (a decorticate posture) shown below

Abnormal extension	2	Extends to pain (a decerebrate posture) shown below

None	1	Doesn't respond; just lies flaccid
Total score		

Speech

Listen to how well the patient expresses thoughts. Does he choose the correct words, or does he seem to have problems finding or articulating words?

It's hard to say

To assess for dysarthria (difficulty forming words), ask the patient to repeat the phrase 'No ifs, ands, or buts'. Assess speech comprehension by determining the patient's ability to follow instructions and cooperate with your examination.

Language changes

Keep in mind that language performance tends to fluctuate with the time of day and changes in physical condition. A healthy person may have language difficulty when ill or fatigued. Increasing speech difficulties may, however, indicate deteriorating neurological status, which warrants further evaluation. The patient may not speak English well, or not at all, so modify your questions, use picture cards or obtain a translator when possible.

When then who

To quickly test your patient's orientation, memory and attention span, use the mental status screening questions. Orientation to time is usually disrupted first; orientation to person, last.

Always consider the patient's environment and physical condition when assessing orientation. For example, a patient admitted to the ED may not be oriented to date because of the rapid activity, events and noise surrounding his transport to the department and the flurry of activity, bright lights and noise in the department itself, but he can still usually remember the year.

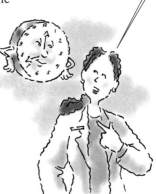

A patient's orientation to time is usually disrupted before his orientation to person.

Thought content

Disordered thought patterns may indicate delirium or psychosis. Assess thought pattern by evaluating the clarity and cohesiveness of the patient's ideas. Is his conversation smooth with logical transitions between ideas? Does he have hallucinations (sensory perceptions that lack appropriate stimuli) or delusions (beliefs not supported by reality)?

Insight on insight

Testing the patient's insight by finding out whether the patient:
- Has a realistic view of himself
- Is aware of his illness and circumstances.

Ask, for example, 'What do you think caused your back pain?' Expect different patients to have different degrees of insight. For instance, a patient may attribute chest discomfort to indigestion rather than acknowledge that he has had a heart attack.

Children

Assessing a child's LOC and mental status requires special consideration as a child may not be at a developmental age so as to respond to questioning as would an adult. It is essential to listen to the parents who can detect subtle changes in the child's condition. When assessing the child, note whether the child is alert and if he interacts with the environment. Medical history or recent signs and symptoms may offer clues to the child's condition, for instance, a post-ictal state following an unwitnessed fit or the child could be drowsy because of undiagnosed diabetic ketoacidosis.

Lost in emotion

Throughout the interview, assess your patient's emotional status. Note his mood, emotional lability or stability and the appropriateness of his emotional responses. Also, assess the patient's mood by asking how he feels about himself and his future. Keep in mind that signs and symptoms of depression in an older adult may be atypical. (See *Depression and older adults*.)

Cranial nerve function

Cranial nerve assessment reveals valuable information about the condition of the central nervous system (CNS), especially the brain stem. The 12 cranial nerves are the primary motor and sensory pathways between the brain and the head and neck. (See *Identifying cranial nerves*, page 278.)

Under pressure

Because of their location, some cranial nerves are more vulnerable to the effects of increasing ICP. Therefore, a neurological screening assessment of the CNS focuses on these key nerves:
- Oculomotor (III)
- Abducens (VI).

Get on some other nerves

The other nerves will be evaluated if the patient's history or symptoms indicate a potential CNS emergency or when performing a complete nervous system assessment.

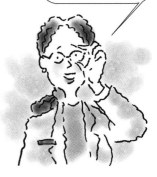

Remember that even healthy patients have different levels of inSIGHT.

Ages and stages

Depression and older adults

Symptoms of depression in older adults may be different from those found in other patients. For example, rather than the usual sad affect seen in patients with depression, older adults may exhibit such atypical signs as decreased function and increased agitation.

Identifying cranial nerves

The cranial nerves have sensory function, motor function or both. They're assigned Roman numerals and written this way: CN I, CN II, CN III and so on. The locations of the cranial nerves as well as their functions are shown below.

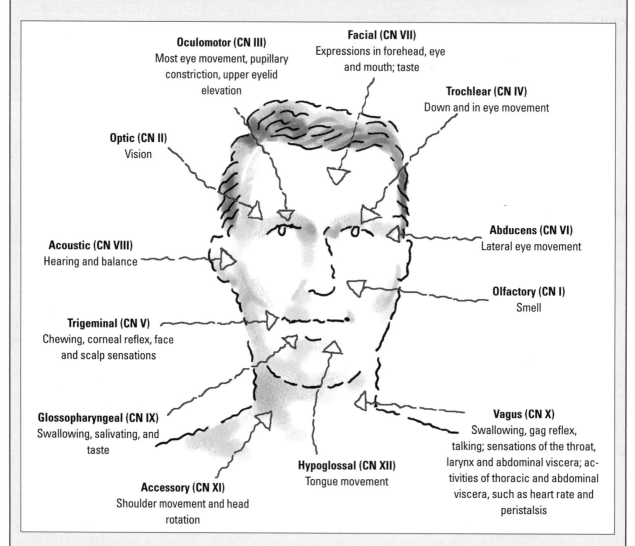

Oculomotor (CN III)
Most eye movement, pupillary constriction, upper eyelid elevation

Facial (CN VII)
Expressions in forehead, eye and mouth; taste

Trochlear (CN IV)
Down and in eye movement

Optic (CN II)
Vision

Acoustic (CN VIII)
Hearing and balance

Abducens (CN VI)
Lateral eye movement

Olfactory (CN I)
Smell

Trigeminal (CN V)
Chewing, corneal reflex, face and scalp sensations

Glossopharyngeal (CN IX)
Swallowing, salivating, and taste

Hypoglossal (CN XII)
Tongue movement

Vagus (CN X)
Swallowing, gag reflex, talking; sensations of the throat, larynx and abdominal viscera; activities of thoracic and abdominal viscera, such as heart rate and peristalsis

Accessory (CN XI)
Shoulder movement and head rotation

See about sight

Next, how do we assess the optic (CN II) and oculomotor (CN III) nerves?
• The optic nerve is assessed by checking visual acuity and visual fields. This can be undertaken using a Snellen eye chart (that starts with large print and moves to small print)

Memory jogger

To help you remember the names of the 12 cranial nerves, use the following mnemonic: *On old Olympus's towering tops, a Finn and German viewed some hops.*

- **On** = **O**lfactory
- **Ol**d = **O**ptic
- **O**lympus's = **O**culomotor
- **T**owering = **T**rochlear
- **T**ops = **T**rigeminal
- **A** = **A**bducens

- **Finn** = **F**acial
- **A**nd = **A**coustic
- **G**erman = **G**lossopharyngeal
- **V**iewed = **V**agus
- **S**ome = **S**pinal accessory
- **H**ops = **H**ypoglossal

- The oculomotor nerve can be assessed by checking pupil size, pupil shape and direct and consensual response to light. When assessing pupil size, look for trends such as a gradual increase in the size of one pupil or appearance of unequal pupils. (See *Recognising pupillary changes*, page 280.)

Funny face

To test the motor portion of the facial nerve (CN VII) to assess for possible stroke or Bell's palsy, the patient will be asked to:
- Wrinkle his forehead
- Raise and lower his eyebrows
- Smile to show his teeth
- Puff out his cheeks.
    Also, with the patient's eyes tightly closed, the examiner will attempt to open the patient's eyelids. Always check for facial symmetry.

Now hear this

To test the vestibular portion of the acoustic nerve, the patient will be observed for nystagmus (a series of involuntary rhythmic oscillations of one or both eyes) and disturbed balance, such as in a cerebellar stroke or Ménière's disease. Note reports of the room spinning or dizziness in your assessment.

Check the pipes

The glossopharyngeal nerve (CN IX) and vagus nerve (CN X) are tested together because their innervation overlaps in the pharynx:
- The glossopharyngeal nerve is responsible for swallowing, salivating and taste perception on the posterior one-third of the tongue
- The vagus nerve controls swallowing and is responsible for voice quality.
    These nerves are assessed by listening to the patient's voice. The gag reflex is tested by the doctor or ENP touching the tip of the tongue blade

Recognising pupillary changes

Use this table as a guide to recognise pupillary changes and identify possible causes.

Pupillary change	Possible causes
Unilateral, dilated (4 mm) fixed, and nonreactive 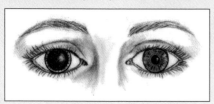	• Uncal herniation with oculomotor nerve damage • Brain stem compression • Increased intracranial pressure • Head trauma with subdural or extradural haematoma • May be normal in some people if eye has been severely damaged or having used eye drops that dilate the pupil such as atropine
Bilateral, dilated (4 mm), fixed and nonreactive 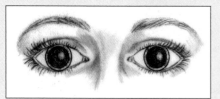	• Severe brain damage • Sympathomimetic intoxication • Anticholinergic poisoning • Cerebral ischaemia or hypoxia
Bilateral, midsize (2 mm), fixed and nonreactive 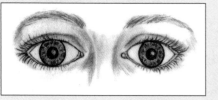	• Midbrain involvement caused by oedema, haemorrhage, infarctions, lacerations or contusions
Bilateral, pinpoint (<1 mm) and usually nonreactive 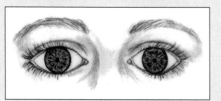	• Lesions of pons, usually after haemorrhage • Opiate overdose
Unilateral, small (1.5 mm) and nonreactive 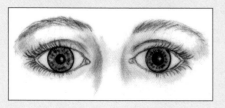	• Disruption of sympathetic nerve supply to the head caused by spinal cord lesion above the first thoracic vertebra

against the posterior pharynx and asking the patient to open wide and say 'ah'. A watch is kept for the symmetrical upwards movement of the soft palate and uvula and the midline position of the uvula. Abnormal findings may indicate stroke, expanding haematoma of the neck, palate infection or airway foreign body.

Shrug it off

To assess for possible stroke or upper spinal cord injury, the spinal accessory nerve (CN XI), which controls the sternocleidomastoid muscles and the upper portion of the trapezius muscles are assessed. This is done by pressing down on the patient's shoulders while he attempts to shrug against this resistance. Note is made of shoulder strength and symmetry while inspecting and palpating the trapezius muscles.

To further test the trapezius muscles, resistance is applied from one side while the patient tries to return his head to midline position.

Test tongue toughness

To assess the hypoglossal nerve (CN XII), these steps are undertaken:
• Asking the patient to stick out his tongue. Looking for any deviation from the midline, atrophy or fasciculations
• Testing tongue strength by asking the patient to push his tongue against his cheek as resistance is applied. Observation of the tongue for symmetry
• Testing the patient's speech by asking him to repeat the sentence, 'Round the rugged rock that ragged rascal ran'.

Sensory function

The sensory system is assessed to evaluate the ability of the:
• Sensory receptors to detect stimulus
• Afferent nerves to carry sensory nerve impulses to the spinal cord
• Sensory tracts in the spinal cord to carry sensory messages to the brain.

This may hurt

To test for pain sensation, the patient is asked to close his eyes; then touch above the area of sensory loss to find the line of demarcation, first with the sharp end of a safety pin and then with the dull end.

Motor function

The doctor or ENP will assess motor function to aid evaluation of these structures and functions:
• Cerebral cortex and its initiation of motor activity by way of the pyramidal pathways
• Corticospinal tracts and their capacity to carry motor messages down the spinal cord

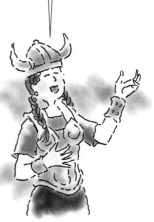

Can you see my uvula movement and position from here? I'll try again – ahhhhh!

- Lower motor neurons and their ability to carry efferent impulses to the muscles
- Muscles and their capacity to carry out motor commands
- Cerebellum and basal ganglia and their capacity to coordinate and fine-tune movement.

Feats of strength

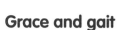

To assess arm muscle strength, the patient is asked to push away from the examiner as resistance is applied. Then the patient is asked to extend both arms, palms up and to close his eyes and maintain this position for 20 to 30 seconds. Observation is made of the arm for downward drifting and pronation.

The patient will be asked to lift his leg off the bed to gauge leg strength.

Grace and gait

The patient's coordination and balance is assessed. A note is made whether the patient can sit and stand without support. If appropriate, observation of the patient walking is undertaken.

While observing the patient, note is made of imbalances and abnormalities. When cerebellar dysfunction is present, the patient has a wide-based, unsteady gait. Deviation to one side may indicate a cerebellar lesion on the side.

Extreme coordination

The extremities are tested for coordination by having the patient touch his nose and then the examiner's outstretched finger as it is moved. The patient will be asked do this faster and faster. His movements should be accurate and smooth.

Cerebellar function is tested further by assessing rapid alternating movements. The patient is asked to use the thumb of one hand to touch each finger of the same hand in rapid sequence and then repeated with the other hand.

Abnormalities can indicate cerebellar disease, stroke, ethanol toxicity or a cerebellar infarct.

Present and absent actions

Motor responses in an unconscious patient may be appropriate, inappropriate or absent. Appropriate responses, such as localisation or withdrawal, mean that the sensory and corticospinal pathways are functioning. Inappropriate responses, such as decorticate or decerebrate posturing, indicate a dysfunction.

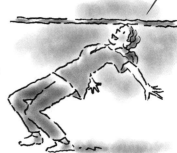

It can be challenging to assess motor responses in a patient who can't follow commands or is unresponsive. It is important to note whether any stimulus produces a response and what that response is.

Superficially speaking

Superficial reflexes can be elicited using light, tactile stimulation such as stroking or scratching the skin.

Because these reflexes are cutaneous, the more they are elicited in succession, the less the response will be. Therefore, observe carefully the first time when these reflexes are stimulated. Superficial reflexes include the plantar, pharyngeal and abdominal reflexes. Here's how they are tested:

• The *plantar reflex* is tested using an applicator stick, tongue blade or key that strokes slowly the lateral side of the patient's sole from the heel to the great toe. The normal response in an adult is plantar flexion of the toes. Upward movement of the great toe and fanning of the little toes – called *Babinski's reflex* – is abnormal. (See *Babinski's reflex in infants*)

• To test the *pharyngeal reflex* of CN IX and CN X, the patient is instructed to open his mouth wide. Then, the back of the pharynx is touched with a tongue blade. Normally, doing so causes the patient to gag

• To test the *abdominal reflex* and intactness of thoracic spinal segments T8, T9 and T10, the tip of the handle on the reflex hammer is used to stroke one side and then the opposite side of the patient's abdomen above the umbilicus. This is repeated on the lower abdomen. Normally, the abdominal muscles contract and the umbilicus deviate towards the stimulated side.

Write it down

The recording of assessment findings is recorded carefully in the patient's notes. Subtle changes in these findings may indicate a worsening condition.

Ages and stages

Babinski's reflex in infants

Babinski's reflex can be elicited in some normal infants – sometimes until age 2 years. However, plantar flexion of the toes is seen in more than 90% of normal infants.

Diagnostic tests

Diagnostic testing may be routine for you, but it can be frightening for the patient. Try to prepare the patient and his family for each test and follow-up monitoring procedure. Some tests can be performed at the patient's bedside but others many require transportation to the X-ray or Imaging department. Early imaging reduces the time lapse between admission and the detection of life-threatening complications. Such early detection is therefore associated with better clinical outcomes.

X-rays

Skull X-ray
Skull X-rays have been largely superseded by computed tomographic (CT) scanning for neurological investigations; however, if a skull X-ray has been

taken it can yield useful information as fractures, especially depressed fractures, maybe detected. Cerebral midline shift can be detected by misalignment of the calcified pineal gland (only in adults).

Spinal X-rays

The doctor may order anteroposterior and lateral spinal X-rays when spinal disease is suspected or when injury to the cervical, thoracic, lumbar or sacral vertebral segments exists. Spinal X-rays are used to detect spinal fracture, displacement and subluxation and destructive lesions, such as primary and metastatic bone tumours. Depending on the patient's condition, other X-ray images may be taken from special angles, such as the open-mouth view (to identify possible odontoid (dens) fracture).

Practice pointers
* Reassure the patient that X-rays are painless
* As ordered, administer an analgesic before the procedure if the patient has existing pain, so he'll be more comfortable
* Remove the patient's cervical collar if cervical X-rays reveal no fracture and the doctor has written an order to remove it.

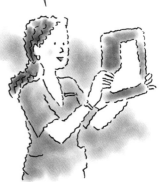

Ready for a real close-up? Spinal X-rays can provide a closer look at damage to the thoracic, lumbar or sacral vertebral segments. Hopefully you won't see a boot!

CT scan

CT scanning combines radiology and computer analysis of tissue density. CT angiogram scanning shows cerebral blood vessels. The CT scan is the primary investigation of choice for acute clinically important brain injuries.

Spine scanning using CT and MRI

CT scanning of the spine is used to assess such disorders as herniated disk, spinal cord tumours, fractures, subluxations and distraction injuries. Magnetic resonance imaging (MRI) scanning of the spine is used to assess herniated discs spinal cord tumours and spinal stenosis.

Brain scanning

CT scanning of the brain is used to detect brain contusion, brain calcifications, cerebral atrophy, hydrocephalus, inflammation, space-occupying lesions (tumours, haematomas and abscesses), foreign bodies and bony displacement. It also detects arteriovenous malformations (AVMs) of the brain, aneurysms, infarctions and blood clots.

Practice pointers
* Provide information and reassurance. Check that consent, where possible, has been gained
* Ensure that a pre-scan checklist has been completed
* Confirm that the patient isn't allergic to iodine or shellfish to avoid an adverse reaction to the contrast medium, if contrast is being used

- If the test calls for a contrast medium, tell the patient that it's injected into an existing I.V. line or that a new line may be inserted. Ensure that the patient has an 18G or larger catheter as close to the heart as possible
- Ensure that pre-procedure tests, including evaluation of renal function (serum creatinine, urea and electrolytes), are available on the patient's chart and have been reviewed; keep in mind that the contrast medium can cause acute renal failure
- Warn the patient and his family that he may feel flushed or notice a metallic taste in his mouth when the contrast medium is injected
- Tell him that the CT scanner rotates around him, and that the table will move in and out of the scanner
- Explain that he must lie still during the test
- Expect the doctor to write an order to increase I.V. flow rate after the test if the patient's oral intake is being restricted or oral intake is contraindicated; otherwise, suggest that the patient drink more fluids to flush the medium out of his body.

Magnetic resonance imaging (MRI)

MRI generates detailed pictures of body structures. The test may involve the use of a contrast medium such as gadolinium. MRI is not currently recommended as a primary investigation for clinically important brain injured patient. It may offer diagnostic and prognostic information for other groups.

Sharper images

Compared with conventional X-rays and CT scans, MRI provides superior visualisation of soft tissues, sharply differentiating healthy, benign, cancerous, injured and oedematous atrophied tissue and clearly revealing blood vessels. In addition, MRI permits imaging in multiple planes, including sagittal and coronal views in regions where bones normally hamper visualisation.

MRI is especially useful for studying the CNS because it can reveal structural abnormalities associated with such conditions as transient ischaemic attack (TIA), tumours, multiple sclerosis, cerebral oedema and hydrocephalus.

Practice pointers

- Check for internal metal, e.g. heart valves, pacemakers cochlear implants or recent surgery, all of which would make MRI contraindicated in the huge magnetic field of the MRI
- Check a detailed history has been undertaken and consent signed
- Most scanners cannot accommodate patients over 20 stone (128 kg)
- Confirm that the patient isn't allergic to the contrast medium
- Explain that the procedure can take up to 1 hour depending on the area being scanned; tell the patient that he must remain still for intervals of 2 to 20 minutes. Check that the patient will be able to maintain the position. Scans take between 10 and 100 minutes in total depending on the area being scanned

- If the test calls for a contrast medium, tell the patient that it's injected into an existing I.V. line or that a new line may be inserted
- Ensure that all metallic items such as hair grips, jewellery (including body-piercing jewellery), watches, eyeglasses, hearing aids and dentures are removed from the patient's body
- Explain that the test is painless, but that the machinery may seem loud and frightening and the tunnel confining. Tell the patient that he'll receive earplugs to reduce the noise. Reassure the patient that he would be able to contact the radiographer during the procedure
- Provide sedation as ordered to promote relaxation during the test
- After the procedure, increase the I.V. flow rate as ordered, or encourage the patient to increase his fluid intake to flush the contrast medium from his system.

Other tests

Lumbar puncture

During lumbar puncture (LP), the doctor inserts a sterile needle into the subarachnoid space of the spinal canal, usually between the third and fourth lumbar vertebrae and draws off or measures the pressure of cerebrospinal fluid (CSF). This test is used to investigate for such conditions as meningitis and sub-arachnoid haemorrhage. It requires sterile technique and careful patient positioning.

Why do it?

Lumbar puncture is used to:
- Detect blood and bacteria in CSF. The CSF should be clear 'gin clear'; cloudy fluid may indicate infection or blood. To distinguish between traumatic contamination during the procedure and blood in the CSF itself, the CSF is examined for a yellow tinge (xanthochromia) that indicates blood breakdown has taken place
- Obtain CSF specimens for laboratory analysis-biochemistry, microbiology, cytology and sugar.

Contraindications and cautions

Lumbar puncture is contraindicated in patients with lumbar deformity or infection at the puncture site. It's performed cautiously. You may see the doctor checking for papilloedema (swelling of the optic disc seen at the back of the eye) in patients with suspected increased ICP, because rapid decrease of pressure that follows withdrawal of CSF can cause tonsillar herniation and medullary compression.

Practice pointers

- Describe what a lumbar puncture is to the patient and his family, explaining that the procedure may cause some discomfort. Check consent has been gained

- Assist in the positioning of the patient on his side in a foetal position on the edge of the bed. The back and the shoulders should be at 90% to the mattress. One pillow is placed under the head and two between the patient's legs
- Reassure the patient that a local anaesthetic is administered before the test. Tell him to report any tingling or sharp pain he feels as the anaesthetic is injected
- Ensure that the patient lies flat on one pillow for 3 to 4 hours after an LP. Monitor the patient for neurological deficits by frequent recordings of GCS, pulse and BP
- Observe for complications, such as headache, fever, back spasms or seizures, according to departmental policy.

Surgical treatment

Life-threatening neurological disorders occasionally require emergency surgery, and the patient will usually have to be transferred to a specialist (tertiary) neurosurgical centre either by road or by air ambulance. Surgery commonly involves *craniotomy*, a procedure to open the skull and expose the brain. *Craniotomy* allows various treatments, such as ventricular shunting, excision of a tumour or abscess, haematoma aspiration and aneurysm clipping (placing one or more surgical clips on the neck of an aneurysm to destroy it). *A burr hole* (drilling a hole in the skull) is an emergency procedure to reduce raised ICP, such as a rapidly expanding extradural haematoma. This procedure is used less now due to improved imaging and diagnosing and faster access to neurosurgical centres.

Drug treatments

For many of your patients with neurological emergencies, medication or drug therapy is essential.
- Thrombolytic therapy is used to treat patients with acute ischaemic stroke
- Anticonvulsants are used to control seizures
- Corticosteroids are used to reduce inflammation.

Other types of drugs commonly used to treat patients with neurological emergencies include:
- Analgesics
- Anticoagulants and antiplatelets
- Anticonvulsants
- Benzodiazepines
- Calcium channel blockers
- Corticosteroids
- Diuretics

- Thrombolytics
- Antipsychotics
- Antibiotics
- Antiparkinson drugs.

Heads up!

When caring for a patient undergoing medication therapy, stay alert for severe adverse reactions and interactions with other drugs. (See *Selected drugs used in neurological emergencies.*)

Common disorders

Head trauma

Head trauma is any traumatic insult to the brain that causes physical, intellectual, emotional, social or vocational changes. Children ages 6 months to 2 years of age and adults ages 15 to 24 years of age are most at risk for head trauma.

To put it bluntly

Head trauma is generally categorised as *blunt trauma* (closed or open) or *penetrating trauma*. Blunt trauma is more common. It typically occurs when the head strikes a hard surface or a rapidly moving object strikes the head. The dura may be intact, and no brain tissue is exposed to the external environment.
    Possible complications include:
- Increased ICP due to oedema or haematoma formation
- Infection (in open wounds)
- Respiratory depression and failure
- Brain herniation and death.

> Extra, extra! Brain exposed in penetrating trauma scandal!

Open and exposed

In penetrating trauma, as the name suggests, an opening in the scalp, skull, meninges or brain tissue exposes the cranial contents to the environment. The risk of infection is high.

On the decline

Mortality from head injury has declined as a result of:
- Advances in preventive measures such as air bags, seat belts and helmet laws
- Quicker emergency response and transport times
- Improved treatment measures.

Selected drugs used in neurological emergencies

Use this table to find out about common neurological drugs and their indications and adverse effects.

Drug	Indications	Adverse effects
Opioid analgesics Morphine	• Severe pain	• Respiratory depression, apnoea, bradycardia, seizures, sedation interference with pupillary responses
Oxycodone, codeine phospate *All counterindicated with raised ICP and head injury.*	• Mild to moderate pain	• Respiratory depression, bradycardia, sedation, constipation, interference with pupillary responses
Anticonvulsants Lorazepam, diazepam, chlormethiazole, phenobarbitone Phenytoin	• Status epilepticus, seizures during neurosurgery • Generalised tonic-clonic seizures, status epilepticus, nonepileptic seizures after head trauma	
Anticoagulants Heparin	• Embolism prophylaxis after cerebral thrombosis in evolving stroke	• Haemorrhage, thrombocytopenia
Antiplatelets Aspirin	• Transient ischaemic attacks, thromboembolic disorders	• GI bleeding, acute renal insufficiency, thrombocytopenia, hepatic dysfunction
Barbiturates Phenobarbital	• All types of seizures except absence seizures and febrile seizures in children; also used for, sedation, and drug withdrawal	• Respiratory depression, apnea, bradycardia, angio oedema, Stevens-Johnson syndrome
Benzodiazepines Diazepam Lorazepam, clonazepam.	• Status epilepticus, anxiety, acute alcohol withdrawal, muscle spasm (can be *given per rectum* also) • Status epilepticus, anxiety, agitation	• Respiratory depression, bradycardia, cardiovascular collapse, drowsiness, acute withdrawal syndrome • Drowsiness, acute withdrawal syndrome
Calcium channel blockers Nimodipine	• Neurological deficits caused by cerebral vasospasm after congenital aneurysm rupture	• Decreased blood pressure, tachycardia, oedema
Corticosteroids Dexamethasone	• Cerebral oedema, severe inflammation related to malignant cerebral tumours or as an adjunct treatment for bacterial meningitis	• Heart failure, cardiac arrhythmias, oedema, circulatory collapse, thromboembolism, pancreatitis, peptic ulceration

(continued)

Selected drugs used in neurological emergencies *(Continued)*

Drug	Indications	Adverse effects
Diuretics		
Mannitol (osmotic)	• Cerebral oedema, increased ICP	• Heart failure, seizures, fluid and electrolyte imbalance
Frusemide (loop)	• Oedema, hypertension	• Renal failure, thrombocytopenia, agranulocytosis, volume depletion, dehydration
Thrombolytics		
Alteplase (recombinant tissue plasminogen activator)	• Acute ischaemic stroke	• Cerebral haemorrhage, spontaneous bleeding, allergic reaction
Serotonin inhibitors		
Sumatriptan	• Acute migraine or cluster-type headache	• Blood pressure alterations

What causes it

Head injury commonly results from:
- Motor vehicle collisions (the most common cause)
- Falls
- Sports-related injuries
- Interpersonal violence.

How it happens

The brain is shielded by the cranial vault (composed of skin, bone, meninges and CSF), which intercepts the force of a physical blow. Below a certain level of force, the cranial vault prevents energy from damaging the brain.

The degree of traumatic head injury is usually proportional to the amount of force reaching the intracranial tissues. In addition, until they're ruled out, you must presume that neck injuries such as a cervical spine fracture are present in patients with traumatic head injuries, so the head and neck will be immobilised usually using a long backboard. Until the neck X-rays are viewed and cleared by the doctor the patient is continued on triple immobilization to protect the spinal cord from further trauma.

Case closed

Blunt trauma is typically a sudden acceleration-deceleration or coup-contrecoup injury. In a coup-contrecoup injury, the head hits a more stationary object or a moving object, injuring cranial tissues near the point of impact (coup); the remaining force then pushes the brain against the opposite side of the skull, causing a second impact and injury on the opposite surface (contrecoup).

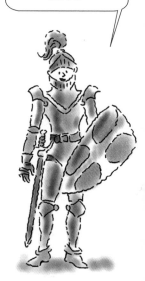

Never fear – the cranial vault is here! It protects the brain from physical blows.

Contusions and lacerations also occur as the brain's soft tissues slide over the rough bone of the skull base. The brain may also endure rotational shear, damaging the upper midbrain and areas of the frontal, temporal, parietal and occipital lobes.

What to look for

Types of head trauma include:
- Concussion
- Contusion
- Extradural haematoma
- Subarachnoid haematoma
- Skull fractures
- Subdural haematoma.

Each type is associated with specific signs and symptoms. (See *Hidden Haematoma* and *Types of head injury*, pages 292–295.)

What tests tell you

These diagnostic tests are used for head injury:
- A CT scan will show a fracture of the cranial vault and shows intracranial haemorrhage from ruptured blood vessels, ischaemic or necrotic tissue, cerebral oedema, a shift in brain tissue and subdural, epidural, and intracerebral haematomas
- MRI can assess diffuse axonal injuries.

How it's treated

Treatment may be surgical or supportive.

It's surgical

Surgical treatment includes:
- Craniotomy (bone of the skull replaced), this includes trepanning or burr holes treatment and decompression craniectomy (bone of the skill removed)
- Evacuation of a haematoma.

Surgery aims to remove fragments driven into the brain and to evacuate haematoma and control bleeding. Such measures reduce the risk of infection and further brain damage due to fractures.

It's supportive

Provide supportive treatment, which includes:
- Close observation to detect changes in neurological status suggesting further damage
- Cleaning and debridement of any wounds associated with skull fractures
- Diuretics, such as mannitol, to reduce cerebral oedema
- Analgesics to relieve complaints of headache, such as codeine phosphate
- Anticonvulsants such as phenytoin to prevent seizures

(Text continues on page 294.)

Ages and stages

Hidden haematoma

An older person with cerebral atrophy can tolerate a larger and lowly developing subdural haematoma for a longer time than a younger person before the haematoma causes neurological changes. Thus, a haematoma in an older adult can become rather large before signs or symptoms occur, even in an acute condition. This can be an easily missed differential diagnosis for patients with sudden onset of confusion.

Types of head injury

The reader is advised to read this information in conjunction with NICE Guidelines (2007) *Head injury: triage, assessment, investigation and early management of head injury in infants, children and adults*.

Here's a summary of the signs and symptoms and diagnostic test findings for different types of head injury.

Type	Description
Closed head injury.	• A blow to the head or a severe shaking causing tearing, shearing or stretching of the nerves at the base of the brain • The skill maybe fractured but there is no penetration of the skull or brain nor any direct connection between the brain and outside • Recovery is usually complete within 24 to 48 hours, but headache can persist for months. • Repeated injuries have a cumulative effect on the brain • Unconsciousness lasts less than 6 hours, frequently only a few minutes.
Cerebral Contusion (bruising of brain tissue).	• Acceleration-deceleration or coup–contrecoup injuries disrupt normal nerve function in bruised area • Injury is directly beneath the site of impact when the brain rebounds against the skull from the force of a blow (a beating with a blunt instrument, for example), when the force of the blow drives the brain against the opposite side of the skull, or when the head is hurled forward and stopped abruptly (as in an car crash when the driver's head strikes the windshield) • Brain continues moving and slaps against the skull (acceleration), then rebounds (deceleration) • Bone may strike bony prominences inside the skull (especially the sphenoidal ridges), causing intracranial haemorrhage that may result in tentorial herniation.
Diffuse axonal injury	• This condition involves severe brain injury with extensive damage to the brain structures, primarily the white matter of the brain • Axon damage in the cerebral hemispheres, corpus callosum and brain stem cause swelling and disconnection • This condition is commonly accompanied by damage to blood vessels and tissues • This condition may be categorised as mild, moderate, or severe.
Extradural (or epidural) haematoma. Subdural haematoma (or haemorrhage).	• Accumulation of blood in the extra dura (between the skull inner surface and the dura mater) • Caused by damage to blood vessels on the surface of the dura mater – often associated with a skull fracture • A collection of blood between the dura mater and the arachnoid mater caused by traumatic damage to the brain and blood vessels is called a sub-dural haematoma • Risk of raised ICP due to this bleeding.

Signs and symptoms	Diagnostic test findings
• Short-term loss of consciousness secondary to disruption of the reticular activating system, possibly due to abrupt pressure changes in the areas responsible for consciousness, changes in polarity of the neurons, ischaemia or structural distortion of neurons • Vomiting from localised injury and brainstem compression • Anterograde and retrograde amnesia (in which the patient can't recall events immediately after the injury or events that led up to the traumatic incident) correlating with severity of injury; all related to disruption of reticular activating system • Irritability or lethargy from localised injury and compression • Behaviour out of character due to focal injury • Complaints of dizziness, nausea, or severe headache due to focal injury and brainstem compression	• Computed tomographic (CT) scan may reveal no sign of open fracture, bleeding or other nervous system lesion.
• Severe scalp wounds from direct injury may or may not be present • Laboured respiration and loss of consciousness secondary to increased pressure from bruising • Drowsiness, confusion, disorientation, agitation, or violence from increased intracranial pressure (ICP) associated with trauma • Hemiparesis related to interrupted blood flow to the site of injury • Decorticate or decerebrate posturing from cortical damage or hemispheric dysfunction • Unequal pupillary response from brain stem involvement.	• CT scan shows changes in tissue density, possible displacement of the surrounding structures, and evidence of ischaemic tissue, haematoma, and fractures.
• *Mild:* Loss of consciousness for 6 to 24 hours with possible decerebrate or decorticate posture; rapid improvement within 24 hours with return to baseline neurological function; possible residual period of amnesia • *Moderate:* Almost immediate and complete loss of consciousness; coma state lasting over 24 hours to days without any lucid intervals; immediate decorticate and decerebrate postures continuing until the patient awakens; residual neurological dysfunction • *Severe:* Nonresolving brain stem impairment; coma state ranging from days to weeks; accompanying autonomic dysfunction.	• CT scan or magnetic resonance imaging (MRI) reveals extent of tissue damage and widespread cerebral oedema.
• Worsening headache from enlarging haematoma • Unilateral pupil abnormality from increased ICP • Gradual or rapidly deteriorating level of consciousness from drowsiness, slow cerebration, and confusion to coma • The rise in pressure caused by this bleeding can lead to significant damage • See above.	• CT scan reveal mass and altered blood flow in the area, confirming a haematoma • CT scan or MRI evidence of or extra dural or subdural mass and brain tissue shifting • See above • The cerebrospinal fluid (CSF) is yellow and has relatively low protein (chronic subdural haematoma).

(continued)

Types of head injury (Continued)

Type	Description
Intracerebral haematoma.	• A collection of blood inside the cranium caused by damage to the brain tissue or the rupture of a blood vessel • Subacute haematomas have a better prognosis because venous bleeding tends to be slower • Depending on the site and amount of bleeding, traumatic or spontaneous disruption of cerebral vessels in brain parenchyma cause neurological deficits • Shear forces from brain movement commonly cause vessel laceration and haemorrhage into the parenchyma • Frontal and temporal lobes are common sites. Trauma is associated with few intracerebral haematomas; most are caused by hypertension. However, patients with severe head injuries almost always have intracerebral bleeds.
Skull fracture.	• Types of skull fractures include: linear, comminuted, and depressed • Fractures of the anterior and middle fossae are associated with severe head trauma and are more common than posterior fossa fractures • A blow to the head causes one or more of the types. This condition may not be problematic unless the brain is exposed or bone fragments are driven into neural tissue or the dura is torn.

• Respiratory support, including mechanical ventilation and endotracheal (ET) tube intubation, for any patient with a GCS score of 8 or less or respiratory failure from brain stem involvement.

Practice pointers
• Assess ABCDE
• Maintain a patent airway. Monitor oxygen saturation levels through pulse oximetry and arterial blood gas (ABG) analysis as ordered
• Institute cardiac monitoring and be alert for cardiac changes or arrhythmias
• Any patient with a GCS score of less than or equal to 8 should have an ET tube and mechanical ventilation in place
• Observe for, record, and report in detail any seizure observed
• In a moderate injury, an oral gastric tube maybe ordered to decompress the stomach. Use of a nasogastric tube must be avoided in neurological cases such as basal skull fractures when there is a risk of a direct communication between the brain and CSF and the nasogastric tube as it passes through the nose
• Initially, monitor vital signs continuously and check for additional injuries; continue to check vital signs and neurological status, including LOC and pupil size, every 15 minutes. (See *After a head injury*)

Signs and symptoms	Diagnostic test findings
• Unresponsive immediately or may experience a lucid period before lapsing into a coma from increasing ICP and mass effect of haemorrhage • Possible motor deficits and decorticate or decerebrate responses from compression of corticospinal tracts and brain stem.	• CT scan identifies the bleeding site.
• May not produce symptoms, depending on underlying brain trauma. • Discontinuity and displacement of bone structure with severe fracture • Motor sensory and cranial nerve dysfunction with associated facial fractures • Persons with anterior fossa basilar skull fractures may have periorbital bruising (raccoon eyes), anosmia (loss of smell due to first cranial nerve involvement) and pupil abnormalities (second and third cranial nerve involvement) • CSF rhinorrhea (leakage through the nose), CSF otorrhea (leakage from the ear), haemotympanium (blood accumulation at the tympanic membrane), bruising over the mastoid bone (Battle sign), and facial paralysis (seventh cranial nerve injury) accompany middle fossa basilar skull fractures • Signs of medullary dysfunction, such as cardiovascular and respiratory failure, accompanying posterior fossa basilar skull fracture.	• CT scan and MRI reveal swelling and intracranial haemorrhage from ruptured blood vessels • CT scan may reveal a fracture.

Education edge

After a head injury

The patient with a head injury may be discharged from the ED once the GCS is 15 (or has returned to normal arousal). There are some basic principles. Firstly, the patient and his family need verbal instructions on how to monitor the patient at home and when the patient should seek medical care. They will also be given take away written guidance (a head injury card): these will be available in a selection of languages.

The following is included in your discharge teaching:

• Ensure that a *responsible person*, such as a family member, will be with the patient at home for the next 24 hours
• *Monitoring patient's neurological status.* Observing for headache, confusion, difficulty walking or with balance, changes in level of consciousness, seizures or passing out, vomiting (especially projectile), any changes in vision, unequal pupils, weakness in one or both arms or legs, lethargy, irritability, difficulty arousing, failure to feed or continuous crying. Any clear fluid from the nose or ears. Any new bleeding from the ears or the nose
• Advise the family member *to notify* their general practitioner or bring the patient back to the ED if any of these signs and symptoms occur.

- Maintain spinal immobilisation until spinal injury has been ruled out
- Assess haemodynamic parameters to help evaluate cerebral perfusion pressure (CPP).

Metabolic medicine

- Observe the patient closely for signs of hypoxia or increased ICP, such as headache, dizziness, irritability, anxiety and such changes in behaviour as agitation
- Administer medications as ordered. If necessary, use continuous infusions of such agents as midazolam, fentanyl or morphine to reduce metabolic demand and the risk of increased ICP
- Carefully monitor the patient for CSF leakage. Check the bed sheets for a blood-tinged spot surrounded by a lighter ring (halo sign). Elevate the head of the bed 30 degrees
- Position the patient so that secretions drain properly. If you detect CSF leakage from the nose, place a gauze pad under the nostrils. Don't use suctioning or packing through the nose. If CSF leaks from the ear, position the patient so his ear drains naturally (do not plug the ear).

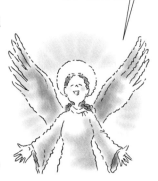

Sometimes it's divine, but after head trauma a halo signals CSF leakage.

Increased ICP

ICP refers to the pressure exerted within the intact skull, a rigid structure, by the three components of intracranial volume, which are:

 Blood

 CSF

 Brain tissue.

Tip the scales

Normally the body can maintain a balance of intracranial volume. However, any condition that alters the normal balance of intracranial components can increase ICP. Significant or rapid elevations in ICP aren't well tolerated by the brain and may result in herniation.

What causes it

Increased ICP can be caused by any condition that decreases any of the three components of the intracranial vault. Some causes may include:
- Haemorrhage
- Cerebral oedema
- Hydrocephalus
- Space-occupying lesions (tumours, including cerebral secondaries, abscesses, cysts, foreign bodies and AVMs).

How it happens

Under normal circumstances, a change in the volume of one of the intracranial contents triggers a reciprocal change in one or more of the components to maintain a consistent pressure. When this balance becomes altered, ICP increases. Initially, the body compensates by regulating the volume of the three substances via:
- Displacing CSF into the spinal canal
- Increasing absorption or decreasing production of CSF
- Limiting blood flow to the head
- Forcing brain tissue out of the skull.
  When these compensatory mechanisms become overtaxed, small changes in volume lead to big changes in pressure.

What to look for

Signs and symptoms of increased ICP can be subtle early on. Typically, signs and symptoms are manifested in the patient's LOC, pupils, motor responses and vital signs.

Early symptoms
- Worsening GCS
- Headache
- Increased blood pressure (intermittently)
- Nausea and vomiting
- Muscle weakness or motor changes on the side opposite the lesion, and positive pronator drift
- Varied LOC (initially) (the patient may become restless, anxious or quiet, or you may note that he needs increased stimulation to be aroused)
- Skin can become flushed and dry.

Further compromise
- Hemiparesis
- Hemiplegia
- Increased systolic blood pressure, profound bradycardia and abnormal respirations
- Can't be aroused (as ICP continues to increase)
- Pupillary changes (may reveal constriction of one pupil and not the other, a sluggish reaction by both pupils, pupillary changes only on one side and unequal pupils)
- Seizures.

Severe increased ICP
- Bradycardia
- Systolic hypertension
- Hyperthermia
- Widened pulse pressure
- Profound weakness
- Pupils fixed and dilated

- Very high urinary output (diabetes insipidus) due to pituitary gland damage
- Doll's eye reflex (when the head is moved the eyes do not move) and indicates brain death.

What tests tell you

The patient with increased ICP typically undergoes diagnostic testing to determine the underlying cause of the problem. Such tests may include computed tomography or MRI to evaluate for haematomas, lesions, ischaemic tissue or fractures.

How it's treated

Treatment focuses on correcting the underlying problem and controlling ICP and may include:
- I.V. normal saline. Head injury patients are not at risk of hypovolaemic shock due to the relatively small volume of blood within the skull. The IV fluid infusion when the patient is hypertensive will be restricted (25 to 50 ml/hour for adults) so not to compound cerebral oedema and ICP. However, if the patient becomes hypotensive then IV fluids will be increased to maintain a systolic blood pressure of at least 90 mm Hg to maintain CPP
- Osmotic diuretics.

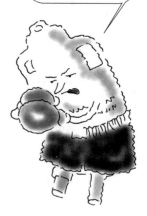

I.V. saline solution can help knock out increased ICP.

What to do – *ABCDE*
- Maintain a patent airway. Monitor pulse oximetry and give oxygen to maintain blood oxygen saturation within prescribed target range
- ABG analysis as ordered
- Institute cardiac monitoring and be alert for cardiac changes or arrhythmias
- Initially, monitor vital signs, including pulse oximetry, continuously and continue to check vital signs and neurological status (GCS), including LOC and pupil size, every 15 minutes
- Assess haemodynamic parameters to aid in evaluating CPP
- Administer medications as ordered. If necessary, use continuous infusions of such agents as fentanyl, or morphine, to reduce metabolic demand
- If an ICP monitoring system is inserted, continuously monitor ICP waveforms and pressure
- Elevate the head of the bed 30 degrees (if no spinal injury)
- Institute seizure precautions as necessary. Use safety precautions to minimise the risk of injury
- Explain all procedures and treatments to the patient and his family
- Prepare to transfer the patient to a specialist neurosurgical unit or to the ICU when indicated.

What to avoid

- Avoid extreme hip and knee flexion because these actions can increase intra-abdominal and intrathoracic pressures
- Minimise procedures that might increase ICP, such as suctioning

- Avoid tight ETT ties as these can restrict venous drainage and also cause damage to the skin.

Seizures

Seizures are paroxysmal events associated with abnormal electrical discharges of neurons in the brain. They aren't an actual disorder but, rather, an indication of an underlying problem. Seizure disorder, or *epilepsy*, is a condition of the brain characterised by recurrent seizures. However, many seizures aren't a part of a seizure disorder but may result from isolated events such as fever, toxin exposure, alcohol withdrawal or a head injury.

Primary and secondary

Primary seizure disorder or epilepsy is idiopathic without apparent structural changes in the brain. Secondary epilepsy, characterised by structural changes or metabolic alterations of the neuronal membranes, causes increased automaticity.

Who's affected...

Epilepsy is a relatively widespread condition, affecting around 456,000 people in the UK. The condition usually begins during childhood but it can start at any age. Around one in every 280 children is affected by epilepsy.

...and how

Complications of epilepsy may include hypoxia or anoxia due to airway occlusion, traumatic injury, brain damage and depression and anxiety.

What causes it

In about one-half of seizure disorder cases, the cause is unknown. Some possible causes are:
- Anoxia
- Birth trauma (such as inadequate oxygen supply to the brain, blood incompatibility or haemorrhage)
- Infectious diseases (meningitis, encephalitis or brain abscess)
- Head injury or trauma
- Perinatal infection.

How it happens

Some neurons in the brain may depolarise easily or be hyperexcitable, firing more readily when stimulated than normally happens. On stimulation, the electric current spreads to surrounding cells, which fire in turn. The impulse thus cascades to:
- One area of the brain (a partial seizure)
- Both sides of the brain (a generalised seizure)
- Cortical, subcortical and brain stem areas.

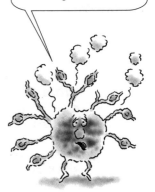

Boy, am I burned out. When neurons get hyperexcited, we fire more readily than usual, causing cells to retaliate and leading to seizures.

Increase O$_2$ or else

The brain's metabolic demand for oxygen increases dramatically during a generalised seizure. If this demand isn't met, hypoxia and brain damage result.

Firing of inhibitory neurons causes the excited neurons to slow their firing and eventually stop. Without this inhibitory action, the result is status epilepticus (continuous seizures or seizures occurring one right after another). Without treatment, the resulting anoxia is fatal.

What to look for

The hallmark of a seizure disorder is recurring seizures, which can be classified as partial or generalised. Some patients are affected by more than one type. (See *Identifying types of seizures*.)

What tests tell you

Here are possible primary diagnostic results of tests for seizure disorders:
- CT scan to show density readings of the brain and may indicate abnormalities in internal brain structures such as a tumour or cyst
- MRI may indicate abnormalities in internal brain structures
- Electroencephalogram is used to confirm the diagnosis of epilepsy by providing evidence of the continuing tendency to have seizures.

How it's treated

Generally, treatment consists of drug therapy specific to the type of seizures. The goal is to reduce seizures using a combination of the fewest drugs.

For tonic-clonic seizures

The most commonly prescribed drugs for generalised tonic-clonic seizures (alternating episodes of muscle spasm and relaxation) include phenytoin, carbamazepine, phenobarbitone and primidone.

Surgery and emergencies

If drug therapy fails, treatment may include surgical removal of a focal lesion or neural pathway in an attempt to stop seizures.

Continuous

In some cases, a patient may experience continuous seizures or recurrent seizures lasting at least 20 to 30 minutes. If these seizures occur, immediate intervention is necessary. (See *Status epilepticus*, page 302.)

What to do
- ABCDE
- Ensure patient safety
- Protect the patient's airway but never place anything in the patient's mouth
- Administer oxygen as needed
- Obtain a blood glucose level as indicated
- Initiate I.V. access
- Administer naloxone if opioid toxicity is suspected

Identifying types of seizures

Use these guidelines to understand different seizure types. Keep in mind that some patients may be affected by more than one type.

Partial seizures

Arising from a localised area in the brain, they may spread to the entire brain, causing a generalised seizure. Types include *Jacksonian*, *sensory*, *complex partial* and *secondarily generalised*.

Jacksonian seizures

These begin as localised motor seizures with stiffening or jerking in one extremity, and a tingling sensation in the same area. The patient seldom loses consciousness unless the seizure progresses to a generalised tonic-clonic seizure.

Sensory seizure

Symptoms include hallucinations, flashing lights, tingling sensations, vertigo, déjà vu and smelling a foul odour.

Complex partial seizure

Signs and symptoms vary but usually include purposeless behaviour, such as a glassy stare, picking at clothes, aimless wandering, lip-smacking or chewing motions and unintelligible speech.

An aura may occur first, and seizures may last a few seconds to 20 minutes. Afterwards, mental confusion may last for several minutes. The patient has no memory of his actions during the seizure.

Secondarily generalised partial seizure

This can be simple or complex and can progress to a generalised seizure. An aura may occur first, with loss of concentration immediately or 1 to 2 minutes later.

Generalised seizures

Types include: absence, myoclonic, clonic, tonic, generalised tonic-clonic and atonic.

Absence seizure

Absence seizure *(petit mal seizure)* is most common in children. It usually begins with a brief change in the level of consciousness, signalled by blinking or rolling of the eyes, a blank stare and slight mouth movements. The patient retains his posture and continues preseizure activity without difficulty.

Such seizures last 1 to 10 seconds. If not properly treated, seizures can recur up to 100 times per day and progress to a generalised tonic-clonic seizure.

Myoclonic seizure

This is marked by brief, involuntary muscle jerks of the body or extremities and typically occurs in early morning.

Clonic seizure

This is characterised by bilateral rhythmic movements.

Tonic seizure

This is characterised by a sudden stiffening of muscle tone, usually of the arms, but may also include the legs.

Generalised tonic-clonic seizure

Typically begins with a loud cry caused by air rushing from the lungs and through the vocal cords. The patient falls to the ground, losing consciousness. The body stiffens (tonic phase) and then alternates between episodes of muscle spasm and relaxation (clonic phase). Tongue biting, incontinence, laboured breathing, apnoea and cyanosis may also occur.

The seizure stops in 2 to 5 minutes. Afterwards, the patient regains consciousness but is somewhat confused. He may have difficulty talking and may have drowsiness, fatigue, headache, muscle soreness and arm or leg weakness. He may fall into a deep sleep afterwards.

Atonic seizure

This is characterised by a general loss of postural tone and temporary loss of consciousness. It occurs in children and is sometimes called a *drop attack* because the child falls.

Stay on the ball

Status epilepticus

Always an emergency

Status epilepticus is accompanied by a continuous generalised tonic-clonic seizure. It can result from withdrawal of antiepileptic medications, hypoxic or metabolic encephalopathy, acute head trauma or septicaemia secondary to encephalitis, meningitis, toxins or hypothermia.

Act fast

Emergency treatment usually consists of lorazepam or diazepam. I.V. dextrose 50% is given when seizures are secondary to hypoglycaemia and I.V. thiamine in patients with chronic alcoholism or those who are undergoing withdrawal.

- Record and report a detailed description of the seizure.
- Administer diazepam or lorazepam I.V., or rectally as ordered, to control seizures
- Institute cardiac monitoring and be alert for cardiac changes or arrhythmias
- Monitor a patient receiving anticonvulsants for signs of toxicity, such as nystagmus, ataxia, lethargy, dizziness, drowsiness, slurred speech, irritability, nausea and vomiting
- When administering phenytoin I.V., use a large vein; administer it according to the guidelines (not more than 150 mg/phenytoin equivalent/ minute). Monitor vital signs continuously during the infusion and for 10 to 20 minutes after the infusion is complete. Be alert for signs of hypotension
- If the patient has a history of anticonvulsant medication use, drug blood levels will be taken.

Tonic-clonic interventions

If the patient has a generalised tonic-clonic seizure, follow these steps:
- Avoid restraining the patient during a seizure
- Help the patient to a lying position if not already in that position, loosen any tight clothing and place something flat and soft, such as a pillow, under his head
- Clear the area of hard objects
- Don't force anything into the patient's mouth
- Turn the patient's head or turn him on his side to allow secretions to drain
- After the seizure, reassure the patient that he's okay, orient him to time and place and tell him that he had a seizure.

Spinal cord injury

Spinal injuries include fractures, contusions and compressions of the vertebral column. They usually result from trauma to the head or neck. Fractures of the 5th, 6th or 7th cervical; 12th thoracic and 1st lumbar vertebrae are most common.

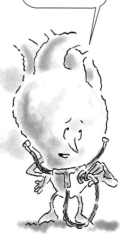

Be alert for cardiac changes after seizures.

Dangerous damage

The real danger with spinal injury is spinal cord damage due to cutting, pulling, swelling, twisting and compression. Spinal cord injury can occur at any level, and the damage it causes may be partial or involve the entire cord. Complications of spinal cord injury include neurogenic shock and spinal shock.

What causes it

The most serious spinal cord trauma typically results from motor vehicle collisions, falls, sports injuries, dives into shallow water and gunshot or stab wounds. Less serious injuries commonly occur from lifting heavy objects and minor falls. Spinal cord dysfunction may also result from hyperparathyroidism and neoplastic lesions.

How it happens

Spinal cord trauma results from deforming forces. Types of trauma include:
- Hyperextension
- Hyperflexion
- Rotational twisting, which adds shearing forces
- Vertebral compression from downward force from the top of the cranium or from the sacrum upward, along the vertical axis, and through the vertebra.

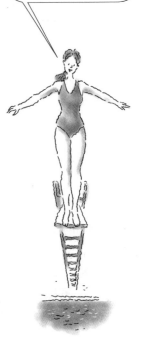

Look out below! Diving into shallow water is a top cause of serious spinal cord trauma.

During spinal cord trauma
- An injury causes microscopic haemorrhages in the gray matter and pia-arachnoid, or macroscopic damage, tearing, compression and disruption
- The haemorrhages gradually increase in size until all of the gray matter is filled with blood, which causes necrosis
- From the gray matter, the blood enters the white matter, where it impedes circulation within the spinal cord
- Resulting oedema causes compression and decreases the blood supply
- The spinal cord loses perfusion and becomes ischaemic. The oedema and haemorrhage are usually greatest in the two segments above and below the injury
- The oedema temporarily adds to the patient's dysfunction by increasing pressure and compressing the nerves. For example, oedema near the 3rd to 5th cervical vertebrae may interfere with respiration.

After acute trauma
- In the white matter, circulation usually returns to normal within 24 hours after injury if the cord wasn't transected
- In the gray matter, an inflammatory reaction prevents restoration of circulation
- Phagocytes appear at the site within 35 to 48 hours after injury
- Macrophages engulf degenerating axons and collagen replaces the normal tissue
- Scarring and meningeal thickening leaves the nerves in the area blocked or tangled.

What to look for

In your assessment, look for:
- History of trauma, a neoplastic lesion, or an infection that could produce a spinal abscess
- Muscle spasm and back or neck pain that worsens with movement; in cervical fractures, pain that causes point tenderness; in dorsal and lumbar fractures, pain that may radiate to other areas, such as the legs
- Sensory loss ranging from mild paraesthesia to quadriplegia and shock, if the injury damages the spinal cord; in milder injury, symptoms that may be delayed several days or weeks
- Bruising, pain, oedema, guarding, tenderness and crepitus over the spine and paraspinal area
- Loss of the bulbocavernous reflex with complete cord transection as evidenced by a lack of anal sphincter response when a finger placed in the rectum and then the clitoris or glans is tugged (or when an indwelling urinary catheter is pulled)
- Loss of rectal tone
- Cough tenderness (coughing can induce neck pain)
- Feeling of hot water or an electric shock running down the patient's back
- Mouth breathing because of a loss of diaphragmatic control
- Arms folded across the chest in a guarded position or outstretched above the head, which may indicate a C5 to C6 injury.

Specifically speaking

Specific signs and symptoms depend on the type and degree of injury. (See *Types of spinal cord injury*.)

What tests tell you

Diagnoses of acute spinal cord injuries are based on the results of these diagnostic tests:
- Plain radiograph (X-ray) is the initial investigation of choice and can reveal fractures
- Depending on the patient a CT scan maybe preferable, if there are areas of concern or uncertainty clinically or after the plain radiograph. A CT scan shows the location of the fracture, site of compression, spinal cord oedema and a possible spinal cord mass
- An MRI can be used and can add important information about disc injuries and soft tissue injuries associated with bony injuries
- Neurological evaluation is used to locate the level of injury and detect cord damage.

How it's treated

The primary treatment after spinal injury is immediate immobilisation to stabilise the spine and prevent further cord damage. Other treatment is supportive.

Cervical injuries require immobilisation, using head support on both sides of the patient's head, a hard cervical collar or skeletal traction with skull tongs, a halo device or surgical fixations.

Types of spinal cord injury

Spinal cord injury may be classified as complete or incomplete. Incomplete injury may be an anterior cord syndrome, central cord syndrome or Brown-Séquard syndrome, depending on which area of the cord is affected. To help you assess your patient, here are the characteristic signs and symptoms of each.

Types	Description	Signs and symptoms
Complete injury	• All tracts of the spinal cord completely disrupted • All functions involving the spinal cord below the level of injury lost • Complete and permanent loss	• Loss of motor function (quadriplegia or tetraplegia) with cervical cord transection; paraplegia with thoracic cord transaction • Muscle flaccidity • Loss of all reflexes and sensory function below the level of injury • Bladder and bowel atony • Paralytic ileus • Loss of vasomotor tone in lower body parts with low and unstable blood pressure • Loss of perspiration below the level of injury • Dry, pale skin • Respiratory impairment
Incomplete injury: Central cord syndrome	• Centre position of cord affected • Typically from cervical hyperextension injury	• Motor deficits greater in upper than in lower extremities • Variable degree of bladder dysfunction
Incomplete injury: Anterior cord syndrome	• Occlusion of anterior spinal artery • Occlusion from pressure of bone fragments	• Loss of motor function below the level of injury • Loss of pain and temperature sensations below the level of injury • Intact touch, pressure, position, and vibration senses
Incomplete injury: Brown–Séquard syndrome	• Hemisection of cord affected (damage to cord on only one side) • Most common in stabbing and gunshot wounds	• Ipsilateral paralysis or paresis below the level of injury • Ipsilateral loss of touch, pressure, vibration, and position sense below the level of injury • Contralateral loss of pain and temperature sensations below the level of injury

What to do
- Immediately stabilise the patient's spine. As with all spinal injuries, suspect cord damage until proven otherwise. Use a rigid cervical collar, lateral head immobiliser and backboard
- If the patient has a helmet in place, remove it if possible, according to departmental guidelines. Ensure that at least two persons are present during the removal
- Check the patient's airway and his respiratory rate and rhythm
- Evaluate the patient's LOC
- Perform a neurological assessment to establish baseline motor and sensory status and continually reassess neurological status for changes
- Assess respiratory status closely at least every hour initially. Obtain baseline tidal volume, pulse oximetry and capnography, and reassess frequently. Breath sounds will be auscultated and secretions checked and removed as necessary.

- Monitor oxygen saturation levels and administer supplemental oxygen as indicated
- Begin cardiac monitoring and assess cardiac status frequently, at least every hour initially. Monitor blood pressure and hemodynamic status frequently
- If your patient becomes hypotensive, prepare to administer fluids and vasopressors
- Administer methylprednisolone as ordered if the patient's injury has occurred within the past 8 hours
- Anticipate gastric tube insertion and low intermittent suctioning. Assess the abdomen for distension.

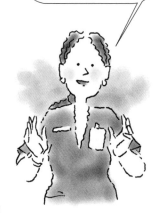

Immediate immobilisation after the injury helps prevent further spinal cord damage.

Distension prevention

- Insert an indwelling urinary catheter as ordered. To prevent bladder distension, monitor intake and output
- Institute measures to keep the patient warm, such as applying warmed blankets, keeping the patient covered when possible and administering warmed I.V. fluids
- Begin measures to prevent skin breakdown due to immobilisation
- Obtain and monitor laboratory and diagnostic test results, including urea and electrolytes, blood sugar, creatinine levels, full blood count (FBC) and urinalysis
- Assess for signs of neurogenic shock, such as bradycardia, pink and warm skin below the injury and cold and pale skin above it, and for signs of spinal shock, such as flaccid paralysis and loss of deep tendon and perianal reflexes
- Prepare the patient for surgical stabilisation if necessary
- Provide emotional support to the patient and his family.

Stroke and Transient Ischaemic Attack (TIA)

Symptoms of stroke include numbness, weakness or paralysis, slurred speech, blurred vision, confusion and severe headache. Stroke is defined by the World Health Organization as a clinical syndrome consisting of 'rapidly developing clinical signs of focal (at times global) disturbance of cerebral function, lasting more than 24 hours or leading to death with no apparent cause other than that of vascular origin'. A TIA is defined as stroke symptoms and signs that resolve within 24 hours. However, the individual patient's presentation may not be as clear cut as these definitions would indicate.

Stroke

Stroke is a sudden impairment of cerebral circulation in one or more blood vessels. Stroke interrupts or diminishes oxygen supply and commonly causes serious damage or necrosis in the brain tissues.

The sooner the better

The sooner circulation returns to normal after a stroke, the better your patient's chances are for a complete recovery. However, about one-half of patients who survive a stroke remain permanently disabled and experience a recurrence within weeks, months or years.

Number three

Stroke is third most common cause of death in the UK after heart disease and cancer. An estimated 150,000 people have a stroke in the UK each year with over 67,000 deaths due to stroke.

What causes it

Stroke typically results from one of three causes:

Thrombosis of the intracranial vessels, occluding blood flow or the cerebral arteries supplying the brain

Embolism from thrombus outside the brain, such as in the heart, aorta or common carotid artery

Haemorrhage from an intracranial artery or vein, such as from hypertension, ruptured aneurysm, AVM, trauma or haemorrhagic disorder.

Risk factor facts

Risk factors that predispose a patient to stroke include:
• Cardiac disease, including arrhythmias, coronary artery disease, myocardial infarction, dilated cardiomyopathy and valvular disease
• Cigarette smoking
• Diabetes
• Familial hyperlipidemia
• Family history of stroke
• History of TIA (See *TIA and the older adult*)
• Hypertension
• Increased alcohol intake
• Obesity and a sedentary lifestyle
• Use of hormonal contraceptives.

How it happens

Regardless of the cause, the underlying event leading to stroke is oxygen and nutrient deprivation in the brain cells. Here's what happens:
• Normally, arterial flow is interrupted and autoregulatory mechanisms maintain cerebral circulation until collateral circulation develops to deliver blood to the affected area
• If the compensatory mechanisms become overworked or cerebral blood flow remains impaired for more than a few minutes, oxygen deprivation leads to infarction of brain tissue
• The brain cells cease to function because they can't engage in anaerobic metabolism or store glucose or glycogen for later use.

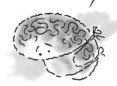

It's sad, but true; one-half of all stroke survivors remain permanently disabled.

Ages and stages

TIA and the older adult

To help assess for a history of transient ischaemic attack (TIA), ask your patient about recent falls – especially frequent falls. Doing so is important because the older adult is less likely to forget about or minimise frequent falls than he is to report other signs of a TIA.

Ischaemic stroke

Here's what happens when a thrombotic or embolic stroke causes cerebral ischaemia:
• Some of the neurons served by the occluded vessel die from lack of oxygen and nutrients
• Cerebral infarction then occurs, in which tissue injury triggers an inflammatory response that in turn increases ICP
• Injury to the surrounding cells disrupts metabolism and leads to changes in ionic transport, localised acidosis, and free radical formation
• Calcium, sodium and water accumulate in the injured cells, and excitatory neurotransmitters are released
• Consequent continued cellular injury and swelling set up a cycle of further damage.

Haemorrhagic Stroke

Here's what happens when a haemorrhage causes a stroke:
• Impaired cerebral perfusion causes infarction, and the blood acts as a space-occupying mass, exerting pressure on the brain tissues
• The brain's regulatory mechanisms attempt to maintain equilibrium by increasing blood pressure to maintain CPP. The increased ICP forces CSF out, thus restoring equilibrium
• If the haemorrhage is small, the patient may have minimal neurological deficits. If the bleeding is heavy then ICP increases rapidly and impedes and compromises cerebral perfusion. Even if the pressure returns to normal, many brain cells die
• Initially, the ruptured cerebral blood vessels may constrict to limit the blood loss. This vasospasm then compromises further blood flow, leading to more ischaemia and cellular damage
• If a clot forms in the vessel, decreased blood flow also promotes ischaemia. If the blood enters the subarachnoid space, meningeal irritation occurs
• Blood cells that pass through the vessel wall into the surrounding tissue may break down and block the arachnoid villi, causing hydrocephalus.

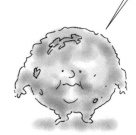

Cellular swelling is one consequence of ischaemic stroke.

What to look for

Clinical features of stroke vary, depending on the artery affected (and, consequently, the portion of the brain it supplies), the severity of the damage and the extent of collateral circulation that develops to help the brain compensate for decreased blood supply. (See *Managing stroke*, pages 310–311). Conduct the *FAST* test:
• Facial weakness
• Arm weakness
• Speech problems
• Test all three

Exclude hypoglycaemia. Conduct the ROSIER (Recognition of Stroke in the Emergency Room) test. (See *Stroke signs and symptoms*, page 312.)

Left is right and right is left

A stroke in the left hemisphere produces symptoms on the right side of the body; in the right hemisphere, symptoms on the left side. Common signs and symptoms of stroke include sudden onset of:
• Hemiparesis on the side opposite the affected side of the brain (may be more severe in the face and arm than in the leg)
• Unilateral sensory defect (such as numbness or tingling) generally on the same side as the hemiparesis (left middle cerebral artery stroke)
• Slurred or indistinct speech or the inability to understand speech
• Blurred or indistinct vision, double vision or vision loss in one eye (usually described as a curtain coming down or 'grey-out' of vision)
• Mental status changes or history or presentation of loss of consciousness (particularly if associated with one of the above symptoms)
• Very severe headache with haemorrhagic stroke (subarachnoid haemorrhage stroke)
• Maybe a seizure has been witnessed.

> Blurred vision, slurred speech and hemiparesis are just three stroke symptoms.

What tests tell you

Here are some test findings that help diagnose a stroke:
• CT scanning discloses structural abnormalities, oedema and lesions, such as non-haemorrhagic infarction and aneurysms. Results are used to differentiate a stroke from other disorders, such as a tumour and haematoma. Patients with TIA generally have a normal CT scan. CT scanning shows evidence of haemorrhagic stroke immediately and of ischaemic (thrombotic or embolic) stroke within 72 hours after the onset of symptoms. CT scans should be obtained immediately ideally but within 1 hour of the patient arriving in the ED, and results should be ideally but certainly within 45 minutes of arrival to determine whether haemorrhage is present. (If haemorrhagic stroke is present, thrombolytic therapy is contraindicated)
• Cerebral angiography shows details of disruption or displacement of the cerebral circulation by occlusion or haemorrhage.

> Give me a CT scan and a DSA! These two tests can help you diagnose a stroke today!

Go with the flow

• Brain scan shows ischaemic areas but may not be conclusive for up to 2 weeks after stroke
• No laboratory tests confirm the diagnosis of stroke, but some tests aid diagnosis and some are used to establish a baseline for thrombolytic treatment. A blood glucose test shows whether the patient's symptoms are related to hypoglycaemia. Haemoglobin level and haematocrit may be elevated in severe occlusion. Baselines obtained before thrombolytic therapy begins include U & Es, FBC, platelet count, PTT, PT and fibrinogen levels.

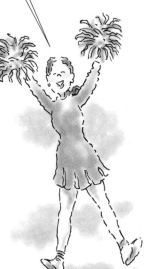

(Text continues on page 313.)

Managing stroke

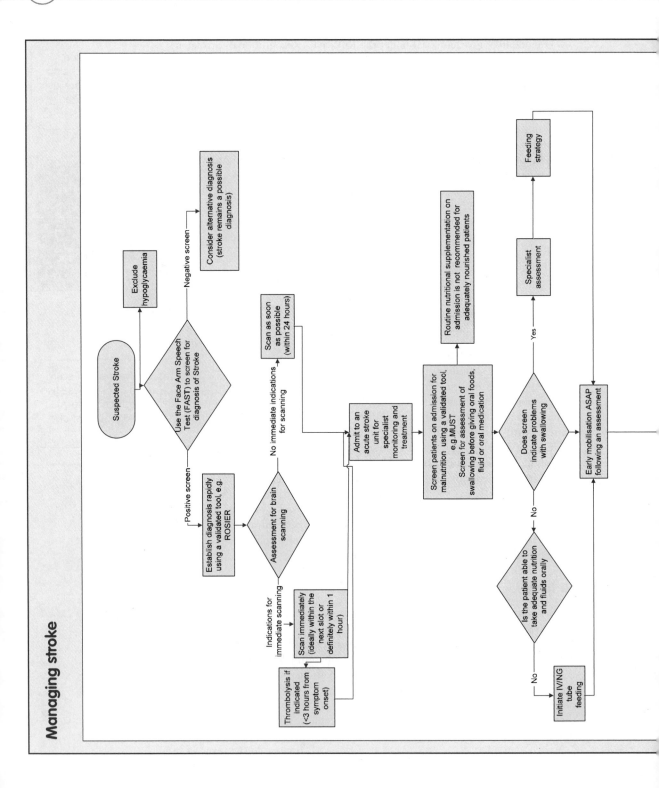

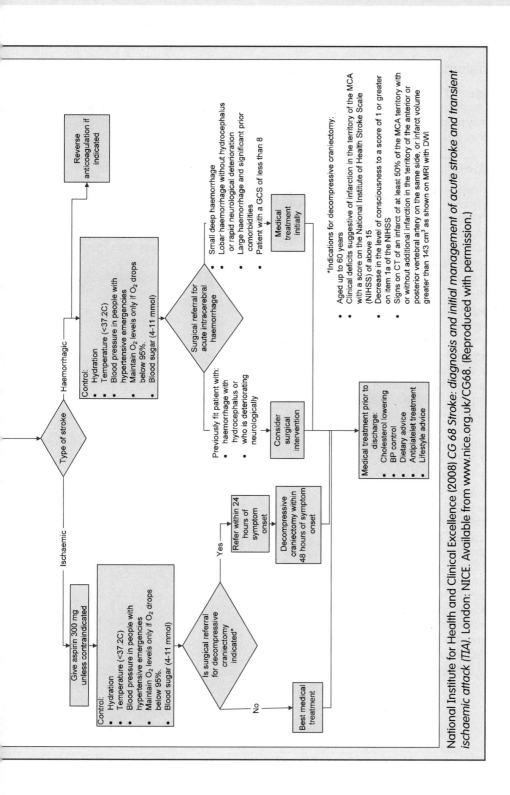

National Institute for Health and Clinical Excellence (2008) *CG 68 Stroke: diagnosis and initial management of acute stroke and transient ischaemic attack (TIA)*. London: NICE. Available from www.nice.org.uk/CG68. (Reproduced with permission.)

Stroke signs and symptoms

With stroke, functional loss reflects damage to the area of the brain that's normally perfused by the occluded or ruptured artery. Although one patient may experience only mild hand weakness, another may develop unilateral paralysis.

Hypoxia and ischaemia may produce oedema that affects distal parts of the brain, causing further neurological deficits. Here are the signs and symptoms that accompany stroke at different sites.

Site	Signs and symptoms	Site	Signs and symptoms
Middle cerebral artery	• Aphasia • Dysphasia • Dyslexia (reading problems) • Dysgraphia (inability to write) • Visual field cuts • Hemiparesis on the affected side, which is more severe in the face and arm than in the leg	Vertebral or basilar artery	• Mouth and lip numbness • Dizziness • Weakness on the affected side • Vision deficits, such as colour blindness, lack of depth perception and diplopia • Poor coordination • Dysphagia • Slurred speech • Amnesia • Ataxia
Internal carotid artery	• Headaches • Weakness • Paralysis • Numbness • Sensory changes • Vision disturbances such as blurring on the affected side • Altered level of consciousness • Bruits over the carotid artery • Aphasia • Dysphagia • Ptosis (dropping of the eyelid)	Posterior cerebral artery	• Visual field cuts • Sensory impairment • Dyslexia • Coma • Blindness from ischaemia in the occipital area
Anterior cerebral artery	• Confusion • Weakness • Numbness on the affected side (especially in the arm) • Paralysis of the contralateral foot and leg • Incontinence • Poor coordination • Impaired motor and sensory functions • Personality changes, such as flat affect and distractibility		

How stroke is treated

The goal is to begin treatment within 60 minutes after your patient arrives in the ED.

Drugs of choice

Thrombolytics (also called *fibrinolytics*) are the drugs of choice in treating a stroke patient. The patient must first meet certain criteria to be considered for this type of treatment. (See *Who's suited for thrombolytic therapy?* page 314)

Drugs for management

Drug therapy for the management of stroke includes:
- Thrombolytics for emergency treatment of ischaemic stroke
- Aspirin as an antiplatelet agent to prevent recurrent ischaemic stroke
- Benzodiazepines to treat patients with seizure activity.

Drugs that may be used

- Antihypertensives and antiarrhythmics to treat patients with risk factors for recurrent stroke
- Corticosteroids to minimise associated cerebral oedema
- Analgesics to relieve the headaches that may follow a haemorrhagic stroke.

Under the knife

Depending on the cause and extent of the stroke, the patient may undergo:
- Craniotomy to remove a haematoma
- Carotid endarterectomy to remove atherosclerotic plaques from the inner arterial wall
- Extracranial bypass to circumvent an artery that's blocked by occlusion or stenosis.

Practice pointers
- Assess ABCDE
- Ensure that the patient's airway, breathing and circulation are adequate
- Secure and maintain the patient's airway and anticipate the need for ET intubation and mechanical ventilation
- Evaluate the patient and complete an initial stroke-screening tool, such as the ROSIER scale. Report findings and facilitate rapid and appropriate care of the patient. Rapid brain imaging is required, so appropriate treatment can be undertaken
- Monitor oxygen saturation levels via pulse oximetry and ABG levels as ordered. Administer supplemental oxygen as ordered to maintain oxygen saturation within prescribed levels following British Thoracic Society guidelines

Stay on the ball

Who's suited for thrombolytic therapy?

Once you've assessed, call for the best – the stroke team if your hospital has one! They'll be able to provide further evaluation.

Not every stroke patient is a candidate for thrombolytic therapy. Each is evaluated to see whether established criteria are met.

Criteria that must be present

Criteria that must be present for a patient to be considered for thrombolytic therapy include:
- Age 18 or older
- Acute ischaemic stroke associated with significant neurological deficit
- Onset of symptoms less than 3 hours before treatment begins

Criteria that must *not* be present

In addition to meeting the above criteria, *the patient must not:*
- Show evidence of intracerebral haemorrhage during pretreatment evaluation
- Exhibit evidence of subarachnoid haemorrhage during pretreatment evaluation even if computed tomographic (CT) scan is normal
- Have a history of recent (within 3 months) intracranial or intraspinal surgery, serious head trauma or previous stroke
- Have a history of intracranial haemorrhage

- Have uncontrolled hypertension at the time of treatment (blood pressure remaining at greater than 185 mm Hg systolic and greater than 110 mm Hg diastolic)
- Have experienced a seizure at the onset of stroke
- Have active internal bleeding or acute trauma
- Have an intracranial neoplasm, arteriovenous malformation or aneurysm
- Have known bleeding diathesis involving, but not limited to:
  - Current use of oral anticoagulants, such as warfarin, International Normalised Ratio greater than 1.7, or prothrombin time greater than 15 seconds
  - Receipt of heparin within 48 hours before the onset of stroke and an elevated partial thromboplastin time
  - Platelet count less than 100,000/ml
- Have a CT scan showing a multilobar infarction
- Have experienced arterial puncture at a noncompressible site within the last 7 days
- Have anticonvulsants to treat patients with seizures or to prevent them after the patient's condition has stabilised

- Place the patient on a cardiac monitor, and monitor for cardiac arrhythmias. Order a 12-lead ECG
- Assess the patient's neurological status frequently; at least every 15 to 30 minutes initially, then hourly as indicated. Observe for signs of increased ICP
- Obtain laboratory studies as ordered, such as FBC, PT, International Normalised Ratio and PTT
- Prepare to administer an anti-hypertension drug, such as labetalol, to maintain the patient's blood pressure at less than 185 mm Hg systolic and less than 110 mm Hg diastolic
- Assess haemodynamic status frequently. Give fluids as ordered and monitor I.V. infusions to avoid overhydration, which may increase ICP
- Assess the patient receiving thrombolytic therapy for signs and symptoms of bleeding every 15 to 30 minutes and institute bleeding precautions. Monitor results of coagulation studies
- Your ED may have a stroke protocol and can call on a stroke team composed of specially trained practitioners who respond to potential stroke patients; ideally patients are admitted directly there. They will then evaluate the patient and complete a neurological assessment using a tool such as the 15-item neurologic examination National Institutes of Health Stroke Scale (NIHSS).

Anticonvulsant, antiplatelet, anticoagulation

- Monitor the patient for seizures and administer anticonvulsants as ordered
- Institute safety precautions to prevent injury
- If the patient had a TIA, administer antiplatelet agents. Administer anticoagulants such as heparin if he shows signs of stroke progression, unstable signs of stroke (such as TIA) or evidence of embolic stroke. Monitor coagulation studies closely
- If the patient has had an ischaemic stroke, prepare to administer intravenous rt-PA alteplase but only under the direct instruction of a neurologist
- Initiate steps to prevent skin breakdown
- Provide meticulous eye and mouth care
- Maintain communication with the patient. If he's aphasic, set up a simple method of communicating
- Provide psychological support
- Anticipate transfer to the ICU or interventional radiology as appropriate.

Subarachnoid haemorrhage

Subarachnoid haemorrhage refers to bleeding that occurs into the subarachnoid space. CSF normally occupies this space. This major complication is associated with cerebral aneurysms.

It's cerebral

A cerebral aneurysm is a weakness in the wall of a cerebral artery that causes the area of the artery to dilate or bulge. The most common form is a *berry aneurysm*, a saclike outpouching in a cerebral artery. Cerebral aneurysms usually arise at an arterial junction in the circle of Willis, the circular anastomosis forming the major cerebral arteries at the base of the brain.

Women more prone

The incidence of cerebral aneurysm is slightly higher in women than in men, especially those in their late 40s or early to mid-50s, but a cerebral aneurysm can occur at any age in either gender.

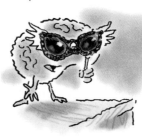

Did you say sub-arachnid? I'm scared of spiders!

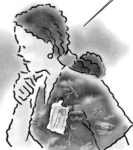

No, I said subarachnoid, as in haemorrhage, which might be scarier!

What causes it

The major cause of a subarachnoid haemorrhage is rupture of a cerebral aneurysm. A cerebral aneurysm may result from a congenital defect, such as an AVM, from a degenerative process or both. The most common cause is trauma.

How it happens

Subarachnoid haemorrhage happens when blood flow exerts pressure against a weak arterial wall, stretching it like an overblown balloon and making it likely to rupture. Rupture is followed by haemorrhage, in which blood spills into the subarachnoid space normally occupied by CSF. Sometimes, blood also spills into brain tissue, where a clot can cause potentially fatal increased ICP and brain tissue damage. Spasm of the cerebral arteries can compound the damage. There is also a risk of a re-bleed.

What to look for

Occasionally, your patient may exhibit signs and symptoms due to blood oozing into the subarachnoid space. These signs and symptoms, which may have persisted for several days, include:
• Headache
• Intermittent nausea and vomiting
• Neck rigidity
• Photophobia
• Stiff back and legs.

Without warning

Aneurysm rupture usually occurs abruptly and without warning, causing:
• Sudden, severe headache from increased pressure due to bleeding into a closed space. Patients often describe this sudden severe headache as being like a 'thunderclap'

Grading cerebral aneurysm rupture

The severity of cerebral aneurysm symptoms varies from patient to patient, depending on the site and amount of bleeding. Five grades characterise ruptured cerebral aneurysm:
- *Grade I: minimal bleeding* – The patient is alert, with no neurological deficit; he may have a slight headache and nuchal rigidity
- *Grade II: mild bleeding* – The patient is alert, with a mild to severe headache and nuchal rigidity; he may have third-nerve palsy
- *Grade III: moderate bleeding* – The patient is confused or drowsy, with nuchal rigidity and, possibly, a mild focal deficit
- *Grade IV: severe bleeding* –The patient is stuporous, with nuchal rigidity and, possibly, mild to severe hemiparesis
- *Grade V: moribund (usually fatal)* – If the rupture is nonfatal, the patient is in a deep coma or decerebrate.

- Nausea and projectile vomiting related to increased ICP
- Altered LOC (possibly including deep coma, depending on the severity and location of bleeding) due to increased pressure caused by increased cerebral blood volume
- Meningeal irritation due to bleeding into the meninges and resulting in neck rigidity, back and leg pain, fever, restlessness, irritability, occasional seizures, photophobia and blurred vision
- Hemiparesis, hemisensory defects, dysphagia and vision defects due to bleeding into the brain tissues
- Diplopia, ptosis (dropping of the eyelid), dilated pupil and inability to rotate the eye caused by compression on the oculomotor nerve if the aneurysm is near the internal carotid artery.

Making the grade

Typically, the severity of a ruptured intracranial aneurysm is graded according to the patient's signs and symptoms. (See *Grading cerebral aneurysm rupture*.)

What tests tell you
The following tests aid in the diagnosis of cerebral aneurysm:
- Cerebral angiography confirms a cerebral aneurysm that isn't ruptured and reveals altered cerebral blood flow, vessel lumen dilation and differences in arterial filling
- CT scan reveals evidence of aneurysm and possible haemorrhage
- Lumbar puncture and analysis of CSF will reveal blood in the CSF
- MRI is used to detect vasospasm and locate the bleeding.

How it's treated
Emergency treatment begins with oxygenation and ventilation. Then, to reduce the risk of rebleeding, the neurosurgeon or neuroradiologist

may attempt to repair the aneurysm. Surgical repair usually includes clipping, ligating or wrapping the aneurysm neck with muscle and sealing. Nimodipine may be given to reduce the risk of cerebral arterial spasm.

Being conservative

The patient may receive conservative treatment when surgical correction poses too much risk, such as with an older person or when the patient has heart, lung or other serious disease, when the aneurysm is in a dangerous location or when vasospasm necessitates a delay in surgery.

What to do

• Establish and maintain a patent airway and anticipate the need for supplementary oxygen or mechanical ventilatory support. Monitor blood gases
• Initiate cardiac monitoring and be alert for cardiac changes and arrhythmias
• Position the patient to promote pulmonary drainage and prevent upper airway obstruction. If intubated, preoxygenate with 100% oxygen before suctioning
• Impose aneurysm precautions (such as bed rest, limited visitors, and avoidance of coffee and physical activity) to minimise the risk of rebleeding and avoid increased ICP
• Monitor LOC and vital signs frequently. Avoid taking temperatures rectally
• Accurately measure intake and output.

Watch out

• Be alert for danger signs and symptoms that may indicate an enlarging aneurysm, rebleeding, intracranial clot, increased ICP or vasospasm. These signs and symptoms include decreased LOC, unilateral enlarged pupil, onset or worsening of hemiparesis or motor deficit, increased blood pressure, slowed pulse rate, worsening of headache or sudden onset of a headache, renewed or worsened nuchal rigidity and renewed or persistent vomiting
• If the patient develops vasospasm – evidenced by focal motor deficits, increasing confusion and worsening headache – initiate hypervolemic-haemodilution therapy as ordered, such as the administration of normal or hypertonic saline, whole blood, packed red cells, albumin plasma protein fraction and crystalloid solution. The calcium channel blocker nimodipine may reduce smooth-muscle spasm and maximise perfusion during spasm. During therapy, assess the patient for fluid overload
• Turn the patient often and institute measures to reduce the risks associated with bed rest.

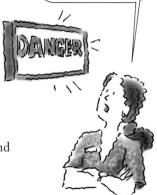

These danger signs may indicate an enlarging aneurysm or other problems.

DANGER

Rebound effects

- Inform the patient and his family about the condition, planned treatments and possible complications
- Prepare the patient for transfer to specialist unit, or the ICU, as appropriate; provide preoperative teaching if the patient's condition permits.

Quick quiz

1. Which finding would lead the nurse to suspect that a patient with spinal cord injury is experiencing spinal shock?
    A. Orthostatic hypotension.
    B. Bradycardia.
    C. Flaccid paralysis.
    D. Lack of sweating below the level of injury.

Answer: C. Signs of spinal shock include flaccid paralysis, loss of deep tendon and perianal reflexes and loss of motor and sensory function.

2. A patient with a head injury is admitted to the ED. Emergency response personnel report that the patient suffered a brief period of loss of consciousness after the injury but is now lucid and complaining of vomiting and a severe headache. Which condition would the nurse suspect?
    A. Concussion.
    B. Skull fracture.
    C. Subdural haematoma.
    D. Diffuse axonal injury.

Answer: A & B. A brief period of loss of consciousness followed by a lucid period and complaints of vomiting and a severe headache may indicate a concussion or skull fracture.

3. During a neurological examination, the patient can't raise his eyebrows or close his eyes tightly against resistance. Which cranial nerve might be damaged?
    A. CN II.
    B. CN V.
    C. CN VII.
    D. CN XII.

Answer: C. The facial nerve, CN VII, controls facial expression and taste in the anterior two-thirds of the tongue.

4. Rapid identification of stroke can lead to appropriate treatment quickly. Which of these tests are used to assess stroke?
    A. ROSIER.
    B. FAST.
    C. NIHSS.
    D. All of the above.

Answer: D. FAST is used often in the pre-hospital setting; ROSIER during the ED assessment: and NIHSS by the Stroke Team.

Scoring

☆☆☆   If you answered all four questions correctly, pat yourself on the back! You're a neurological emergency know-it-all.

☆☆   If you answered three questions correctly, stand tall! You're emerging as an emergency expert.

☆   If you answered fewer than three questions correctly, don't worry! Just 'head' back to the beginning of the chapter and try again.

9 Gastrointestinal emergencies

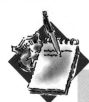

Just the facts

In this chapter, you'll learn:

♦ Emergency assessment of the gastrointestinal (GI) system

♦ Diagnostic tests and procedures for GI emergencies

♦ GI disorders in the emergency department (ED) and their treatments

Understanding GI emergencies

Being able to identify subtle changes in a patient's GI system can mean the difference between effective and ineffective emergency care. GI signs and symptoms can have many baffling causes. When your patient comes to the ED with a GI emergency, your assessment can be used to determine whether the patient's signs and symptoms are related to his current medical problem or indicate a new problem.

When faced with an emergency involving the GI system, you must assess the patient thoroughly, although you will be guided by your level of practice and local policies of assessment and investigations. You should stay alert for subtle changes that may indicate a potential deterioration the patient. A thorough assessment forms the basis for your interventions, which then must be instituted quickly to minimise what can be life-threatening risks to the patient.

Assessment

Unless the patient requires immediate stabilising treatment found in the primary survey, begin by taking a thorough health history. Then probe further by conducting a thorough physical examination by inspection, auscultation, percussion and palpation.

If you can't interview the patient because of his condition, you may gather the patient's history from his family members or his medical record.

In some cases, you may need to ask the paramedic team that transported him to the ED.

Health history

Begin by introducing yourself and explaining what happens during the health history and physical examination. Then obtain information about the patient's chief complaint, medications used, family history and lifestyle patterns. Conduct this part of the assessment as privately as possible because the patient may feel embarrassed when talking about GI function.

Chief complaint
A patient with a GI problem can complain of:
• Altered bowel habits
• Heartburn
• Nausea
• Pain
• Vomiting.
   To investigate these and other signs and symptoms, ask about the onset, duration and severity of each. Inquire about the location of the pain, precipitating factors, alleviating factors and associated symptoms. (See *Asking the right questions*.)

Previous health status

To determine if the patient's problem is new or recurring, ask about GI illnesses, such as an ulcer, gallbladder disease, inflammatory bowel disease and GI bleeding. Also ask if he has had abdominal surgery or trauma.

Further questions

Ask the patient additional questions, such as:
• Are you allergic to any foods or medications?
• Have you noticed a change in the colour, amount and appearance of your stool? Have you ever seen blood in your stool?
• Have you recently travelled abroad? (This question applies if the patient seeks care for diarrhoea, because diarrhoea, hepatitis and parasitic infections can result from ingesting contaminated food or water)
• Ask him about his dental history. Poor dentition may impair his ability to chew and swallow food.

Medications used
Ask the patient if he's taking medication. Several drugs, including aspirin, nonsteroidal anti-inflammatory drugs (NSAIDs), analgesics and some antihypertensives, can cause nausea, vomiting, diarrhoea, constipation and other GI problems. Be sure to ask about laxative use because habitual laxative intake can cause constipation.

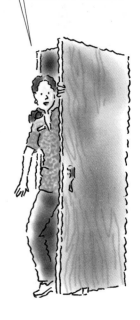

A patient may be embarrassed to talk about GI function, so make your health history assessment as private as possible.

Asking the right questions

When assessing a patient with GI-related signs and symptoms, be sure to ask the right questions. To establish a baseline for comparison, ask about the patient's current state of health, including questions about the onset, duration, quality, severity and location of problems as well as precipitating factors, alleviating factors and associated symptoms.

Onset

How did the problem start? Was it gradual or sudden? With or without previous symptoms? What was the patient doing when he noticed it? If he has diarrhoea, has he been travelling? If so, when and where?

Duration

When did the problem start? Has the patient had the problem before? Has he had abdominal surgery? If yes, when? If he's in pain, find out when the problem began. Is the pain continuous, intermittent or colicky (cramplike)?

Quality

Ask the patient to describe the problem. Has he ever had it before? Was it diagnosed? If he's in pain, find out whether the pain feels sharp, dull, aching or burning.

Severity

Ask the patient to describe how badly the problem bothers him – for example, have him rate it on a pain scale of 0 to 10. Does it keep him from his normal activities? Has it improved or worsened since he first noticed it? Does it wake him at night? If he's in pain, does he double over from it?

Location

Where does the patient feel the problem? Does it spread, radiate or shift? Ask him to point to where he feels it the most.

Precipitating factors

Does anything seem to bring on the problem? What makes it worse? Does it occur at the same time each day or with certain positions? Does the patient notice it after eating or drinking certain foods or after certain activities?

Alleviating factors

Does anything relieve the problem? Does the patient take any prescribed or over-the-counter medications for relief? Has he tried anything else for relief?

Associated symptoms

What else bothers the patient when he has the problem? Has he had nausea, vomiting, dry heaves, diarrhoea, constipation, bloating or flatulence? Has he lost his appetite or lost or gained any weight? If so, how much? When was the patient's last bowel movement? Was it unusual? Has he seen blood in his vomitus or stool? Has his stool changed in size or colour or included mucus? Ask the patient whether he can eat normally and hold down foods and liquids. Also ask about alcohol consumption.

Family history

Because some GI disorders are hereditary, ask the patient whether anyone in his family has had a GI disorder, including:

- Colon cancer
- Crohn's disease
- Diabetes
- Stomach ulcer
- Ulcerative colitis.

Sociological factors

Psychological and sociologic factors can profoundly affect health. To determine factors that may have contributed to your patient's problem, ask about his occupation, home life, financial situation, stress level and recent life changes.

Be sure to ask about alcohol, recreational drugs, caffeine and tobacco use as well as food consumption, exercise habits and oral hygiene. Also ask about sleep patterns, such as hours of sleep and whether sleep is restful.

Cultural factors may affect a patient's dietary habits; so ask about any dietary restrictions the patient has, such as following a vegetarian diet.

Physical examination

You will be guided by your level of practice and local policies of assessment and investigations.

Physical examination of the GI system usually includes evaluation of the mouth, abdomen, liver, rectum and spleen. Before beginning your examination, gain consent, explain the techniques you'll be using and warn the patient that some procedures might be uncomfortable. Perform the examination in a private, quiet, warm and well-lit room.

Assessing the mouth

Use inspection and palpation to assess the oral cavity:
• First, inspect the patient's mouth and jaw for asymmetry and swelling. Check his bite, noting any misalignment of his teeth from an overbite or underbite. If the patient has dentures, do they fit? Are they intact or broken?
• Inspect the inner and outer lips, teeth and gums with a penlight. Note bleeding, gum ulcerations and missing, displaced or broken teeth. Palpate the gums for tenderness and the inner lips and cheeks for lesions
• Assess the tongue, checking for coating, tremors, swelling and ulcerations. Note unusual breath odours
• Lastly, examine the pharynx, looking for uvular deviation, tonsillar abnormalities, lesions, plaques and exudate.

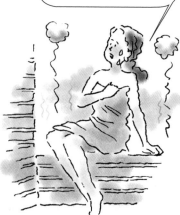

Keeping the room, your hands and your stethoscope warm (but not this warm) can ease patient discomfort during abdominal examination.

Assessing the abdomen

To ensure an accurate assessment, be sure to:
• Cover the patient appropriately to maintain dignity
• Keep the room warm because chilling can cause abdominal muscles to tense
• Warm your hands and the stethoscope
• Speak softly and encourage the patient to perform breathing exercises or use imagery during uncomfortable procedures
• Assess painful areas last to avoid making the patient tense
• Make sure you avoid embarrassment for the patient by trying to maintain his dignity when you are not examining him.

In order, please

The GI system requires abdominal auscultation before percussion and palpation because the latter can alter intestinal activity and bowel sounds.

So, when assessing the abdomen, perform the four basic steps in the following sequence:

 Inspection

 Auscultation

 Percussion

 Palpation

Abdominal inspection

Before inspecting the abdomen, mentally divide it into four quadrants. This can assist in identifying areas for examination. (See *Identifying abdominal landmarks*, page 326.)

General inspection

Begin by performing a general inspection of the patient:
• Observe the skin, oral mucosa, nail beds and sclera for jaundice or signs of anaemia
• Observe the abdomen for symmetry, checking for bumps, bulges or masses. A bulge may indicate bladder distention or hernia
• Note the patient's abdominal shape and contour. The abdomen should be flat to rounded in people of average weight. A protruding abdomen may be caused by obesity, pregnancy, ascites or abdominal distention. A slender person may have a slightly concave abdomen.

To striae or not to striae

Next, inspect the abdominal skin, which normally appears smooth and intact. Striae, or stretch marks, can be caused by pregnancy, excessive weight gain or ascites. New striae are pink or blue; old striae are silvery white. In patients with darker skin, striae may be dark brown. Note dilated veins. Record the length of any surgical scars on the abdomen.

Note abdominal movements and pulsations. Usually, waves of peristalsis aren't visible unless the patient is very thin, in which case they may be visible as slight wavelike motions. Marked visible rippling may indicate bowel obstruction; report it immediately. In a thin patient, pulsation of the aorta is visible in the epigastric area. Marked pulsations may occur with hypertension, aortic insufficiency and other conditions causing widening pulse pressure.

Abdominal auscultation

Auscultation provides information about bowel motility and the underlying vessels and organs.

Follow the clock

Use a stethoscope to auscultate for bowel and vascular sounds. Lightly place the stethoscope diaphragm in the right lower quadrant, slightly below and to the right of the umbilicus.

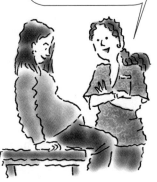

The cause of abdominal bulge is pretty obvious here, but in other patients it may be due to distention or hernia.

Identifying abdominal landmarks

To aid accurate abdominal assessment and documentation of findings, you can mentally divide the patient's abdomen into regions. Use the quadrant method – the easiest and most commonly used method – to divide the abdomen into four equal regions using two imaginary perpendicular lines crossing above the umbilicus.

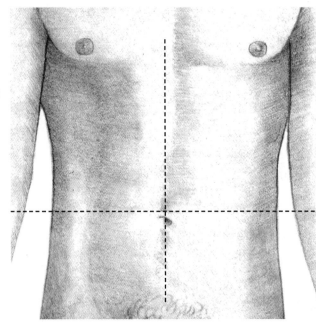

Right upper quadrant
• Liver and gallbladder
• Pylorus
• Duodenum
• Head of pancreas
• Hepatic flexure of colon
• Portions of ascending and transverse colon

Left upper quadrant
• Left liver lobe
• Stomach
• Body of pancreas
• Splenic flexure of colon
• Portions of transverse and descending colon

Right lower quadrant
• Caecum and appendix
• Portion of ascending colon
• Lower portion of right kidney
• Bladder (if distended)

Left lower quadrant
• Sigmoid colon
• Portion of descending colon
• Lower portion of left kidney
• Bladder (if distended)

Do you hear what I hear?

Auscultate in a clockwise fashion in each of the four quadrants, spending at least 2 minutes in each area. Note the character and quality of bowel sounds in each quadrant. In some cases, you may need to auscultate for 5 minutes before you hear sounds. Be sure to allow enough time to listen in each quadrant before you decide that bowel sounds are absent.

Sound class

Bowel sounds are classified as normal, hypoactive or hyperactive:
• *Normal* bowel sounds are high-pitched, gurgling noises caused by air mixing with fluid during peristalsis. The noises vary in frequency, pitch and intensity and occur irregularly from 5 to 34 times per minute. They're loudest before mealtimes. Borborygmus, or stomach growling, is the loud, gurgling, splashing sound heard over the large intestine as gas passes through it

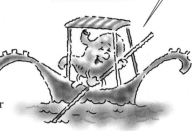

The gurgling, the splashing – nothing makes me happier than a normal bowel sound!

- *Hypoactive* bowel sounds are heard infrequently. They're associated with bowel obstruction, or peritonitis and indicate diminished peristalsis. Paralytic ileus, torsion of the bowel or use of opioids and other medications can decrease peristalsis
- *Hyperactive* bowel sounds are loud, high-pitched, tinkling sounds that occur frequently and may be caused by diarrhoea, constipation or laxative use.

Sound off

Next, use the bell of the stethoscope to auscultate for vascular sounds. Normally, you should detect no vascular sounds. Note a bruit, venous hum or friction rub. (See *Interpreting abnormal abdominal sounds*, page 328.)

Abdominal percussion

Use abdominal percussion to determine the size and location of abdominal organs and detect excessive accumulation of fluid and air. Begin percussion in the right lower quadrant and proceed clockwise, covering all four quadrants. Keep the approximate locations of the patient's organs in mind as you progress. Use direct or indirect percussion:
- In *direct* percussion, strike your hand or finger directly over the patient's abdomen
- With *indirect* percussion, use the middle finger of your dominant hand or a percussion hammer to strike a finger resting on the patient's abdomen.

Percussion precaution

Don't percuss the abdomen of a patient with an abdominal aortic aneurysm or a transplanted abdominal organ. Doing so can precipitate a rupture or organ rejection.

Tympany and dullness

Normally, you should hear two sounds during percussion of the abdomen: (1) tympany and (2) dullness. When you percuss over hollow organs, such as an empty stomach or bowel, you should hear a clear, hollow sound like a drum beating. This sound, *tympany*, predominates because air is normally present in the stomach and bowel. The degree of tympany depends on the amount of air and gastric dilation.

When you percuss over solid organs, such as the liver, kidney or faeces-filled intestines, the sound changes to dullness. Note where percussed sounds change from tympany to dullness, which may indicate a solid mass or enlarged organ.

Abdominal palpation

Abdominal palpation includes light and deep touch to determine the size, shape, position and tenderness of major abdominal organs and detect masses and fluid accumulation. Palpate all four quadrants, leaving painful and tender areas for last.

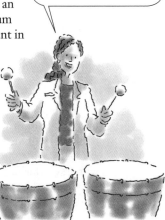

Tympany should be the predominant sound you hear when percussing the abdomen. And now for my drum roll…

Interpreting abnormal abdominal sounds

This chart lists abnormal abdominal sounds along with the location and possible cause of each.

Sound and description	Location	Possible cause
Abnormal bowel sounds		
Hyperactive sounds (unrelated to hunger)	Any quadrant	Diarrhoea, laxative use or early intestinal obstruction
Hypoactive, then absent sounds	Any quadrant	Paralytic ileus or peritonitis
High-pitched tinkling sounds	Any quadrant	Intestinal fluid and air under tension in a dilated bowel
High-pitched rushing sounds coinciding with abdominal cramps	Any quadrant	Intestinal obstruction
Systolic bruits		
Vascular blowing sounds resembling cardiac murmurs	Over abdominal aorta Over renal artery Over iliac artery	Partial arterial obstruction or turbulent blood flow Renal artery stenosis Iliac artery obstruction
Venous hum		
Continuous, medium-pitched tone created by blood flow in a large engorged vascular organ such as the liver	Epigastric and umbilical regions	Increased collateral circulation between portal and systemic venous systems, such as in cirrhosis
Friction rub		
Harsh, grating sound like two pieces of sandpaper rubbing together	Over liver and spleen	Inflammation of the peritoneal surface of the liver, such as from a tumour

Light palpation

Use light palpation to identify muscle resistance and tenderness as well as the location of some superficial organs. To do so, gently press your fingertips 1.5 to 2 cm (½″ to ¾″) into the abdominal wall. Use the lightest touch possible because too much pressure blunts your sensitivity.

Deep palpation

Use deep palpation by pressing the fingertips of both hands about 3.5 cm (½″) into the abdominal wall. Move your hands in a slightly circular fashion so that the abdominal wall moves over the underlying structures.

Deep palpation may evoke rebound tenderness when you suddenly withdraw your fingertips, a possible sign of peritoneal inflammation. Rebound tenderness is a painful procedure and should not be carried out where there is sufficient evidence from the history and the rest of the examination for an acute abdomen, for example, altered bowel sounds, guarding, tenderness, temperature and vomiting.

Percussing the liver

Begin percussing the abdomen along the right midclavicular line, starting below the level of the umbilicus. Move upward until the percussion notes change from tympany to dullness, usually at or slightly below the costal margin. Mark the point of change with a felt-tip pen.

Then percuss downward along the right midclavicular line, starting above the nipple. Move downward until percussion notes change from normal lung resonance to dullness, usually at the 5th to 7th intercostal space. Again, mark the point of change with a felt-tip pen. Estimate liver size by measuring the distance between the two marks.

Anatomic landmarks for liver percussion

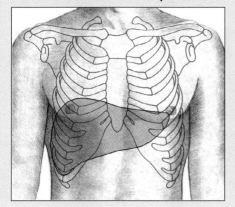

Hand position for liver percussion

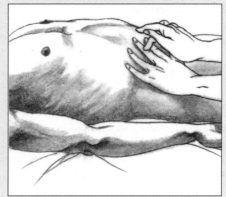

Assessing the liver

You can estimate the size and position of the liver through percussion and palpation.

Percussion discussion

Percussing the liver allows you to estimate its size. Hepatomegaly is commonly associated with hepatitis and other liver disease. Liver borders may be obscured and difficult to assess. (See *Percussing the liver*.)

Palpation problem

It's usually impossible to palpate the liver in an adult patient. If palpable, the liver border feels smooth and firm, with a rounded, regular edge. A palpable liver may indicate hepatomegaly. To palpate for hepatomegaly:

☝ Start at the lower left quadrant

✌ Have the patient take a deep breath and hold it while you palpate using the tips of your fingers

🖐 Slowly move your hand up towards the costal margin and palpate while the patient exhales.

Assessing the rectum

A rectal examination may be part of your GI assessment, although, to maintain dignity and repeated procedures, this procedure may be performed by the doctor who has accepted the care of the patient. Explain the procedure to reassure the patient.

Perianal is primary

To perform a rectal examination, first inspect the perianal area following these steps:
• Put on gloves and spread the buttocks to expose the anus and surrounding tissue, checking for fissures, lesions, scars, inflammation, discharge, rectal prolapse and external haemorrhoids
• Ask the patient to strain as if he's having a bowel movement; this may reveal internal haemorrhoids, polyps or fissures.

Rectum is next

After examining the perianal area, palpate the rectum:
• Place the patient in the left lateral position
• Apply a water-soluble lubricant to your gloved index finger. Tell the patient to relax and explain to him that he'll feel some pressure
• Insert your finger into the rectum towards the umbilicus. To palpate, rotate your finger. The walls should feel soft and smooth without masses, faecal impaction or tenderness
• Remove your finger from the rectum and inspect the glove for stool, blood or mucus. Test faecal material adhering to the glove for occult blood.

Faecal studies

Normal stool appears brown and formed but soft. These abnormal findings may indicate a problem:
• Narrow, ribbonlike stool signals spastic or irritable bowel, partial bowel obstruction or rectal obstruction
• Constipation may be caused by diet or medications
• Diarrhoea may indicate spastic bowel or viral infection
• Mixed with blood and mucus, soft stool can signal bacterial infection; mixed with blood or pus, colitis
• Yellow or green stool suggests severe, prolonged diarrhoea; black stool suggests GI bleeding or intake of iron supplements or raw-to-rare meat. Tan or white stool shows hepatic duct or gallbladder-duct blockage, hepatitis or cancer. Red stool may signal colon or rectal bleeding; however, drugs and foods can also cause this colouration
• Most stool contains 10% to 20% fat. A higher fat content can turn stool pasty or greasy, a possible sign of intestinal malabsorption or pancreatic disease.

Bristol Stool Chart

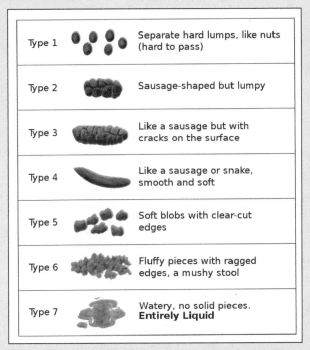

Type 1		Separate hard lumps, like nuts (hard to pass)
Type 2		Sausage-shaped but lumpy
Type 3		Like a sausage but with cracks on the surface
Type 4		Like a sausage or snake, smooth and soft
Type 5		Soft blobs with clear-cut edges
Type 6		Fluffy pieces with ragged edges, a mushy stool
Type 7		Watery, no solid pieces. **Entirely Liquid**

Reproduced with permission from Lewis SJ, Heaton KW (1997). Stool form scale as a useful guide to intestinal transit time. *Scand J Gastroenterol* **32**(9):920–924.

The Bristol Stool Chart could be used to classify the form of faeces. The chart places the faeces into seven types (see *Bristol Stool Chart*):
- Type 1: Separate hard lumps, like nuts (hard to pass)
- Type 2: Sausage-shaped but lumpy
- Type 3: Like a sausage but with cracks on its surface
- Type 4: Like an Italian sausage or snake, smooth and soft
- Type 5: Soft blobs with clear cut edges (passed easily)
- Type 6: Fluffy pieces with ragged edges, a mushy stool
- Type 7: Watery, no solid pieces. Entirely liquid

Types 1 and 2 indicate constipation, with 3 and 4 being the 'ideal stools', as they are the easiest to pass, and 5–7 being further tending towards diarrhoea or urgency.

Practice pointers
- Collect the stool specimen in a clean, dry container, and immediately send it to the laboratory
- Don't use stool that has been in contact with toilet-bowl water or urine.

Assessing the spleen

Unless the spleen is enlarged, it isn't palpable. To attempt to palpate the spleen, stand on the patient's right side. Use your left hand to support his posterior left lower rib cage, and ask him to take a deep breath. Then with your right hand on his abdomen, press up and towards the spleen.

Stop in the name of spleen

If you do feel the spleen, stop palpating immediately because compression can cause rupture.

Diagnostic tests

Many tests provide information to guide your care of a patient with a GI emergency. Even if you don't participate in testing, you should know why the test was ordered, what the results mean, and what your responsibilities are before, during and after the test. Diagnostic tests commonly ordered in the ED include abdominal and chest X-ray, computed tomography (CT) scan, focused ultra sound scan, magnetic resonance imaging (MRI).

Abdominal X-ray

An abdominal X-ray, also called *kidney-ureter-bladder* (KUB) *radiography* is used to detect and evaluate tumours, kidney stones, abnormal gas collection and other abdominal disorders. The test consists of two X-rays: one taken with the patient supine (lying down with the face up) and a chest X-ray taken while he stands (erect).

Reading the rays

On X-ray, air appears black, fat appears gray and bone appears white. Although a routine X-ray doesn't reveal most abdominal organs, it does show the contrast between air and fluid. For example, intestinal blockage traps large amounts of detectable fluids and air inside organs. When an intestinal wall tears, air leaks into the abdomen and becomes visible on X-ray.

Practice pointers
• Explain the procedure to the patient and gain consent
• Radiography requires no special pretest or posttest care. It's usually done on the ED trolley using portable X-ray equipment or X-ray table.

CT scan

A CT is a scanner using X-rays interpreted by a computer and manipulated to form three-dimensional images. It can provide images of the pancreas biliary tract, liver, spleen, GI tract, kidneys, ureter and bladder. The test can be done with or without a contrast medium, but contrast is preferred unless the patient is allergic to contrast media.

Scads of scans

CT scan is used to:
- Distinguish between obstructive and nonobstructive jaundice
- Identify abscesses, cysts, haematomas, tumours and pseudocysts
- Evaluate the cause of weight loss and look for occult malignancy
- Diagnose and evaluate pancreatitis.

Practice pointers
- Gain consent, explain the procedure to the patient and tell him that he should lie still, relax and breathe normally or as instructed during the test. Explain that, if the doctor orders an I.V. contrast medium, he may experience discomfort from the needle puncture, a localised feeling of warmth on injection, wetting sensation and sometimes a metallic taste at the back of the mouth
- Ascertain when the patient last ate or drank; restrict food and fluids as soon as possible, but continue any drug regimen as ordered
- Confirm if the patient has an allergy to iodine or shellfish. Nowadays, modern technology has improved, and the chances of the patient having a reaction to the dye is slim. However, if he has a seafood or dye allergy, a pretest preparation maybe required, and steroid cover will be prescribed to reduce the risk of a reaction to the dye. Report immediately any adverse reactions, such as nausea, vomiting, dizziness, headache and urticaria
- If the patient is nil-by-mouth, increase the I.V. fluid rate as ordered after the procedure to flush the contrast medium from his system. Monitor serum creatinine and blood urea nitrogen levels for signs of acute renal failure, which may be caused by the contrast medium.

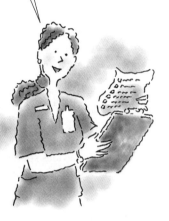

CT scans evaluate everything from A to P – abscesses to pancreatitis – and more.

Focused ultrasound

A focused ultrasound (FAST) scan is currently considered to be a safe, noninvasive, accurate and cost-effective investigation. It allows the diagnosis of potentially life-threatening haemorrhage and can assist in making decisions to determine the need for transfer to the operating room, CT scanner or angiography suite. The equipment can pick up images within the abdomen that can be represented on a monitor screen. These images are detected and transported from a transducer, based with lubricating gel, which is placed in contact with the abdomen and can be moved to look at any particular content of the abdomen.

The information obtained from different reflections is recomposed back into a picture on a monitor screen. Abnormalities can be assessed and measurements of organs can be made accurately on the images displayed on the screen. Such measurements form the foundation of the assessment.

Practice pointers
- Explain the procedure to the patient and tell him that he should lie still, relax and breathe normally during the test
- Ascertain when the patient last ate or drank, but continue any drug regime as ordered
- Confirm if the patient has an allergy
- A full bladder is often required for the procedure
- Explain that there may be some discomfort from pressure on the full bladder
- Explain that the conducting gel is non-staining but may feel slightly cold and wet and that there is no sensation at all from the ultrasound waves
- Offer wipes/tissue to wipe off the gel.

MRI

MRI is used to examine the liver and abdominal organs. It's useful in evaluating liver disease by characterising tumours, masses or cysts found on previous studies. An image is generated by energising protons in a strong magnetic field. Radio waves emitted as protons return to their former equilibrium and are recorded. No ionising radiation transmits during the scan.

MRI mire

Disadvantages of MRI include the closed, tubelike space required for the scan. Newer MRI centres offer a less confining 'open-MRI' scan. In addition, the test can't be performed on patients with body jewellery, implanted devices such as cardiac pacemakers but metal prostheses can be scanned provided it has been embedded for up to 90 days.

Practice pointers
- Explain the procedure to the patient and stress the need to remove metal objects such as jewellery before the procedure
- Generally, you'll accompany the patient to the MRI suite. If he becomes claustrophobic during the test, administer mild sedation as ordered.

Treatments

GI emergencies present many treatment challenges because they stem from various mechanisms occurring separately or simultaneously, including tumours, hyperactivity and hypoactivity, malabsorption, infection and inflammation, vascular disorders, intestinal obstruction, and degenerative disease. Treatment options include drug therapy and GI intubation.

Drug therapy

Drug therapy may be used for disorders, such as acute GI bleeding, peptic ulcer disease, and hepatic failure. Some of the most commonly used drugs include antacids, antidiuretic hormone, antiemetics, histamine-2 (H_2) receptor antagonists and proton pump inhibitors.

How fast?

Some of these drugs, such as antacids and antiemetics, provide relief immediately. Other drugs, such as ammonia detoxicants and H_2-receptor antagonists, may take several days or longer to alleviate the problem. (See *Watch out for sedatives* and *Common GI drugs*, pages 336–337.)

Common disorders

GI disorders commonly encountered in the ED include abdominal trauma, acute GI bleeding, appendicitis, cholecystitis, diverticulitis and bowel obstruction.

Abdominal trauma

Abdominal trauma is associated with a high rate of morbidity and mortality. It can occur as a single event or be associated with multiple injuries, further compounding their seriousness.

What causes it

Abdominal trauma is commonly classified as *penetrating* or *blunt*, depending on the type of injury.

An explosive situation

Penetrating abdominal trauma involves an injury by a foreign object, such as a knife (the most common cause of stabbing injury), bullet (the most common cause of missile injury), pitchfork or other pointed object that penetrates the abdomen.

Typically, penetrating abdominal trauma is fairly limited, usually involving isolated organs and lacerated tissues. In some cases, however, extensive tissue damage can occur if a bullet explodes in the abdominal cavity.

To put it bluntly

Blunt abdominal trauma results from sudden compression or positive pressure inflicted by a direct blow to the organ and surrounding tissue. Blunt abdominal trauma commonly occurs in motor vehicle collisions, assaults and falls.

Blunt abdominal trauma can cause extensive injury to the peritoneum and abdominal organs. The liver and spleen are the two organs most commonly injured from blunt abdominal trauma. The other organs, such as the stomach, intestines and pancreas, as well as the diaphragm and vascular structures, can also be injured, although these injuries are less common.

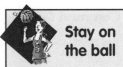

Stay on the ball

Watch out for sedatives

Administer sedatives cautiously in a patient with underlying liver disease. Be sure to establish a baseline for the patient's level of consciousness (LOC) before administering the medication to ensure valid assessments of the patient's LOC after the medication has been given.

Common GI drugs

This chart lists common GI drugs along with their indications and adverse reactions.

Drugs	Indications	Adverse reactions
Ammonia detoxicant		
Lactulose	• To prevent and treat portosystemic encephalopathy in patients with severe hepatic disease (increasing clearance of nitrogenous products and decreasing serum ammonia levels through laxative effects) • Laxative to treat constipation	Abdominal cramps, diarrhoea, flatulence
Antacids		
Aluminium hydroxide	• Antacid used for heartburn, acid indigestion and adjunct therapy with peptic ulcer disease	Constipation, intestinal obstruction, encephalopathy
Aluminium hydroxide and magnesium hydroxide (Gaviscon)	• Antacid used for heartburn, acid indigestion and adjunct therapy with peptic ulcer disease	Diarrhoea, hypermagnesemia in patients with severe renal impairment
Calcium carbonate (Caltrate)	• Antacid used for heartburn, acid indigestion and adjunct therapy with peptic ulcer disease • Calcium supplement	Nausea, vomiting, possibly hypercalcemia (with excessive use)
Antidiuretic hormone		
Vasopressin (Pitressin)	• Injection administered I.V. used as treatment in acute, massive GI haemorrhage (such as peptic ulcer disease, ruptured oesophageal varices and Mallory-Weiss syndrome)	Angina, cardiac arrhythmias (bradycardia, heart block), cardiac arrest, water intoxication, seizures, bronchospasms, coronary thrombosis, possibly mesenteric and small bowel infarction with mesenteric artery intra-arterial infusion
Antiemetics		
Metoclopramide (Maxolon)	• Prevention and treatment of nausea and vomiting especially in gastro-intestinal disorders	Restlessness, anxiety, depression, seizures, drowsiness, diarrhoea.
Histamine-2 receptor antagonists		
Cimetidine	• Treatment of duodenal and gastric ulcers, gastro-oesophageal reflux disease. • Prevention of gastric ulcers	Headache, rash, diarrhoea, dizziness

Common GI drugs *(Continued)*

Drugs	Indications	Adverse reactions
Ranitidine (Zantac)	• Treatment of duodenal and gastric ulcers, • Prevention of gastric ulcers	Malaise, reversible confusion, depression or hallucinations, blurred vision, jaundice, leukopenia, angioedema
Proton pump inhibitors		
Lansoprazole (zoton), Omeprazole (losec), Pantoprazole (Protium)	• Treatment of duodenal and gastric ulcers, erosive oesophagitis, *Helicobacter pylori* eradication • Prophylaxis for gastric stress ulcer (in critically ill patients)	Diarrhoea, abdominal pain, nausea, constipation, blurred vision, depression, dizziness, dry mouth

How it happens

Injuries to the abdomen usually involve one or more of these conditions:
• Hypovolaemia resulting from massive fluid or blood loss, especially if the spleen is injured
• Hypoxaemia resulting from damage to the diaphragm or associated chest trauma
• Respiratory or cardiac failure resulting from associated chest injury.

Tissue damage caused by penetrating trauma, such as an impaled object or foreign body, is related to the object size as well as the depth and velocity of penetration. For example, penetrating abdominal trauma from a bullet has many variables; the extent of injury depends on the distance at which the weapon was fired, the type of ammunition, the velocity of the ammunition and the entrance and (if present) exit wounds.

Other considerations

Additional factors to consider when assessing the extent of abdominal trauma from a bullet include: type of weapon; calibre, barrel and length of the gun; and powder composition. An intact bullet causes less damage than a bullet that explodes on impact. A bullet that explodes within the abdomen may break up and scatter fragments, burn tissue, fracture bone, disrupt vascular structures or cause a bullet embolism.

Trauma physics

Injury resulting from blunt abdominal trauma is related to the amount of force, compression, and cavitation. Blunt force that strikes the abdomen at high velocity transfers that force to underlying organs and tissue. The direct impact of force is transmitted internally, and the energy dissipates to internal structures.

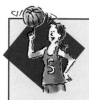

Stay on the ball

Identifying injuries to the liver and spleen

The liver and spleen are the two organs most commonly injured from abdominal trauma.

Spleen signs

When performing your assessment, suspect injury to the spleen if your patient:
- Has a history of blunt trauma to the left upper quadrant
- Complains of pain or exhibits bruising in the left upper quadrant
- Demonstrates a positive Kehr's sign (evidence of left shoulder pain due to irritation of the diaphragm with blood from the peritoneum)

Liver look-fors

Suspect a liver injury if your patient:
- Has a history of direct trauma to the right upper quadrant (between the eighth rib and central abdominal area)
- Has pain or bruising over the right upper quadrant
- Complains of referred pain to the right shoulder
- Demonstrates haemodynamic instability

Memory jogger

To help remember what information to obtain during assessment of the patient with abdominal trauma, use the acronym **SAMPLE:**
- **S**igns and symptoms
- **A**llergies
- **M**edications
- **P**ast medical history
- **L**ast meal
- **E**vents leading to injury

Have a look-see

When assessing the patient with abdominal trauma, be alert for:
- Bruising, abrasions and lacerations of the abdomen. (See *Identifying injuries to the liver and spleen*)
- Bruising along the area of the seat belt line
- Obvious wounds, such as gunshot wounds or stab wounds
- Change in bowel sounds (the presence of bowel sounds in the chest suggests diaphragmatic rupture and should be reported immediately)
- Pain, rigidity, tenderness or guarding on palpation.

What tests tell you

Diagnostic testing depends on the patient's condition and extent of injuries. In addition, diagnostic tests performed are based on the area affected by the trauma. Some possible diagnostic tests include:
- CT scan, which may reveal haemorrhage, haematomas or skeletal injuries
- Ultrasonography, which may show free fluid in the abdominal cavity
- Peritoneal lavage to detect blood in the peritoneal cavity
- Abdominal and chest X-rays to detect fluid, free air, ileus or rupture of the diaphragm
- Pelvic X-rays, which may demonstrate bony abnormalities.
  Other tests that may be performed include:
- Arterial blood gas (ABG) analysis to evaluate respiratory and acid-base status
- Full blood count (FBC) to evaluate degree of blood loss

- Coagulation studies to determine the patient's clotting ability
- Serum electrolyte levels to determine possible imbalances.

How it's treated

Treatment of abdominal trauma focuses on immediately stabilising the patient; assessing and maintaining his airway, breathing and circulation (ABCs); assessing LOC and preparing him for transport and possible surgery.

If the patient has a wound, treatment may include controlling bleeding, usually by applying firm, direct pressure and cleaning the wound. Pain medication and antibiotic therapy are instituted as indicated. In addition, I.V. therapy is started to ensure fluid balance and maintain the patient's haemodynamic status.

What to do

- Assess the patient's primary and secondary survey, including ABCDEs and initiate emergency measures if necessary; administer supplemental oxygen as ordered
- Monitor vital signs and note significant changes
- Assess oxygen saturation and cardiac rhythm for arrhythmias. Assess neurologic status, including LOC and pupillary and motor response
- Obtain blood studies, including type and crossmatch
- Insert two large-bore I.V. catheters and infuse prescribed normal saline or lactated Ringer's solution as ordered
- Quickly and carefully assess the patient for other areas of trauma
- Assess wounds and provide wound care as appropriate. Cover open wounds and control bleeding by applying pressure
- Assess for increased abdominal distention
- Administer blood products as appropriate
- Monitor for signs of hypovolaemic shock
- Provide pain medication, as appropriate
- Prepare the patient and family for diagnostic testing and possible surgery
- Provide reassurance to the patient and his family.

Acute GI bleeding

GI bleeding can occur anywhere along the GI tract. Although GI bleeding stops spontaneously in most patients, acute bleeding accounts for significant morbidity and mortality.

Maybe multiple morbidities

Many patients who require emergency care experience upper GI bleeding. Additionally, they may have underlying comorbidities that contribute to the risk of upper GI bleeding, such as:
- Coronary artery disease
- History of myocardial infarction

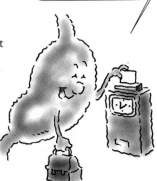

Most GI bleeding clocks out on its own, but the kind that sticks around carries a risk of morbidity and mortality.

- Renal failure
- History of chronic liver damage secondary to alcohol abuse or hepatitis
- History of radiation therapy
- Chronic pain condition, such as arthritis, requiring treatment with NSAIDs.

What causes it

Upper GI bleeding includes bleeding in the oesophagus, stomach and duodenum. Bleeding below the Treitz ligament is considered lower GI bleeding; the most common site is in the colon.

Upper causes

Causes of upper GI bleeding include:
- Angiodysplasias
- Arteriovenous malformations (AVMs)
- Erosive gastritis
- Oesophagitis
- Mallory-Weiss tear (gastroesophageal laceration)
- Peptic ulcer disease
- Rupture of oesophageal varices.

Lower causes

The most common causes of lower GI bleeding include:
- Diverticulitis
- Haemorrhoids
- Inflammatory bowel disease
- Neoplasm
- Polyps.

How it happens

In GI bleeding, the patient experiences a loss of circulating blood volume, regardless of the cause of bleeding. Because the arterial blood supply near the stomach and oesophagus is extensive, bleeding can lead to a rapid loss of large amounts of blood, subsequent hypovolaemia and shock. Here's what else happens:
- Loss of circulating blood volume leads to a decreased venous return
- Cardiac output and blood pressure decrease, causing poor tissue perfusion. In response, the body compensates by shifting interstitial fluid to the intravascular space
- The sympathetic nervous system is stimulated, resulting in vasoconstriction and increased heart rate
- The renin-angiotensin-aldosterone system is activated, leading to fluid retention and increasing blood pressure
- If blood loss continues, cardiac output decreases, leading to cellular hypoxia. Eventually, all organs fail due to hypoperfusion.

What to look for

Because GI bleeding can occur anywhere along the GI tract, assessment is crucial to determine the level and possible location of bleeding.

Source signs

The appearance of blood in tube drainage, vomitus and stool indicates the source of GI bleeding:
• *Haematemesis* (bright-red blood in NG tube drainage or vomitus) typically indicates an upper GI source. However, if the blood has spent time in the stomach where it was exposed to gastric acid, the drainage or vomitus resembles coffee grounds
• *Haematochezia* (bright-red blood from the rectum) typically indicates a lower GI source of bleeding. It may also suggest an upper GI source if the transit time through the bowel was rapid
• *Melaena* (black, tarry, sticky stool) usually indicates an upper GI bleeding source. However, it can result from bleeding in the small bowel or proximal colon.

Signs and symptoms

Typically, the patient exhibits signs and symptoms based on the amount and rate of bleeding. With acute GI bleeding and blood loss >30% of the patient's blood volume, he exhibits signs and symptoms of hypovolaemic shock (see Chapter 4), including:
• Apprehension
• Cool, clammy skin
• Respiratory rate
• Sweating
• Hypotension
• Pallor
• Restlessness
• Syncope
• Tachycardia.

What tests tell you

These findings aid in diagnosing acute GI bleeding:
• FBC reveals the amount of blood loss
• ABG analysis can indicate metabolic acidosis from haemorrhage and possible hypoxaemia
• 12-lead electrocardiogram (ECG) may reveal evidence of cardiac ischaemia secondary to hypoperfusion
• Abdominal X-ray may indicate air under the diaphragm, suggesting ulcer perforation
• Admission for angiography may aid in visualising the bleeding site
• Admission for upper GI endoscopy reveals the source of oesophageal or gastric bleeding.

How it's treated

Treatment goals include stopping the bleeding and providing fluid replacement while maintaining the patient's function. Treatment may include:
- Respiratory support
- Fluid volume replacement with crystalloid solutions initially, followed by colloids and blood component therapy
- May require insertion of nasogastric tube (unless the patient has oesophageal varices) and gastric pH monitoring
- Drug therapy, such as antacids, H_2-receptor antagonists and proton pump inhibitors
- Endoscopic or surgical repair of bleeding sites.

What to do

- Ensure the patient's airway is patent
- Keep Nil By Mouth (NBM)
- Type and crossmatch at least 2 units of blood
- Start at least two large-bore I.V. lines (16G or 14G preferred). Assess the patient for blood loss and begin fluid replacement therapy as ordered, initially delivering crystalloid solutions such as normal saline or lactated Ringer's solution, followed by blood component products
- May require central venous pressure line for administering fluids
- May require urinary catheterisation for monitoring fluid balance
- Monitor cardiac and respiratory status and assess LOC at least every 15 minutes until the patient's condition stabilises and then as indicated by his status.

Don't forget

- Administer supplemental oxygen as ordered. Monitor and record oxygen saturation levels
- Monitor the patient's skin colour and capillary refill for signs of hypovolaemic shock
- Obtain serial haemoglobin and haematocrit levels. Administer albumin or blood as ordered
- Monitor the patient's intake and output closely, including all losses from the GI tract. Check all stools and gastric drainage for occult blood
- Assess the patient's abdomen for bowel sounds and gastric pH as ordered
- Provide appropriate emotional support to the patient
- Prepare the patient for endoscopic repair or surgery, if indicated. Anticipate transfer of the patient to the critical care unit.

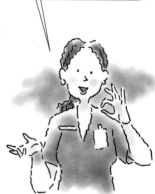

Just a little bit of emotional support can go a long way for a patient who has suffered dramatic blood loss.

Appendicitis

Appendicitis is the most common major surgical emergency. It occurs when the appendix becomes inflamed. More precisely, this disorder is an inflammation of the vermiform appendix, a small, fingerlike projection attached to the caecum just below the ileocecal valve. Although the appendix has no known function, it does regularly fill and empty itself of food.

What causes it
Appendicitis may be due to:
• Barium ingestion
• Faecal mass
• Mucosal ulceration
• Stricture
• Viral infection.

How it happens
Mucosal ulceration triggers inflammation that temporarily obstructs the appendix. The obstruction blocks mucus outflow. Pressure in the now-distended appendix increases, and the appendix contracts. Bacteria multiply, and inflammation and pressure continue to increase, restricting blood flow to the organ and causing severe abdominal pain.

Inflammation can lead to infection, clotting, tissue decay, and perforation of the appendix. If the appendix ruptures or perforates, the infected contents spill into the abdominal cavity, causing peritonitis, the most common and most dangerous complication.

What to look for
Initially, look for these signs or symptoms:
• Abdominal pain, generalised or localised in the right upper abdomen and eventually localising in the right lower abdomen
• Anorexia
• Boardlike abdominal rigidity
• Nausea and vomiting
• Retractive respirations
• Increasingly severe abdominal spasms and rebound spasms (rebound tenderness on the opposite side of the abdomen suggests peritoneal inflammation).

... and then later

Later, look for these signs or symptoms:
• Constipation (although diarrhoea is also possible)
• Fever of 37.2° to 38.9°C (99° to 102°F)
• Tachycardia
• Sudden cessation of abdominal pain (indicates perforation or infarction of the appendix).

What tests tell you
These tests help diagnose appendicitis:
• White blood cell (WBC) count is moderately elevated, with increased immature cells
• Ultrasound of the abdomen and pelvis can be helpful in diagnosing a nonperforated appendix. A CT scan can help identify an abscess.

Education edge

Teaching the patient with appendicitis

- Explain what happens in appendicitis.
- Help the patient understand the required surgery and its possible complications.
- If time allows, provide preoperative teaching, including coughing and deep breathing exercises.
- Discuss postoperative care and activity limitations. Tell the patient to follow the doctor's orders for driving, returning to work and resuming physical activity.

How it's treated

An appendicectomy is the only effective treatment for appendicitis. If peritonitis develops, treatment involves GI intubation, parenteral replacement of fluids and electrolytes and administration of antibiotics.

What to do

If appendicitis is suspected or you're preparing for an appendicectomy, follow these steps:
- Administer I.V. fluids to prevent dehydration. Never administer enemas because they may rupture the appendix
- Maintain the patient on NBM status, and administer analgesics judiciously because they may mask symptoms of rupture
- Assist the patient into a comfortable position
- Never apply heat to the lower right abdomen or perform palpation; these actions may cause the appendix to rupture
- Provide support to the patient and family; prepare them for surgery as indicated
- Begin educating the patient about his condition and care. (See *Teaching the patient with appendicitis*.)

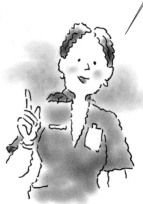

Sometimes there's only one way to go with treatment. In the case of appendicitis, it's surgical removal.

Cholecystitis

Cholecystitis refers to an acute or chronic inflammation of the gallbladder, usually associated with a gallstone impacted in the cystic duct, causing painful gallbladder distention. The acute form is most common during middle age, whereas the chronic form is more common in the elderly. Prognosis is good with treatment.

What causes it

The exact cause of cholecystitis is unknown. However, certain risk factors have been identified, including:
- High-calorie, high-cholesterol diet associated with obesity
- Elevated oestrogen levels from hormonal contraceptives, postmenopausal therapy or pregnancy

- Diabetes mellitus, ileal disease, haemolytic disorders, liver disease or pancreatitis
- Genetic factors
- Weight-reduction diets with severe calorie restriction and rapid weight loss.

How it happens

Certain conditions (such as age, obesity and oestrogen imbalance) cause the liver to secrete bile that's abnormally high in cholesterol or that lacks the proper concentration of bile salts. Excessive water and bile salts are reabsorbed, making the bile less soluble. Cholesterol, calcium and bilirubin then precipitate into gallstones.

What to look for

In acute cholecystitis, look for:
- Classic attack signs and symptoms with severe mid-epigastric or right upper quadrant pain radiating to the back or referred to the right scapula, commonly after meals rich in fats
- Recurring fat intolerance
- Belching that leaves a sour taste in the mouth
- Flatulence
- Indigestion
- Diaphoresis
- Nausea
- Chills and low-grade fever
- Possible jaundice and clay-coloured stools with common duct obstruction
- Local and rebound tenderness.

What tests tell you

These tests help diagnose cholecystitis:
- Ultrasonography reveals calculi in the gallbladder with 96% accuracy. Percutaneous transhepatic cholangiography distinguishes between gallbladder disease and cancer of the pancreatic head in patients with jaundice
- CT scan may identify ductal stones
- Endoscopic retrograde cholangiopancreatography (ERCP) visualises the biliary tree after endoscopic examination of the duodenum, cannulation of the common bile and pancreatic ducts and injection of a contrast medium
- Cholescintigraphy/magnetic resonance cholangiopancreatography (MRCP) detects obstruction of the cystic duct.

Bad to the stone

- If stones are identified in the common bile duct by radiologic examination, a therapeutic ERCP may be performed before cholecystectomy to remove the stones
- Oral cholecystography shows calculi in the gallbladder and biliary duct obstruction

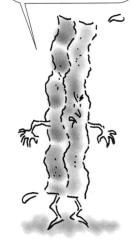

Okay, so I'm part of a high-calorie, high-cholesterol diet. There are other risk factors for cholecystitis, you know!

- Laboratory tests showing an elevated icteric index and elevated total bilirubin, urine bilirubin and alkaline phosphatase levels support the diagnosis
- WBC count is slightly elevated during a cholecystitis attack
- Serum amylase levels distinguish gallbladder disease from pancreatitis
- Serial enzyme tests and an ECG should precede other diagnostic tests if heart disease is suspected.

How it's treated

- During an acute attack, treatment may include bowel rest, analgesia, insertion of an NG tube and I.V. fluids as well as antibiotic administration
- Surgery is the treatment of choice for cholecystitis. Cholecystectomy (removal of the gallbladder) restores biliary flow. The surgery may be performed conventionally via a large incision, or laparoscopically. The laparoscopic procedure aids in speeding recovery and reducing the risk of infection and herniation
- In patients who are poor surgical candidates for cholecystectomy, a cholecystostomy (incision into the fundus of the gallbladder to remove and drain retained stones or inflammatory debris) or choledochotomy (incision into the common bile duct to remove gallstones or other obstructions) may be performed
- A low-fat diet is prescribed to prevent attacks. Vitamin K is also prescribed for itching, jaundice and bleeding tendencies caused by vitamin K deficiency
- Ursodeoxycholic acid, a drug that dissolves gallstones, provides an alternative for patients who are poor surgical risks or who refuse surgery. However, use of Ursodeoxycholic acid is limited by the need for prolonged treatment (2 years), the incidence of adverse reactions, and the frequency of calculi reformation after treatment
- Lithotripsy, the ultrasonic breakup of gallstones, is usually unsuccessful, and the rate of recurrence after this treatment is significant. The relative ease, short length of stay and cost-effectiveness of laparoscopic cholecystectomy have made dissolution and lithotripsy less viable options.

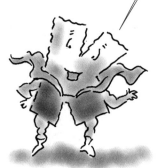

Lack of vitamin K isn't okay; it can lead to itching, jaundice and bleeding tendencies.

What to do

- Monitor the patient's vital signs and intake and output
- Insert an NG tube as ordered
- Administer medications to control complaints of nausea and vomiting
- Give opioid analgesics for pain
- Assist in stabilising the patient's nutritional and fluid balance before surgery
- NBM; determine the time when the patient last ate
- Provide preoperative care including teaching and administration of preoperative medications
- Ensure that an informed consent form has been signed and is on the patient's chart.

Diverticulitis

Diverticulitis is a form of diverticular disease. In diverticular disease, bulging, pouchlike herniations (diverticula) in the GI wall push the mucosal lining through the surrounding muscle. Diverticula occur most commonly in the sigmoid colon, but they may develop anywhere from the proximal end of the pharynx to the anus. Other typical sites are the duodenum, near the pancreatic border or the ampulla of Vater, and the jejunum.

Diverticula in the stomach are rare and are usually a precursor to peptic or neoplastic disease. Diverticular disease of the ileum (Meckel's diverticulum) is the most common congenital anomaly of the GI tract. Diverticular disease has two clinical forms:

 Diverticulosis – diverticula that are present but produce no symptoms

 Diverticulitis – inflamed diverticula that may cause potentially fatal obstruction, infection and haemorrhage.

What causes it
The exact cause of diverticular disease is unknown, but it may result from:
- Diminished colonic motility and increased intraluminal pressure
- Defects in colon wall strength.

How it happens
Diverticula probably result from high intraluminal pressure on an area of weakness in the GI wall where blood vessels enter. Diet may be a contributing factor because insufficient fibre reduces faecal residue, narrows the bowel lumen and leads to high intra-abdominal pressure during defaecation.

Packed in the sac

In diverticulitis, undigested food and bacteria accumulate in the diverticular sac. This accumulation causes the formation of a hard mass that cuts off the blood supply to the thin walls of the sac, making them more susceptible to attack by colonic bacteria. Inflammation follows and may lead to perforation, abscess, peritonitis, obstruction or haemorrhage. Occasionally, the inflamed colon segment adheres to the bladder or other organs and causes a fistula.

What to look for
- Meckel's diverticulum usually produces no symptoms
- In diverticulosis, recurrent left lower abdominal quadrant pain is relieved by defaecation or passage of flatus. Constipation and diarrhoea alternate
- In diverticulitis, the patient may have moderate left lower abdominal quadrant pain, mild nausea, gas, irregular bowel habits, low-grade fever, leukocytosis, rupture of the diverticula (in severe diverticulitis) and fibrosis and adhesions (in chronic diverticulitis).

Education edge

Teaching the patient with diverticulitis

- Explain what diverticula are as well as how they form.
- Make sure the patient understands the importance of dietary fibre and the harmful effects of constipation and straining at stool.
- Encourage increased intake of foods high in digestible fibre.
- Advise the patient to relieve constipation with stool softeners or bulk-forming laxatives, but caution against taking bulk-forming laxatives without plenty of water.

What tests tell you

These tests aid diagnosis of diverticular disease:
- An upper GI series confirms or rules out diverticulosis of the oesophagus and upper bowel
- Barium enema confirms or rules out diverticulosis of the lower bowel
- Biopsy rules out cancer; however, a colonoscopic biopsy isn't recommended during acute diverticular disease because of the strenuous bowel preparation it requires
- Blood studies may show an elevated erythrocyte sedimentation rate in diverticulitis, especially if the diverticula are infected.

How it's treated

Treatment of mild diverticulitis without signs of perforation must prevent constipation and combat infection. It may include bed rest, a liquid diet, stool softeners, a broad-spectrum antibiotic, opioids to control pain and relax smooth muscle and an antispasmodic, such as atropine sulphate or hyoscine butylbromide, to control muscle spasms.

What to do

If the patient with a history of diverticulosis comes to the ED, observe his stool carefully for frequency, colour and consistency; monitor pulse and temperature for changes which may signal developing inflammation or complications. Care of the patient with diverticulitis depends on the severity of symptoms:
- In mild disease, administer medications as ordered. Explain diagnostic tests and preparations for such tests; observe stool carefully and maintain accurate records of temperature, pulse rate, respiratory rate and intake and output. Begin patient teaching for discharge. (See *Teaching the patient with diverticulitis*.)

Severe steps

If the patient's condition is more severe:
- Insert an I.V. line to administer fluids for rehydration
- Maintain the patient on NBM status and anticipate insertion of an NG tube
- Administer antispasmodic agents to reduce colon spasms; give analgesics to manage pain and antibiotics for infection as ordered

• Assess the patient for signs and symptoms of peritonitis, such as tachycardia, hypotension, abdominal rigidity, rebound tenderness and fever
• Watch for signs and symptoms of vasopressin-induced fluid retention (apprehension, abdominal cramps, seizures, oliguria and anuria) and severe hyponatraemia (hypotension; rapid, thready pulse; cold, clammy skin; and cyanosis)
• Prepare the patient for surgery as indicated; provide preoperative teaching and support to the patient and his family.

Bowel obstruction

Bowel obstruction is a blockage that prevents stools from passing through the small or large intestine.

What causes it
It can result from many problems, such as:
• Impacted stools
• Tumours
• Hernia
• Adhesions
• Inflammatory problems.

What happens
The blockage occurs from the food and gas accumulating above the obstruction. The proximal bowel distends, resulting in pain. As the bowel extends it can impair the blood supply to the intestine causing perforation or necrosis of the bowel.

What to look for
Following the systematic approach for assessment:
• Inspect the abdomen for any distention or scars
• Auscultate: Bowel sounds – you may hear high-pitched sounds with a newly diagnosed obstruction. No bowel sounds if the obstruction has been present for some time
• Percussion may elicit tympani – an air-filled peritoneal cavity
• Palpate for tenderness, guarding or any masses
• Abdominal pain
• Dehydration
• Bloating
• Vomiting
• Constipation or diarrhoea.

What tests tell you
There isn't one specific test that will confirm the extent of bowel obstruction but the following tests may aid diagnosis:
• Blood testing for dehydration or infection
• Erect chest and abdominal X-ray
• Abdominal CT

- Sometimes gastrografin studies are performed (a dye containing iodine used to clearly show X-ray images of a body part that needs investigating).

How it's treated

Some obstructions may resolve without any intervention. However, many obstructions will require treatment which may include:
- Assessing the ABCs especially if the patient is vomiting
- Administering prescribed analgesia, antibiotics and stool softener
- Inserting a nasogastric tube and maintaining NBM status
- Administering prescribed intravenous fluids
- Preparing the patient for surgery as indicated; provide preoperative teaching and support to the patient and his family.

Quick quiz

1. The priority for a patient with abdominal pain is:
   A. Pain relief.
   B. Surgery.
   C. Something to eat.
   D. Assessment of their airway, breathing and circulation.

Answer: D. Although the patient will require analgesia their most important priority is to assess their airway breathing and circulation first.

2. Auscultation of a patient's abdomen reveals hypoactive bowel sounds. You should interpret this sign as indicating:
   A. Turbulent blood flow in the arteries.
   B. Inflammation of the peritoneal surface.
   C. Diminished peristaltic activity.
   D. Obstruction in the intestine.

Answer: C. Hypoactive bowel sounds indicate that peristalsis is slowed or diminished and are associated with ileus, bowel obstruction, peritonitis or use of such medications as opioids.

3. Which sign or symptom would you be least likely to observe in a patient with acute cholecystitis?
   A. Fever >38.6°C (101.4°F).
   B. Right upper quadrant pain radiating to the back and/or shoulder.
   C. Belching that leaves a sour taste in the mouth.
   D. Recurrent fat intolerance.

Answer: B. In cholecystitis, the patient usually has right upper quadrant pain that radiates to the back or shoulder, a history of fat intolerance and belching that leaves a sour taste in the mouth. The patient may have a fever, but it's usually low-grade.

4. Which intervention would be appropriate for a patient diagnosed with appendicitis?
  A. Maintaining the patient on NBM status.
  B. Applying a heating pad to the abdomen.
  C. Administering an enema before surgery.
  D. Giving frequent doses of opioid analgesics.

Answer: A. For the patient with appendicitis, you should maintain the patient on NBM status and administer I.V. fluids. In addition, analgesics are given cautiously because they may mask the signs and symptoms of rupture. Heat and enemas are never used because they could lead to rupture.

Scoring

☆☆☆ If you answered all four questions correctly, you deserve a gourmet meal! You're an abdominal genius!

☆☆ If you answered three questions correctly, read up and try again! Your hunger for GI information makes it easy to swallow.

☆ If you answered fewer than three questions correctly, you may be fact-starved. Chew over the chapter and then take the test again.

Genitourinary, gynaecological and childbirth emergencies

10

Just the facts

In this chapter, you'll learn:

♦ Emergency assessment of the genitourinary (GU) and reproductive systems

♦ Diagnostic tests and procedures for GU and gynaecological emergencies

♦ GU and gynaecological disorders and their treatments in the emergency department

♦ How to deal with emergency childbirth

♦ How to care for the patient who has been sexually assaulted

Genitourinary and reproductive emergencies

The genitourinary (GU) and reproductive systems are closely related, and identifying subtle changes within them can mean the difference between effective and ineffective emergency care.

An emergency involving the urinary or reproductive system can have far-reaching consequences. In addition to affecting the system itself, it can trigger problems in other body systems and affect the patient's quality of life, self-esteem and sense of well-being.

Despite these dangers, many patients are reluctant to discuss their problems or have intimate areas of their bodies examined. Your challenge is

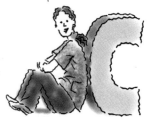

Compassion and comfort are two Cs that will put GU emergency patients right at ease.

to perform skilled, sensitive assessment. To do so, you must put the patient at ease; if you appear comfortable discussing the problem, the patient will feel encouraged talking openly.

Assessment

When your patient comes to the emergency department (ED) with a GU or gynaecological emergency, your assessment can help determine whether the symptoms are related to a current medical problem or indicate a new one. You need to assess the patient thoroughly, always being alert for subtle changes that may indicate a potential deterioration in condition.

Unless the patient requires immediate stabilising treatment, begin by taking a comprehensive patient history. Then probe further by conducting a thorough physical examination.

Peruse the record

If you can't interview the patient because of the presenting condition, gather information from medical records. In some cases, you may need to ask the patient's family or paramedic team that transported the patient to the ED.

The genitourinary system

The urinary system consists of the kidneys, ureters, bladder and urethra. Remember sex differences; for the male patient, the urethral meatus is also part of the reproductive system, carrying semen as well as urine. The male reproductive system also includes the penis, scrotum, testicles, epididymis, vas deferens, seminal vesicles and prostate gland.

For the female patient, the reproductive system consists of the external genitalia (collectively called the *vulva* – mons pubis, labia majora, labia minora, clitoris, vagina, urethral meatus and Skene's and Bartholin's glands) and the internal genitalia (vagina, uterus, ovaries and fallopian tubes). To care effectively for the patient effectively you need good knowledge of the anatomy and physiology of these systems. *Anatomy and Physiology Made Incredibly Easy* in the same series as this book can give you suitable underpinning knowledge.

Health history

Focus on the chief complaint when gathering your patient's health history and then explore the patient's previous health status. If appropriate you may need to explore further by assessing their sexual-reproductive history. Ask patients to describe symptoms in their own words, encouraging free and open speech. As you obtain a history, remember that the patient may feel uncomfortable discussing urinary or reproductive problems. (See *Putting your patient at ease*, page 354.)

Putting your patient at ease

Here are some tips for helping your patient feel more comfortable during the health history:

- Make sure that the room is private and that you won't be interrupted
- Tell the patient that all answers will remain confidential, and phrase your questions tactfully
- Start with less sensitive topic areas and work up to more sensitive clinical assessment information
- Don't rush or omit important facts because the patient seems embarrassed.

- Be especially tactful when assessing sensitive issues
- When asking questions you should phrase your questions carefully and offer reassurance as needed
- Consider the patient's educational and cultural background. If the patient uses slang or euphemisms to talk about sexual organs or function, make sure you're both talking about the same thing.

Chief complaint

Because the locations of the urinary and reproductive systems are so close, you and the patient may have trouble differentiating signs and symptoms. Even if the patient's complaint seems minor, investigate it; ask about its onset, duration, aggravating factors, alleviating factors, severity and the measures taken to treat it.

Current health status

Ask the patient about current problems and medications:

- Does the patient have diabetes which increases the risk of a urinary tract infection (UTI), cardiovascular disease (which can alter kidney perfusion) or hypertension (which can contribute to renal failure and nephropathy)?
- Has the patient noticed a change in the colour or odour of urine?
- Is there pain or burning during urination or problems with incontinence or frequency?
- Does the patient have allergies? Allergic reactions can cause tubular damage; a severe anaphylactic reaction can cause temporary renal failure and permanent tubular necrosis
- Make a list of all the prescribed medications the patient takes, including contraception and hormones, herbal preparations and over-the-counter drugs. Some drugs can affect the appearance of urine; nephrotoxic drugs can alter urinary function.

Be sure to weed out information about existing conditions, especially diabetes, cardiovascular disease or hypertension.

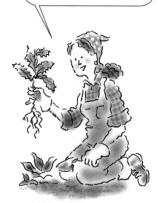

Previous health status

Past illnesses and pre-existing conditions can affect a patient's GU and reproductive health:

- Has the patient ever had a kidney or bladder infection or an infection of the reproductive system?
- Has the patient ever had kidney or bladder trauma, surgery, congenital problems or kidney stones?
- Has the patient ever been catheterised?

Also ask about the patient's family history to get information about the risk of developing kidney failure or kidney disease.

Common complaints

The most common complaints associated with GU problems involve output changes, such as polyuria, oliguria and anuria. Patients also commonly report complaints related to voiding pattern changes, including:
- Hesitancy
- Frequency
- Urgency
- Dysuria
- Nocturia
- Incontinence
- Urine colour changes
- Pain.

Common complaints associated with male reproductive problems include penile discharge, scrotal or inguinal masses or pain and tenderness. For women, common reproductive complaints include vaginal discharge, abnormal uterine bleeding and prolapses.

Sexual-reproductive history

Many patients feel uncomfortable answering questions about their sexual health or reproductive history. To establish a rapport, begin with less personal questions.

Female patients

With female patients start by asking about the menstrual cycle:
- How old was she when she began to menstruate? In girls, menses generally starts by age 15. If it hasn't and if no secondary sex characteristics have developed, the patient should be evaluated by the doctor
- How long does her menses usually last and how often does it occur? When was her last menstrual period? The normal cycle for menstruation is one menses every 21 to 38 days. The normal duration is 2 to 8 days
- Does she have cramps, spotting or an unusually heavy or light flow? Does she use tampons? Spotting between menses, or *metrorrhagia*, may be normal in patients taking low-dose hormonal contraceptives or progesterone or a peri-menopause; otherwise, spotting may indicate infection, cancer or some other abnormality.

Pregnancy clues

- Be extremely sensitive to any questions regarding pregnancy as the patient may not wish her family to know she is (or might be) pregnant or that she has had a baby before or has been pregnant in the past
- What kind of contraception, if any, does she use?
- Is the patient possibly pregnant now?
- Might she be experiencing a miscarriage of pregnancy or an ectopic pregnancy?

- Ask the patient if she has ever been pregnant. If so:
  - How many times has she been pregnant and how many times did she give birth?
  - Has she had any miscarriages or therapeutic abortions?
  - Did she have a vaginal or caesarean birth?

Comfort zone

When the patient seems comfortable, where appropriate ask about:
- Sexual practices
- Whether she uses protection (oral contraception, condoms)
- Pain with intercourse
- Sexually transmitted infection (STI) history and precautions taken to prevent STI contraction
- Human immunodeficiency virus (HIV) status
- Date of last intercourse
- Date and results of last cervical smear test
- Vaginal discharge
- External lesions
- Itching.
  If the patient is sexually active, talk to her about the importance of safer sex and the prevention of STIs.
  If your patient is postmenopausal, ask for the date of her last menses. To find out more about her menopausal symptoms, ask if she's having hot flushes, night sweats, mood swings, flushing or vaginal dryness or itching.

Male patients
Ask the male patient about his past medical history. Also ask about:
- Has he ever experienced trauma to his penis or scrotum?
- Was he ever diagnosed with an undescended testicle?
- Has he had a vasectomy?
- Has he ever been diagnosed with a low sperm count?
- If he participates in sports, how does he protect himself from possible genital injuries?
- Number of current and past sexual partners
- STI history and precautions taken to prevent STI contraction
- HIV status. (See *Don't forget to ask the older person*)
- Contraception measures.

Physical examination

Physical examination of the GU system usually includes inspection, auscultation, percussion and palpation. (See *Percussing the kidney and bladder*.) Reproductive system examination involves inspection and palpation. You will need to see what the practice in your department is as some of these techniques are only practiced by medical staff, Emergency Nurse Practitioners (ENPs) or other nurses who have undertaken advanced examination skills training.

Ages and stages

Don't forget to ask the older person

Older people who are sexually active with multiple partners have as high a risk for developing a sexually transmitted disease as younger adults. However, because of decreased immunity, poor hygiene, poor symptom reporting and, possibly, several concurrent conditions, they may seek treatment for different symptoms.

Percussing the kidney and bladder

The kidneys and bladder are percussed using the techniques described here.

Kidney percussion

With the patient sitting upright, each costovertebral angle (the angle over each kidney whose borders are formed by the lateral and downward curve of the lowest rib and the vertebral column) is percussed. To perform mediate percussion, the left palm is placed over the costovertebral angle and is stroked gently with the right fist. To perform immediate percussion, the fist is stroked gently over each costovertebral angle. Usually, the patient will feel a thudding sensation or pressure during percussion.

Bladder percussion

Using mediate percussion, the area over the bladder is percussed, beginning 5 cm above the symphysis pubis. To detect differences in sound, percussion moves toward the bladder's base. Percussion usually produces a tympanic sound. (Over a urine-filled bladder, it produces a dull sound.)

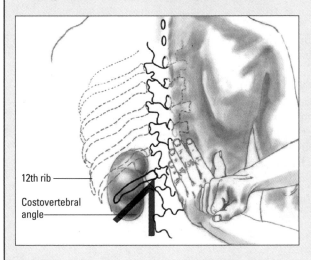

12th rib
Costovertebral angle

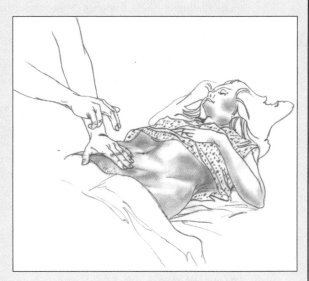

At ease, please

Before starting, the techniques to be used must be explained and the patient warned that some procedures may be uncomfortable and the patient's consent gained. The examination is performed in a private, quiet, warm, well-lit room.

Renal red flags

The physical examination begins with assessing ABCDE. These observations will provide clues about renal dysfunction. For example, a patient's vital signs might reveal hypertension, which can cause renal dysfunction if it isn't controlled.

Behavioural hints

Observing the patient's behaviour can give you clues about mental status. Kidney dysfunction can cause such symptoms as trouble concentrating, memory loss and disorientation. Progressive, chronic kidney failure can cause lethargy, confusion, disorientation, stupor, seizures and coma.

It's in the skin

The patient's skin is observed. A person with decreased renal function may be pale because of a low haemoglobin level or may even have *uraemic frost* (snow-like crystals on the skin from metabolic wastes). Also look for signs of fluid imbalance, such as dry mucous membranes, sunken eyeballs, oedema or ascites.

Inspection

Inspection usually includes examination of the abdomen and external genitalia for swelling, tumours or any abnormality.

Leading off: The abdomen

The patient is asked to empty the bladder and then helping the patient into the supine position with arms at the sides. To maintain patient dignity expose only the areas being examined.

First, the patient's abdomen is inspected. When supine, the abdomen should be symmetrical and smooth, flat or concave. The skin should be free from lesions, bruises, discolourations and prominent veins.

Abdominal distention with tight, glistening skin and *striae* – silvery streaks caused by rapidly developing skin tension are observed for. These are signs of ascites, which may accompany nephrotic syndrome. This syndrome is characterised by oedema, increased urine protein levels and decreased serum albumin levels.

Lastly, inspect the external genitalia for inflammation or discharge from the urethral meatus.

Auscultation

The renal arteries in the left and right upper abdominal quadrants are auscultated by pressing the stethoscope bell lightly against the abdomen and instructing the patient to exhale deeply. Auscultation begins at the midline and works to the left; then return to the midline and then works to the right. Systolic bruits or other abnormal sounds are listened for, which may indicate a significant problem. For example, a systolic bruit may signal renal artery stenosis.

Percussion

Kidney percussion checks for costovertebral angle tenderness that occurs with inflammation. To percuss over the kidneys, the patient is asked to sit up. The ball of the practitioner's nondominant hand is placed on the patient's back at the costovertebral angle of the 12th rib. The ball of that hand is struck with the ulnar surface of the other hand; using just enough force to cause a painless but perceptible thud.

Palpating the kidneys

To palpate the kidneys, the patient will lie in a supine position. To palpate the right kidney, the practitioner stands on the patient's right side. The left hand is placed under the back and the right hand on the abdomen.

The patient is instructed to inhale deeply, so the kidney moves downward. As the patient inhales, the left hand is pressed up and pressed down with the right, as shown.

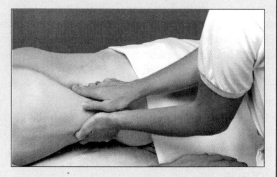

As the kidneys are percussed, pain or tenderness is checked for; its presence suggests a kidney infection. Both sides of the body need to be percussed to assess both kidneys.

Bladder up

To percuss the bladder, the patient is asked to empty the bladder if he hasn't done so already. The patient then lies in the supine position. Starting at the symphysis pubis the percussion moves upward toward the bladder and over it. We expect to hear tympany – a dull sound signals retained urine.

Palpation

Because the kidneys lie behind other organs and are protected by muscle, they normally aren't palpable unless they're enlarged. However, in very thin patients the lower end of the right kidney as a smooth round mass that drops on inspiration may be felt. (See *Palpating the kidneys*.)

Normally I hide behind other organs, but every once in a while, I've got to stand up and be palpated!

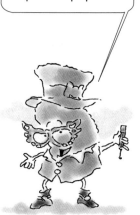

Diagnostic tests

Many tests provide information to guide your care of a GU or gynaecology emergency patient. Even if you don't conduct the test you should know why the test was ordered, what the results mean and what your responsibilities are before, during and after the test.

Common diagnostic tests carried out in the Emergency department include, blood studies, ultrasound, kidney-ureter-bladder (KUB) CT scan, urine studies and pregnancy testing. Once admitted to the ward or to specialist units other tests will include I.V. urography (IVU), computed tomography (CT) scan, magnetic resonance imaging (MRI), laparoscopy, percutaneous renal biopsy, renal angiography and renal scan.

Blood studies

Blood studies used to diagnose and evaluate GU function include:
• Full blood count (FBC) to evaluate white blood cell (WBC) count, red blood cell (RBC) count, haemoglobin level and haematocrit
• Urea and electrolyte (U&Es) measurements to evaluate calcium, phosphorus, chloride, potassium and sodium levels
• Serum osmolality, creatinine clearance and urea clearance measurements and serum creatinine, serum protein and uric acid levels. (See *Interpreting blood studies*)
• Blood (or urine) studies for beta human chorionic gonadotropin (BHCG), the pregnancy hormone, to exclude pregnancy or miscarriage

Practice pointers

• The patient is informed that the test requires a blood sample and consent is gained
• Check the patient's medication history for drugs that might influence test results.

Ultrasonography

Ultrasonography (ultrasound) uses high-frequency sound waves to reveal internal structures; it can involve the abdomen, pelvis or specifically the renal structures. This test provides information about internal structures of the abdomen, pelvis and, more specifically, the kidney's size, shape and position. It's also used to detect pregnancy.

Practice pointers

• Tell the patient that he'll be prone (the renal examination position) or supine during the test
• Explain that a technician will spread coupling oil or gel on his skin and then move a probe or transducer against the skin and across the area being tested
• If a pelvic ultrasound is being done, make sure that the patient has a full bladder, which is used as landmark for defining pelvic organs.

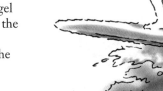

Whoa, dude! Ultrasonography uses high-frequency sound waves to reveal internal structures.

Urine studies

Urine studies, such as urinalysis and urine osmolality, can indicate acute renal failure, renal trauma, UTI and other disorders. Urine testing can also indicate pregnancy (ensure that you have the patient's consent before undertaking a pregnancy test). Urinalysis can indicate renal or systemic disorders, warranting further investigation. A random urine specimen is used. (See *What urinalysis findings mean*, pages 362–363.)

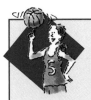

Stay on the ball

Interpreting blood studies

Here's how you may interpret the results of blood studies used in diagnosing problems of the genitourinary system.

Complete blood count

An increased white blood cell count may indicate urinary tract infection, peritonitis (in peritoneal dialysis patients) or kidney transplantation infection and rejection.

RBC count, Hb level and HCT decrease in a patient with chronic renal insufficiency resulting from decreased erythropoietin production by the kidneys. HCT also provides an index of fluid balance because it indicates the percentage of RBCs in the blood.

Blood urea nitrogen

Increased blood urea nitrogen levels may indicate glomerulonephritis, extensive pyogenic infection, oliguria (from mercuric chloride poisoning or post traumatic renal insufficiency), tubular obstruction or other obstructive uropathies. Because nonrenal conditions can also cause these levels to increase, interpret in conjunction with serum creatinine levels.

Electrolytes

Because the kidneys regulate fluid and electrolyte balance, a critically ill patient with renal disease may experience significant serum electrolyte imbalances. The most commonly measured electrolytes are:

- *Calcium and phosphorus* – Calcium and phosphorus levels have an inverse relationship; when one increases, the other decreases. In renal failure, the kidneys aren't able to excrete phosphorus, resulting in hyperphosphatemia and hypocalcemia.
- *Chloride* – Chloride levels relate inversely to bicarbonate levels, reflecting acid-base balance. In renal disease, elevated chloride levels suggest metabolic acidosis. Hyperchloremia occurs in renal tubular necrosis, severe dehydration and complete renal shutdown. Hypochloremia may also occur with pyelonephritis.
- *Potassium* – Hyperkalaemia occurs with renal insufficiency or acidosis. In renal shutdown, potassium may rapidly increase to life-threatening levels. Hypokalaemia may reflect renal tubular disease.
- *Sodium* – Sodium helps the kidneys regulate body fluid. Renal disease may result in the loss of sodium through the kidneys.

Serum creatinine

The serum creatinine level reflects the glomerular filtration rate (GFR). Renal damage is indicated more accurately by increases in serum creatinine than by the level of urea and nitrogen.

Serum osmolality

An increase in serum osmolality with a simultaneous decrease in urine osmolality indicates diminished distal tubule responsiveness to circulating antidiuretic hormone.

Serum proteins

Levels of the serum protein albumin may decline sharply from its loss in the urine during nephritis or nephrosis, which in turn causes oedema. Nephrosis may also cause total serum protein levels to decrease.

Uric acid

Because uric acid clears from the body by glomerular filtration and tubular secretion, elevated levels may indicate impaired renal function; below-normal levels may indicate defective tubular absorption.

What urinalysis findings mean

Test	Normal values or findings	Abnormal findings	Possible causes of abnormal findings
Colour and odour	• Straw colour	Clear to black	Dietary changes; use of certain drugs; metabolic, inflammatory or infectious disease
	• Slightly aromatic odour	Fruity odour	Diabetes mellitus, starvation, dehydration
	• Clear appearance	Turbid appearance	Renal infection
Specific gravity	• 1.005 to 1.030, with slight variations from one specimen to the next	Below-normal specific gravity	Diabetes insipidus, glomerulonephritis, pyelonephritis, acute renal failure, alkalosis
		Above-normal specific gravity	Dehydration, nephrosis
		Fixed specific gravity	Severe renal damage
pH	• 4.5 to 8.0	Alkaline pH (above 8.0)	Fanconi's syndrome (chronic renal disease), urinary tract infection (UTI), metabolic or respiratory alkalosis
		Acidic pH (below 4.5)	Renal tuberculosis, phenylketonuria, acidosis
Protein	• No protein	Proteinuria	Renal disease (such as glomerulosclerosis, acute or chronic glomerulonephritis, nephrolithiasis, polycystic kidney disease and acute or chronic renal failure)
Ketones	• No ketones	Ketonuria	Diabetes mellitus, starvation, conditions causing acutely increased metabolic demands and decreased food intake (such as vomiting and diarrhoea)
Glucose	• No glucose	Glycosuria	Diabetes mellitus
Red blood cells (RBCs)	• 0 to 3 RBCs/high-power field	Numerous RBCs	UTI, obstruction, inflammation, trauma or tumour; glomerulonephritis; renal hypertension; lupus nephritis; renal tuberculosis; renal vein thrombosis; hydronephrosis; pyelonephritis; parasitic bladder infection; polyarteritis nodosa; haemorrhagic disorder
Epithelial cells	• Few epithelial cells	Excessive epithelial cells	Renal tubular degeneration
White blood cells (WBCs)	• 0 to 4 WBCs/high-power field	Numerous WBCs	UTI, especially cystitis or pyelonephritis
		Numerous WBCs and WBC casts	Renal infection (such as acute pyelonephritis and glomerulonephritis, nephrotic syndrome, pyogenic infection and lupus nephritis)

(continued)

What urinalysis findings mean (Continued)

Test	Normal values or findings	Abnormal findings	Possible causes of abnormal findings
Casts	• No casts (except occasional hyaline casts)	Excessive casts	Renal disease
		Excessive hyaline casts	Renal parenchymal disease, inflammation, glomerular capillary membrane trauma
		Epithelial casts	Renal tubular damage, nephrosis, eclampsia, chronic lead intoxication
		Fatty, waxy casts	Nephrotic syndrome, chronic renal disease, diabetes mellitus
		RBC casts	Renal parenchymal disease (especially glomerulonephritis), renal infarction, subacute bacterial endocarditis, sickle cell anaemia, blood dyscrasias, malignant hypertension, collagen disease
Crystals	• Some crystals	Numerous calcium oxalate crystals	Hypercalcaemia
		Cystine crystals (cystinuria)	Inborn metabolic error
Yeast cells	• No yeast cells	Yeast cells in sediment	External genitalia contamination, vaginitis, urethritis, prostatovesiculitis
Parasites	• No parasites	Parasites in sediment	External genitalia contamination
Creatinine clearance	• Males: 14 to 26 mg/kg/ 24 hours • Females: 11 to 20 mg/ kg/24 hours	Above-normal creatinine clearance	Little diagnostic significance
		Below-normal creatinine clearance	Reduced renal blood flow (associated with shock or renal artery obstruction), acute tubular necrosis, acute or chronic glomerulonephritis, advanced bilateral renal lesions (as in polycystic kidney disease, renal tuberculosis and cancer), nephrosclerosis, heart failure, severe dehydration

Concentrate, concentrate

Urine osmolality is used to evaluate the diluting and concentrating ability of the kidneys and varies greatly with diet and hydration status. The ability to concentrate urine is one of the first functions lost in renal failure.

Practice pointers
• Before collecting urine for pathological investigation, such as culture and sensitivity, collect a random urine specimen from an indwelling urinary catheter or a mid stream urine and send the specimen to the laboratory immediately
• If testing for pregnancy, follow the manufacturers' information closely
• For urine osmolality and routine testing collect a random urine sample.

Treatments

GU and gynaecological emergencies present many treatment challenges because they stem from various mechanisms occurring separately or simultaneously. Common treatments include drug therapy and nonsurgical and surgical procedures.

Drug therapy

Ideally, drug therapy should be effective and not impair urologic function. However, because GU disorders can affect the chemical composition of body fluids and the pharmacokinetic properties of many drugs, standard regimens of some drugs may require adjustment. For example, dosages of drugs that are mainly excreted by the kidneys unchanged or as active metabolites may require adjustment to avoid nephrotoxicity.

Drug therapy for GU disorders can include:
• Antibiotics
• Urinary tract antiseptics
• Diuretics.

In addition, electrolytes and replacements may be necessary depending on the underlying cause of the GU dysfunction.

Drug therapy for gynaecological disorders commonly includes antibiotics and analgesics for pain.

Urinary catheterisation

Catheterisation – the insertion of a drainage device into the urinary bladder – may be intermittent or continuous.

Intermittent catheterisation drains urine remaining in the bladder after voiding. It's used for patients with urinary incontinence, urethral strictures, cystitis, prostatic obstruction, neurogenic bladder or other disorders that interfere with bladder emptying. It may also be used postoperatively.

Indwelling urinary catheterisation helps relieve bladder distention caused by such conditions as urinary tract obstruction and neurogenic bladder. It allows continuous urine drainage in patients with a urinary meatus swollen from local trauma or childbirth as well as from surgery. Catheterisation can also provide accurate monitoring of urine output when normal voiding is impaired.

Practice pointers

• Ensure that catheterisation is carried out in accordance with agreed local protocols, procedures and guidelines. For instance in the UK male catheterisation usually requires the completion of a distinct training programme. EDs may have their own policies related to chaperone use and if persons of different gender to the patient can carry out catheterisation
• Thoroughly review the procedure with the patient and reassure him that although catheterisation may produce slight discomfort, it shouldn't be painful. Explain that you'll stop the procedure if he experiences severe discomfort

- Assemble the necessary equipment, including a sterile catheterisation package
- Choose the right type (short- or long-term use) and right size and length of catheter. Catheter size is noted by its 'Charriere' (ch) size – as a general guide 12 to 14 ch for male and female urethral catheterisations
- Perform the catheterisation using an aseptic technique and inflate the balloon using sterile water ensuring that you follow the manufacturer's instructions carefully
- During catheterisation, note difficulty or ease of insertion, patient discomfort and the amount and nature of urine drainage
- During urine drainage, monitor the patient for pallor, sweating and painful bladder spasms. If these occur, clamp the catheter tubing for 10 to 15 minutes. When symptoms resolve, resume drainage and recording output. See the information on catheterisation on the Skills for Health Website http://www.skillsforhealth.org.uk.

Fluid watch

- Frequently assess and record the patient's intake and output. Encourage fluid intake to maintain continuous urine flow through the catheter and decrease the risk of infection and clot formation
- To help prevent infection, avoid separating the catheter and tubing join unless absolutely necessary
- Closely assess the patient for signs and symptoms of UTI and for signs of catheter obstruction.

Surgical procedures

Suprapubic catheterisation surgery may be necessary when conservative measures fail to control the patient's problem.

Suprapubic catheterisation

Suprapubic catheterisation is a type of urinary diversion connected to a closed drainage system that involves transcutaneous insertion of a catheter through the suprapubic area into the bladder. Typically, suprapubic catheterisation provides temporary urinary diversion after certain gynaecological procedures, bladder surgery or prostatectomy and relieves obstruction from calculi, severe urethral strictures or pelvic trauma. Less commonly, it may be used to create a permanent urinary diversion, thereby relieving obstruction from an inoperable tumour. This is usually carried once the patient is admitted but may be done in the ED.

Practice pointers

- It will be explained to the patient that the doctor will insert a soft plastic tube through the skin of the abdomen and into the bladder and then connect the tube to an external collection bag
- It is explained that the procedure is done under local anesthesia, causes little or no discomfort and takes 15 to 45 minutes

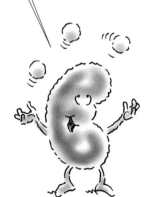

Suprapubic catheterisation provides a temporary urinary diversion. Well, not THIS type of diversion.

- The patient's consent is gained
- The insertion site is assessed closely
- To ensure adequate drainage and tube patency, the suprapubic catheter is checked at least hourly for the first 24 hours after insertion. Making sure that the collection bag is below bladder level to enhance drainage and prevent backflow, which can lead to infection
- The catheter is taped securely into place on the abdominal skin to reduce tension and prevent dislodgment. To prevent kinks in the tube, curving the tube gently helps but don't bend it
- Assess dressings frequently and change as necessary. Observe the skin around the insertion site for signs of infection and encrustation.

Common disorders

GU and gynaecological disorders commonly encountered in the ED include UTI, pyelonephritis kidney trauma, renal calculi, testicular torsion, emergency child birth, ovarian cyst, ectopic pregnancy, abortion, Pelvic Inflammatory Disease (PID) and sexual assault such as rape.

Urinary tract infection (UTI)

UTI typically refers to infection of the lower urinary tract. Lower UTIs commonly respond readily to treatment, but recurrence and resistant bacterial flare-up during therapy are possible. Lower UTIs are nearly 10 times more common in women than in men and affect 1 in 5 women at least once. Lower UTIs also occur in relatively large percentages in sexually active teenage girls. Lower UTIs fall into two types:

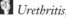 *Cystitis*, which is an inflammation of the bladder that usually results from an ascending infection

Urethritis, which is an inflammation of the urethra.

What causes it
UTI may be caused by:
- Infection by gram-negative enteric bacteria, such as *E. coli*, *Klebsiella*, *Proteus*, *Enterobacter*, *Pseudomonas* or *Serratia*
- Simultaneous infection with multiple pathogens in a patient with neurogenic bladder
- Indwelling urinary catheter
- Fistula between the intestine and the bladder

How it happens
Recent studies suggest that infection results from a breakdown in local defense mechanisms in the bladder that allows bacteria to invade the bladder mucosa and multiply. These bacteria can't be readily eliminated by normal micturition.

What to look for

Characteristic signs and symptoms include:

- Urinary urgency and frequency
- Dysuria
- Bladder cramps or spasms
- Itching
- Feeling of warmth during urination
- Nocturia
- Possible haematuria
- Fever
- Urethral discharge in males.

Other common features include lower back pain, malaise, confusion, nausea, vomiting, abdominal pain or tenderness over the bladder, chills and flank pain.

What tests tell you

- A mid-stream urinalysis reveals a bacteria count of 100,000/ml, confirming UTI. Lower counts don't necessarily rule out infection, especially if the patient is urinating frequently, because bacteria require 30 to 45 minutes to reproduce in urine. Culture and sensitivity testing determine the exact organism and the appropriate antimicrobial drug
- A blood test or stained smear rules out STI
- Testing once admitted using Voiding Cystourethrography or Excretory Urography may detect congenital anomalies.

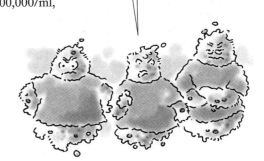

Looks like your bladder defenses broke down. Tough break; we're moving in and bringing a UTI with us.

Practice pointers

To ensure that your mid-stream urine sample is as clean as possible, ensure that you:

- Gain informed consent
- Wash and dry your hands and wear gloves and an apron
- Ask the patient to begin passing urine and collect the urine during mid-stream using a sterile universal specimen container or if a female from a sterile receiver
- Send the correctly labeled specimen to the laboratory promptly, i.e. within 2 hours (24 hours if refrigerated at 4°C). Record in patient's notes.

How it's treated

A 7- to 10-day course of an appropriate antibiotic is usually the treatment of choice for an initial lower UTI. After 3 days of antibiotic therapy, urine culture should show no organisms. If the urine isn't sterile, bacterial resistance has probably occurred, making the use of a different antimicrobial necessary. Antibiotic therapy with Amoxicillin or Trimethoprim may be effective in women with acute uncomplicated UTI. A urine culture taken 1 to 2 weeks later indicates whether the infection has been eradicated.

Education edge

UTI teaching tips

Follow these guidelines below when teaching your patient with a urinary tract infection (UTI):

- Explain the nature and purpose of antibiotic therapy. Emphasise the importance of completing the prescribed course of therapy and, with long-term prophylaxis, of adhering strictly to the ordered dosage
- Urge the patient to drink plenty of water (at least eight glasses per day). Instruct the patient to avoid alcohol while taking antibiotics. Fruit juices, especially cranberry juice, and oral doses of vitamin C may help acidify urine and enhance the action of the medication

- Suggest warm baths for relief of perineal discomfort. If baths aren't effective, apply heat sparingly to the perineum but be careful not to burn the patient
- Teach the patient about general perineal hygiene measures, such as wiping from front to back, avoiding bubble baths and douching and wearing cotton-lined underwear
- Recurrent infections caused by renal calculi, chronic prostatitis or a structural abnormality may require surgery. If there are no predisposing conditions, long-term, low-dose antibiotic therapy is preferred.

What to do

- Assess the patient's vital signs and obtain a mid-stream urine specimen for urinalysis and culture and sensitivity
- Encourage fluid intake; if necessary, administer I.V. fluids
- Initiate antimicrobial therapy as ordered
- Provide comfort measures, such as a warm bath and warm compresses
- Prepare the patient for discharge. Instruct her about the medication regimen and measures to promote infection resolution and prevent recurrence. (See *UTI teaching tips*.)

Pyelonephritis

One of the most common renal diseases, acute pyelonephritis is a sudden bacterial inflammation. It primarily affects the interstitial area, the renal pelvis and, less commonly, the renal tubules. With treatment and continued follow-up care, the prognosis is good; extensive permanent damage is rare. (See *Understanding chronic pyelonephritis*.)

What causes it

The two causes of pyelonephritis are:

 Bacterial infection

 Haematogenous or lymphatic spread.

Understanding chronic pyelonephritis

Chronic pyelonephritis, or persistent inflammation of the kidneys, can scar the kidneys and may lead to chronic renal failure. Its cause may be bacterial, metastatic or urogenous. This disease occurs most commonly in patients who are predisposed to recurrent acute pyelonephritis such as those with urinary obstructions or vesicoureteral reflux.

Signs and symptoms

Patients with chronic pyelonephritis may have a childhood history of unexplained fevers or bed-wetting. Signs and symptoms include flank pain, anaemia, low urine specific gravity, proteinuria, leukocytes in urine and, especially in late stages, hypertension. Uraemia rarely develops from chronic pyelonephritis unless structural abnormalities exist in the urinary system. Bacteriuria may be intermittent. When no bacteria are found in the urine, diagnosis depends on excretory urography (where the renal pelvis may appear small and flattened) and renal biopsy.

Treatment

Treatment requires control of hypertension, elimination of the existing obstruction (when possible) and long-term antimicrobial therapy.

Risk factors include:
- Diagnostic and therapeutic use of instruments, such as in catheterisation, cystoscopy or urologic surgery
- Inability to empty the bladder
- Urinary stasis
- Urinary obstruction
- Sexual activity (in women)
- Use of diaphragms and condoms with spermicidal gel
- Pregnancy
- Diabetes
- Other renal diseases
- UTI.

How it happens
Typically, the infection spreads from the bladder to the ureters and then to the kidneys. Bacteria refluxed to intrarenal tissues may create colonies of infection within 24 to 48 hours.

What to look for
- Urinary urgency and frequency
- Pain over one or both kidneys
- Burning during urination
- Dysuria, nocturia, haematuria
- Cloudy urine with an ammonia or fish odour
- Temperature of 38.9°C or higher
- Shaking chills
- Flank pain, including on palpation (costovertebral tenderness)

- Anorexia
- General fatigue.

What tests tell you
- Urinalysis reveals pyuria and, possibly, a few RBCs; low specific gravity and osmolality; slightly alkaline pH; and, possibly, proteinuria, glycosuria and ketonuria
- Urine culture reveals more than 100,000 organisms/μl of urine
- Ultrasound may reveal calculi, tumours or cysts in the kidneys and the urinary tract
- Excretory urography may show asymmetrical kidneys.

How it's treated
Therapy centres on antibiotic therapy appropriate to the specific infecting organism after it has been identified by urine culture and sensitivity studies. When the infecting organism can't be identified, therapy usually consists of a broad-spectrum antibiotic. If the patient is pregnant, antibiotics must be prescribed cautiously. Analgesia may be prescribed.

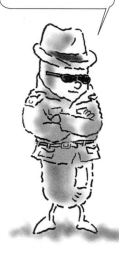

Even when the pyelonephritis perpetrator hasn't been identified, antibiotics usually take care of the problem.

Antibiotic aid
Symptoms may disappear after several days of antibiotic therapy. Although urine usually becomes sterile within 48 to 72 hours, the course of such therapy is 10 to 14 days. Follow-up treatment includes reculturing urine 1 week after drug therapy stops and then periodically for the next year to detect residual or recurring infection. Most patients with uncomplicated infections respond well to therapy and don't suffer re-infection.

Infection from obstruction or vesicoureteral reflux may be less responsive to antibiotics. Treatment may then necessitate surgery to relieve the obstruction or correct the anomaly. Patients at high risk for recurring UTIs and kidney infections, such as those using an indwelling urinary catheter for a prolonged period and those on maintenance antibiotic therapy, require long-term follow-up care.

What to do
- Obtain a mid-stream or catheter urine specimen for culture and sensitivity
- Monitor the patient's vital signs, especially temperature, and administer antipyretics for fever
- Ensure adequate hydration with fluids. Encourage increased fluid intake to achieve a urine output of more than 2,000 ml/day. Don't encourage intake of more than 2 to 3 L because this amount of fluid intake may decrease the effectiveness of antibiotics. If the patient has difficulty with oral fluid intake, expect to administer I.V. fluids
- Prepare the patient for discharge. Review the medication therapy regime and teach recurrence prevention measures. (See *Acute pyelonephritis teaching tips*.)

Education edge
Acute pyelonephritis teaching tips

- Teach the patient about measures to reduce and avoid bacterial contamination, including using proper hygienic toileting practices such as wiping the perineum from front to back after bowel elimination
- Teach the proper technique for collecting a clean-catch urine specimen. Tell the patient to be sure to refrigerate a urine specimen within 30 minutes of collection to prevent overgrowth of bacteria
- Stress the need to complete the prescribed antibiotic therapy even after symptoms subside

- Advise routine checkups for a patient with chronic urinary tract infections
- Teach the patient to recognise signs and symptoms of infection, such as cloudy urine, burning on urination and urinary urgency and frequency, especially when accompanied by a low-grade fever
- Encourage long-term follow-up care for high-risk patients.

Kidney trauma

Kidney trauma can involve damage to minor tissues or, possibly, major vascular structures. Trauma to the kidney can be wide-ranging, from contusions and subcapsular haematomas to fractured kidney, renal artery thrombosis or avulsion of the major renal artery or vein. Kidney trauma may be classified by severity using a grading scale of 1 to 5 or using the categories of minor, major and critical trauma. (See *Staging kidney trauma*, page 372.)

What causes it

Kidney trauma is commonly classified as *penetrating* or *blunt*, depending on the type of injury.

Penetrating kidney trauma involves an injury by a foreign object, such as a bullet (or a bullet fragment or effect of the blast) or knife. A gunshot wound involving the kidney typically results in a complex array of injuries.

Blunt kidney trauma is the cause of approximately 75% of all kidney injuries, most of which result from motor vehicle collisions. Other less common causes include sports injuries, occupational injuries and assaults.

Kidney trauma may also result from iatrogenic causes. These causes may include percutaneous nephrostomy, renal biopsy and extracorporeal shockwave lithotripsy (ESWL).

How it happens

Three mechanisms are responsible for causing blunt kidney trauma:

Direct blow to the flank area

Laceration of the parenchyma from a fractured rib or vertebra

Sudden deceleration leading to shearing and subsequent damage.

Staging kidney trauma

This chart highlights the different classifications of kidney trauma, their locations and types and associated signs and symptoms.

Classification grade and category	Location and type of trauma	Associated signs and symptoms
Grade: 1 Category: Minor	• Contusion (bruising of the renal parenchyma) • Superficial laceration of the renal cortex	• Microscopic or gross haematuria • Urologic studies within normal parameters • Flank tenderness
Grade: 2 Category: Minor	• Laceration of the renal parenchyma measuring less than 1 cm • Nonexpanding haematoma around the kidney	• Microscopic or gross haematuria • Urologic studies within normal parameters • Flank tenderness
Grade: 3 Category: Major	• Laceration of the parenchyma without involvement of the collecting system	• Haematuria • Flank pain • Possible hypotension
Grade: 4 Category: Major	• Major laceration involving the cortex and medulla with continuation through the renal capsule of the kidney – laceration involving the collecting system • Extravasation within and around the kidney • Thrombosis of a segment of the renal artery • Controlled bleeding involving the major renal artery or vein	• Haematuria • Flank pain • Hypovolaemia • Possible hypotension
Grade: 5 Category: Critical	• Shattered kidney with injury and fragmentation (fracture) • Thrombosis of the main renal artery • Avulsion of the main renal artery or vein	• Severe blood loss • Hypovolaemic shock

What to look for

Assessment findings may vary based on the type and extent of kidney trauma. One common finding is haematuria, which may be gross or microscopic. However, the degree of haematuria doesn't correlate with the severity of kidney trauma.

And that's not all

Additional findings may include:
• Abdominal or flank pain
• Tenderness along the back
• Complaints of colicky pain with the passage of clots in the urine
• Haematoma over the flank area, usually in the area of the 11th or 12th rib
• Obvious wounds, bruises or abrasions in the flank area or abdomen
• Turner's sign (bruising of the flanks that can indicate acute pancreatitis)

- Costovertebral angle pain or tenderness
- Palpable mass in the flank or abdominal area
- Signs and symptoms of haemorrhage and hypovolaemic shock, such as pallor, sweating, hypotension, tachycardia and changes in mental status.

What tests tell you

Diagnostic testing depends on the patient's condition and extent of injuries. Some diagnostic tests may include:
- X-ray to identify the path and appearance of the object causing the penetrating trauma and to determine the outline or fragmentation of the kidney
- IVU to stage the degree of kidney injury
- Ultrasound, CT scan and MRI to evaluate kidney structure and identify haematomas, lacerations and vascular disruptions
- Renal angiography to detect arterial injury.
  Other tests include:
- Arterial blood gas analysis to evaluate respiratory and acid-base status secondary to blood loss and shock
- FBC to evaluate the degree of blood loss
- Coagulation studies to determine the patient's clotting ability
- Serum electrolyte level to determine possible imbalances.

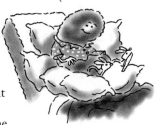

Blunt kidney trauma treatment focuses on bed rest. Sounds good to me!

How it's treated

Treatment of blunt kidney trauma typically focuses on bed rest with frequent assessments and serial specimens for urinalysis. In addition, analgesics are used to manage pain. A penetrating kidney trauma, such as a laceration to the kidney, requires surgical intervention.

Haemodynamics count

A kidney trauma patient who's haemodynamically stable requires close monitoring in the initial period after injury. Surgery is typically performed later, as indicated by the patient's condition.

For a patient who's haemodynamically unstable, has other associated trauma or exhibits shock, treatment focuses on immediate stabilisation; assessing and maintaining airway, breathing and circulation (ABC); and disability (D) assessing level of consciousness (LOC) and exposure (E) – are there other injuries? An exploratory laparotomy is usually performed immediately.

Wound care

If the patient has a wound, treatment may include controlling bleeding – usually by applying firm, direct pressure – and cleaning the wound. Pain medication and antibiotic therapy are instituted as indicated. In addition, I.V. therapy is started to ensure fluid balance and maintain the patient's haemodynamic status.

What to do

- Assess the patient (ABCDE) and initiate emergency measures if necessary; administer supplemental oxygen as ordered in line with British Thoracic Society Guidelines to maintain target oxygen saturations between 94% and 98%
- Monitor the patient's vital signs, usually at least every 15 to 30 minutes and note significant changes
- Assess oxygen saturation and monitor cardiac rhythm for arrhythmias using a cardiac monitor and undertake a 12 lead ECG
- Assess the patient's neurologic status, including LOC and pupillary and motor response
- Obtain blood studies, including type and crossmatch
- Insert two large-bore I.V. catheters and infuse normal saline or Hartmann's solution as ordered
- Quickly and carefully assess for other areas of trauma
- Institute complete bed rest with frequent assessments, such as every 15 to 30 minutes or as indicated by the patient's condition
- Assess wounds and provide wound care as appropriate. Cover open wounds and control bleeding by applying pressure.

Watch and record

- Assess for increased abdominal distention
- Administer blood products as appropriate
- Monitor for signs of hypovolaemic shock (See Chapter 4, *Shock*)
- Provide pain medication, as appropriate
- Prepare the patient and his family for diagnostic testing and possible surgery
- Provide reassurance to the patient and his family.

Renal calculi

Renal calculi may form anywhere in the urinary tract, but usually develop in the renal pelvis or calyces. Such formation follows precipitation of substances normally dissolved in urine (calcium oxalate, calcium phosphate, magnesium ammonium phosphate or, occasionally, urate or cystine). Renal calculi vary in size and may be solitary or multiple. They may remain in the renal pelvis or enter the ureter and may damage renal parenchyma. Large calculi cause pressure necrosis. In certain locations, calculi cause obstruction (with resultant hydronephrosis) and tend to recur. (See *A close look at renal calculi*.)

What causes it

Renal calculi may result from:
- *Dehydration*. Decreased urine production concentrates calculus-forming substances
- *Infection*. Infected, damaged tissue serves as a site for calculus development. Infected calculi (usually magnesium ammonium phosphate

A close look at renal calculi

Renal calculi vary in size and type. Small calculi may remain in the renal pelvis or pass down the ureter as shown below left. A staghorn calculus, shown below right, is a cast in the innermost part of the kidney – the calyx and renal pelvis. A staghorn calculus may develop from a calculus that stays in the kidney.

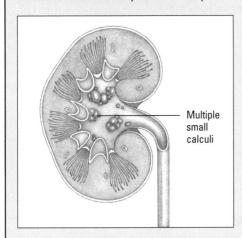

Multiple small calculi

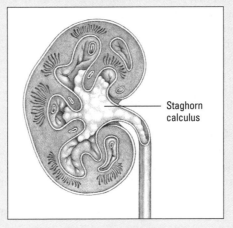

Staghorn calculus

or staghorn calculi) may develop if bacteria serve as the nucleus in calculus formation. Such infections may promote destruction of renal parenchyma
• *Changes in urine pH.* Consistently acidic or alkaline urine provides a favorable medium for calculus formation
• *Obstruction.* Urinary stasis (such as in immobility from spinal cord injury) allows calculus constituents to collect and adhere, forming calculi Obstruction also promotes infection that, in turn, compounds the obstruction
• *Diet.* Increased intake of calcium or oxalate-rich foods encourages calculus formation
• *Immobilisation.* Immobility from spinal cord injury or other disorders allows calcium to be released into the circulation and eventually filtered by the kidneys
• *Metabolic factors.* Hyperparathyroidism, renal tubular acidosis, elevated uric acid levels (usually with gout), defective metabolism of oxalate, genetically defective metabolism of cystine and excessive intake of vitamin D, protein or dietary calcium may predispose a patient to renal calculi.

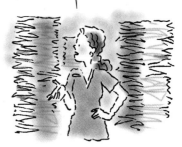

Renal calculi sure are calculating. Just look at all their possible causes!

How it happens

Calculi form when substances that normally dissolve in urine, such as calcium oxalate and calcium phosphate, precipitate. Large, rough calculi may occlude the opening to the ureteropelvic junction. The frequency and force of peristaltic contractions increase, causing pain.

What to look for

Clinical effects vary with size, location and cause of the calculus. Pain is the key symptom. The pain of classic renal colic travels from the costovertebral angle to the flank, the suprapubic region and the external genitalia. The pain fluctuates in intensity and may be excruciating at its peak. If calculi are in the renal pelvis and calyces, pain may be more constant and dull. Back pain occurs from calculi that produce an obstruction within a kidney. Nausea and vomiting usually accompany severe pain.

Other symptoms include:
- Abdominal distention
- Fever and chills
- Haematuria, pyuria and, rarely, anuria
- Restlessness
- Inability to lie in a supine position.

What tests tell you

- Ultrasound reveals most renal calculi
- Calculus analysis shows mineral content
- Excretory urography confirms the diagnosis and determines the size and location of calculi
- Renal ultrasonography may detect obstructive changes such as hydronephrosis
- Urine culture of a midstream specimen may indicate UTI
- Urinalysis results may be normal or may show increased specific gravity and acid or alkaline pH suitable for different types of calculus formation. Other urinalysis findings include haematuria (gross or microscopic), crystals (urate, calcium or cystine), casts and pyuria with or without bacteria and WBCs. A 24-hour urine collection is evaluated for calcium oxalate, phosphorus and uric acid excretion levels
- Other laboratory results support the diagnosis. Serial blood calcium and phosphorus levels detect hyperparathyroidism and show increased calcium levels in proportion to normal serum protein levels. Blood protein levels determine free calcium unbound to protein. Blood chloride and bicarbonate levels may show renal tubular acidosis. Increased blood uric acid levels may indicate gout as the cause.

How it's treated

Because 90% of renal calculi are smaller than 5 mm in diameter, treatment usually consists of measures to promote their natural passage. Along with vigorous hydration, such treatment includes antimicrobial therapy (varying with the cultured organism) for infection, analgesics for pain and diuretics to prevent urinary stasis and further calculus formation (because thiazide diuretics decrease calcium excretion into the urine, which reduces calculus formation).

Prophylaxis to prevent calculus formation includes a low-calcium diet for absorptive hypercalciuria, parathyroidectomy

> Vigorous hydration is a main component of renal calculi treatment – with enough hydration, the little suckers will eventually "go" with your flow.

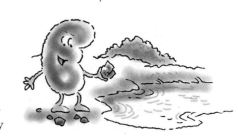

for hyperparathyroidism, allopurinol for uric acid calculi and daily administration of ascorbic acid by mouth to acidify the urine. A calculus that's too large for natural passage may require surgical removal or percutaneous ultrasonic lithotripsy.

What to do
• Promote sufficient intake of fluids to maintain a urine output of 3 to 4 L/day (urine should be very dilute and colourless). If the patient can't drink the required amount of fluid, supplemental I.V. fluids may be given
• Strain all urine through gauze or a tea strainer and save the solid material recovered for analysis
• Administer analgesics as ordered
• Encourage ambulation if appropriate to aid in spontaneous passage of stones
• Record intake, output and weight to assess fluid status and renal function
• If surgery is necessary, reassure the patient by supplementing and reinforcing what the surgeon has told him about the procedure. Explain preoperative and postoperative care.

Testicular torsion

Testicular torsion is the abnormal twisting of the spermatic cord resulting from the rotation of a testis or the *mesorchium*, a fold in the area between the testis and epididymis. It causes strangulation and, if untreated, eventual infarction of the testis.

This condition is almost always unilateral. Although it's most common between ages 12 and 18, it may occur at any age. The prognosis is good with early detection and prompt treatment.

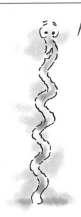

I happen to like my twisty figure, but I don't think a spermatic cord would share my opinion.

What causes it
Testicular torsion is caused in part by abnormalities inside or outside the *tunica vaginalis*, the serous membrane covering the internal scrotal cavity. Normally the tunica vaginalis envelops the testis and attaches to the epididymis and spermatic cord. Testicular torsion can be intravaginal or extravaginal.

Intra vs extra
Intravaginal torsion is caused by:
• Abnormality of the tunica vaginalis and the position of the testis
• Incomplete attachment of the testis and spermatic fascia to the scrotal wall, leaving the testis free to rotate around its vascular pedicle.
Extravaginal torsion is caused by:
• Loose attachment of the tunica vaginalis to the scrotal lining, causing spermatic cord rotation above the testis
• Sudden forceful contraction of the cremaster muscle due to physical exertion or irritation of the muscle

How it happens

In testicular torsion, the testis rotates on its vascular pedicle and twists the arteries and vein in the spermatic cord. This twisting interrupts blood flow to the testis, resulting in vascular engorgement, ischaemia and scrotal swelling.

What to look for

Torsion produces excruciating pain in the affected testis or iliac fossa. Physical examination reveals tense, tender swelling in the scrotum or inguinal canal and hyperemia of the overlying skin. Scrotal swelling is unrelieved by rest or elevation of the scrotum.

What tests tell you

Doppler ultrasonography helps distinguish testicular torsion from strangulated hernia, undescended testes or epididymitis.

How it's treated

If manual reduction or detorsion is unsuccessful, torsion must be surgically corrected within 6 hours after the onset of symptoms to preserve testicular function (70% salvage rate). Treatment consists of immediate surgical repair by *orchiopexy* (fixation of a viable testis to the scrotum) or *orchiectomy* (excision of a nonviable testis). Without treatment, the testis becomes dysfunctional and necrotic after 12 hours.

What to do

- Administer analgesics as ordered to aid pain relief
- Assess vital signs and prepare the patient for surgery
- Provide emotional support to the patient and his family
- Perform preoperative teaching.

Emergency child birth

Emergency child birth or emergency delivery can occur after 24 weeks gestation and refers to a situation in which the neonate's birth is imminent. It's commonly defined as labour completed within less than 3 hours. In such cases, rapid assessment of the mother and fetus is critical. Complicating factors may be that the neonate will need resuscitation and the mother may experience a primary postpartum haemorrhage because of the rapidity of the birth.

What causes it

Emergency child birth may result from various factors. In some situations, it results from precipitous labour in which uterine contractions are so strong and rapid that the woman delivers after only a few of them. Emergency delivery may also occur due to a lack of understanding about labour signs and symptoms. Additionally, it may be necessary when the mother or fetus exhibit signs of compromise for delivery to be expedited.

What to look for

The assessment and management of an emergency delivery should be carried out in a delivery room by an experienced qualified practitioner.

Emergency delivery due to precipitous labour may be identified from a partogram that shows the active phase of dilation at a rate greater than 5 cm/hour in a woman who has never given birth to a child (1 cm every 12 minutes) and greater than 10 cm/hour (1 cm every 6 minutes) in a woman who has multiple deliveries. Additionally, uterine contraction monitoring may reveal hypertonic contractions occurring > than 5 contractions in a 10 minute period.

Vaginal examination may reveal rupture of membranes, with rapid and progressive cervical dilation. Crowning may also be evident.

What you need

- Syringe
- Sterile scissors or scalpel
- Two cord clamps
- Basin
- Fluid absorbent pads
- Sterile gloves
- Clean baby blankets
- Sanitary pad
- Infant stockinette hat
- Identification bands per local policy
- Heated Isolette or warm blankets.

What to do

If a patient requires emergency delivery, contact the senior personnel within the department and fast bleep the obstetrician and midwife and follow these steps:
- Explain to the patient what's happening and what to expect
- Monitor the patient's vital signs and foetal heart rate and pattern closely, reporting any significant changes
- Pulse oximetry. Administer oxygen via face mask as ordered to ensure adequate oxygenation as per BTS guidelines to maintain oxygen saturations, usually 94% to 98%. Be aware that oxygen therapy may be harmful to the fetus if the mother is not hypoxaemic
- Initiate I.V. therapy if ordered to maintain fluid balance
- Put on appropriate attire such as a gown and gloves, adhering to standard precautions and your hospital's policy
- Assist the practitioner with delivery by applying gentle pressure with a sterile towel to the neonate's head as it crowns
- Quickly inspect the neonate's neck area for evidence of the umbilical cord; if present and loose, gently slide it over the neonate's head
- Assist with delivering the remainder of the neonate, providing support to the head and shoulders
- Assess for spontaneous breaths and crying; if they don't occur, gently rub the neonate's back

- Assist with clamping the umbilical cord
- Quickly wrap the neonate in a warmed blanket or place him under a radiant heat source such as an Isolette
- Determine the neonate's Apgar score
- If the neonate is stable, place him on the mother's abdomen
- Assist with delivery of the placenta; after it's delivered, place it in a basin or plastic bag and send it with the mother to the obstetric unit
- Document the time of delivery of the neonate and placenta. Also document the neonate's status and his Apgar score
- Monitor maternal vital signs and vaginal bleeding. Maternal bleeding should slow significantly after the placenta's delivery
- Assess the fundus by gently massaging it while applying moderate suprapubic pressure
- Prepare the mother and her neonate for transfer to the appropriate ward.

The newborn assessment is performed immediately after birth. Respiratory effort, heart rate and skin colour for perfusion are evaluated using the Apgar scoring system. Listen for breath sounds in the mid-axillary area and palpate the pulse at the umbilical stump or apically on the chest.

Use this chart to determine the neonatal Apgar score at 1-minute and 5-minute intervals after birth. For each category listed, assign a score of 0 to 2, as shown. A total score of 7 to 10 indicates that the neonate is in good condition; 4 to 6, fair condition (the neonate may have moderate central nervous system depression, muscle flaccidity, cyanosis and poor respirations); 0 to 3, danger (the neonate needs immediate resuscitation, as ordered).

Sign	Apgar score		
	0	1	2
Heart rate	Absent	Less than 100 beats/minute	More than 100 beats/minute
Respiratory effort	Absent	Slow, irregular	Good crying
Muscle tone	Flaccid	Some flexion and resistance to extension of extremities	Active motion
Reflex irritability	No response	Grimace or weak cry	Vigorous cry
Colour	Pallor, cyanosis	Pink body, blue extremities	Completely pink

Ovarian cyst

An ovarian cyst refers to the development of a saclike structure on the ovary. The sac can contain fluid, semi-fluid or solid material. Cysts may be categorised as *endometrial*, *follicular* or *corpus luteal* depending on the underlying mechanism associated with their development.

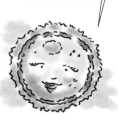

A funny thing happened on the way to the uterus … namely a cyst. What type it is depends on its cause.

What causes it

Ovarian cysts vary in size, consistency and development. The underlying cause of the cyst identifies its type:

- *Endometrial cyst* – results from an overgrowth of endometrial tissue such as endometriosis
- *Follicular cyst* – results from failed follicular rupture from the ovary at ovulation
- *Corpus luteal cyst* – results from the continued presence of a corpus luteum that has failed to atrophy.

How it happens

Within the ovary, the follicle develops because of hormonal influences. At the midpoint of a woman's menstrual cycle, a follicle, now mature, ruptures from the ovary (with follicular cysts, this rupture doesn't occur).

After ovulation, the follicle becomes the corpus luteum and travels to the fallopian tube where it may be fertilised by spermatozoa. If the corpus luteum isn't fertilised, it degenerates (with corpus luteal cysts, this degeneration doesn't occur).

Normally, endometrial tissue is located in the uterine cavity. However, for unknown reasons the tissue sometimes appears outside of the endometrial cavity, commonly around the ovaries. This tissue responds to oestrogen and progesterone secretion and proliferates. Upon menstruation the tissue bleeds and becomes inflamed, leading to fibrosis.

What to look for

Most patients with ovarian cysts may be asymptomatic. Typically, they experience signs and symptoms when rupture, haemorrhage or torsion (twisting) of a cyst occurs. Follicular cysts commonly rupture in the first half of the menstrual cycle with strenuous exercise or sexual intercourse, whereas corpus luteal cysts typically rupture in the last half of the cycle, usually in the weeks before the woman's menses.

If the patient is experiencing symptoms, they may include:

- Pressure or abdominal pain
- Dull ache on the affected side
- Prolonged menstruation
- Mittelschmerz pain (pain with ovulation) with rupture of the cyst.

Pelvic examination may reveal ovarian tenderness and enlargement. With rupture, the patient may exhibit signs and symptoms of hypovolaemic shock, especially with rupture of a blood-filled cyst such as a mature corpus luteal cyst. These symptoms may range from mild to severe, depending on the extent of blood loss.

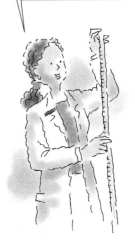

Diagnosing an ovarian cyst relies more on ruling out other conditions than on specific testing.

What tests tell you

There's no specific test used to identify ovarian cysts. Usually, ultrasound is used to rule out other conditions, such as appendicitis, ectopic pregnancy and intraperitoneal bleeding, which demonstrate similar symptoms. In addition, a pregnancy test maybe requested (explicit consent must be gained). Routine diagnostic tests, such as FBC and urinalysis, are done to establish a baseline and rule out other possible disorders.

How it's treated

Treatment for an unruptured cyst includes analgesics for pain management and support for the patient. In most cases, nonopioids, such as nonsteroidal anti-inflammatory drugs (NSAIDs), are used. If necessary, opioids may be given for a short-term pain relief. If the patient has polycystic disease (multiple follicular cysts on both ovaries) typically, surgery isn't required unless the patient exhibits signs and symptoms of hypovolaemic shock.

What to do

- Assess ABCDE
- Be alert for signs and symptoms of haemorrhage and hypovolaemic shock (see Chapter 4, *Shock*)
- Administer analgesics as ordered for pain management
- Provide reassurance and support to the patient; explain that small cysts usually reabsorb on their own
- Review the treatment plan for the patient
- Teach the patient about signs and symptoms of possible torsion (twisting of the ovary)
- Prepare the patient for surgery if indicated.
  If the patient develops hypovolaemic shock:
- Initiate fluid therapy and start an I.V. line if one isn't already in place; administer fluids as ordered
- Obtain a specimen for blood typing and crossmatching.

Ectopic pregnancy

An ectopic pregnancy is the term given the condition where a fertilised egg has lodged in a fallopian tube rather than in the uterus. The classic symptoms are amenorrhoea (absence of periods), vaginal bleeding and abdominal pain. Initially the pain is described as being cramp-like and intermittent and is located in one side of the abdomen. We have an emergency situation if a spontaneous abortion occurs or if the fallopian tube ruptures.

Practice pointers

- Access ABCDE
- The patient will be in constant severe pain. Shoulder pain may indicate a massive haemoperitoneum (blood in the abdominal cavity)
- There may be vaginal bleeding
- High risk for hypovolaemic shock (see Chapter 4, *Shock*).

Miscarriage

A miscarriage is a pregnancy that ends before 24 weeks, which is before most developing babies are able to survive outside the uterus. Third-trimester bleeding presents the biggest risk to the woman due to the large volume of blood present in the woman's body (however, at any stage, there is a risk of severe bleeding and hypovolaemic shock).

Practice pointers

- Assess ABCDE record frequent vital signs and attach a cardiac monitor
- Keep the woman recumbent and lying on her left side
- Pulse oximetry and give oxygen to maintain blood oxygen saturation within prescribed limits in line with British Thoracic Guidelines usually a target saturation of 94% to 98% is required
- I.V. infusion (normal saline) via wide bore I.V. cannula as prescribed
- Bloods taken for cross match, FBC, U&Es
- Place pads externally to catch and observe blood loss
- Do not discard any products of expelled pregnancy
- Offer emotional support and information.

Pelvic inflammatory disease (PID)

PID refers to any acute, sub acute, recurrent or chronic infection of the oviducts and ovaries, with adjacent tissue involvement. It includes inflammation of the cervix (cervicitis), uterus (endometritis), fallopian tubes (salpingitis) and ovaries (oophoritis), which can extend to the connective tissue lying between the broad ligaments (parametritis) (See *Three types of PID*, page 384.)

Early diagnosis and treatment prevent damage to the reproductive system. Complications of PID include infertility and potentially fatal septicaemia, pulmonary emboli and shock. Untreated PID may be fatal.

What causes it?

PID can result from infection with aerobic or anaerobic organisms. About 60% of cases result from overgrowth of one or more of the common bacterial species found in cervical mucus, including staphylococci, streptococci, diphtheroids, *Chlamydiae* and such coliforms as *Pseudomonas* and *Escherichia coli*. PID also results from infection with *Neisseria gonorrhoeae*. Finally, multiplication of typically nonpathogenic bacteria in an altered endometrial environment can cause PID. This multiplication occurs most commonly during parturition.

Upping the ante

These factors increase the patient's chances of developing PID:
- History of STIs
- More than one sexual partner
- Conditions (such as uterine infection) or procedures (such as cone biopsy or cauterisation of the cervix) that alter or destroy cervical mucus, allowing bacteria to ascend into the uterine cavity
- Procedures that risk transfer of contaminated cervical mucus into the endometrial cavity by instrumentation, such as use of a biopsy curette or an irrigation catheter, tubal insufflation, abortion or pelvic surgery

Three types of PID

This chart lists the types of pelvic inflammatory disease (PID), their signs and symptoms and diagnostic test findings.

Type and signs and symptoms	Diagnostic test findings
Cervicitis	
• *Acute:* purulent, foul-smelling vaginal discharge; vulvovaginitis with itching or burning; red, oedematous cervix; pelvic discomfort; sexual dysfunction; metrorrhagia; infertility; spontaneous abortion • *Chronic:* cervical dystocia, laceration or eversion of the cervix, ulcerative vesicular lesion (when cervicitis results from herpes simplex virus type 2)	• Cultures for *Neisseria gonorrhoeae* are positive; with chronic cervicitis, causative organisms are usually *Staphylococcus* or *Streptococcus*. • Cytologic smears may reveal severe inflammation. • If cervicitis isn't complicated by salpingitis, white blood cell (WBC) count is normal or slightly elevated; erythrocyte sedimentation rate (ESR) is elevated. • With acute cervicitis, cervical palpation reveals tenderness.
Endometritis (usually postpartum or postabortion)	
• *Acute:* mucopurulent or purulent vaginal discharge oozing from cervix; oedematous, hyperaemic endometrium, possibly leading to ulceration and necrosis (with virulent organisms); lower abdominal pain and tenderness; fever; rebound pain; abdominal muscle spasm; thrombophlebitis of uterine and pelvic vessels • *Chronic:* recurring acute episodes (usually from having multiple sexual partners and sexually transmitted infections)	• With severe infection, palpation may reveal boggy uterus. • Uterine and blood samples are positive for causative organism, usually *Staphylococcus*. • WBC count and ESR are elevated.
Salpingo-oophoritis	
• *Acute:* sudden onset of lower abdominal and pelvic pain, usually after menses; increased vaginal discharge; fever; malaise; lower abdominal pressure and tenderness; tachycardia; pelvic peritonitis • *Chronic:* recurring acute episodes	• WBC count is elevated or normal. • X-ray may show ileus. • Pelvic examination reveals extreme tenderness. • Smear of cervical or periurethral gland exudate shows gram-negative intracellular diplococci.

• Infection during or after pregnancy
• Infectious focus within the body, such as drainage from a chronically infected fallopian tube, a pelvic abscess, a ruptured appendix, diverticulitis of the sigmoid colon or a tampon left in situ.

How it happens
Various conditions, procedures or instruments can alter or destroy the cervical mucus, which usually serves as a protective barrier. As a result, bacteria enter the uterine cavity, causing inflammation of various structures.

What to look for
Signs and symptoms vary with the affected area and include:
• Profuse, purulent vaginal discharge
• Low-grade fever and malaise (especially if *N. gonorrhoeae* is the cause)

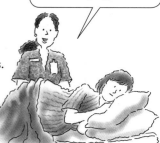

Infection during or after pregnancy is just one factor increasing a patient's risk of developing PID.

- Lower abdominal pain
- Extreme pain on movement of the cervix or palpation of the fallopian tubes and ovaries.

What tests tell you
- Gram stain of secretions from the endocervix helps identify the infecting organism
- Culture and sensitivity testing aid selection of the appropriate antibiotic. Urethral and rectal secretions may also be cultured
- Ultrasonography identifies an adnexal or uterine mass
- Culdocentesis (the extraction of fluid from the rectouterine pouch posterior to the vagina through a needle) obtains peritoneal fluid or pus for culture and sensitivity testing.

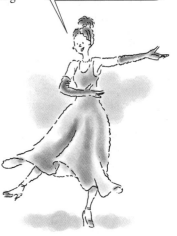

I'm glad to be cultured in this sense, and not in the sense that urethral and rectal secretions are.

How it's treated
Effective management eradicates the infection, relieves symptoms and leaves the reproductive system intact. It includes:
- Aggressive therapy with multiple antibiotics beginning immediately after culture specimens are obtained
- Reevaluation of therapy as soon as laboratory results are available (usually after 24 to 48 hours)
- Supplemental treatment, including bed rest, analgesics and I.V. therapy
- Adequate drainage if a pelvic abscess develops
- NSAIDs for pain relief (preferred treatment); opioids if necessary.

Additional considerations

Treatment for patients suffering from PID as a result of gonorrhea or syphilis includes an antibiotic regime as per current guidelines: this may include Doxycycline, Erythromycin and Benzylpenicillin.

A total abdominal hysterectomy with bilateral salpingo-oophorectomy may be recommended for patients suffering from a ruptured pelvic abscess (a life-threatening complication).

What to do
- Institute aggressive antibiotic therapy as ordered
- Position the patient with the head of the bed elevated approximately 30 to 45 degrees – this helps keep secretions pooled in the lower pelvic area
- Administer analgesics as ordered for pain
- Monitor vital signs for changes, especially in temperature
- Assess the abdomen for rigidity and distention, which are possible signs of developing peritonitis
- Provide frequent perineal care if vaginal drainage occurs
- Support the patient and her family
- Prepare the patient for possible surgery if a ruptured abscess is suspected

Education edge

PID teaching tips

If your patient has pelvic inflammatory disease (PID), cover these important points:

- To prevent recurrence, encourage compliance with treatment and explain the nature and seriousness of PID
- Because PID may cause painful intercourse, advise the patient to consult with her practitioner about sexual activity
- Stress the need for the patient's sexual partner to be examined and treated for infection

- To prevent infection after minor gynaecological procedures, such as dilatation and curettage, tell the patient to immediately report fever, increased vaginal discharge or pain. After such procedures, instruct her to avoid douching and intercourse for at least 7 days.

- If the patient will be discharged, review the medication therapy regimen for outpatient therapy. Provide education related to recurrence prevention. (See *PID teaching tips*.)

Severe situation

If the patient's PID is considered severe, expect the patient to be admitted for I.V. antibiotic administration. Criteria for possible hospitalisation include:
- Child or adolescent age group
- Pregnancy or HIV infection
- Suspected or positive evidence of a pelvic abscess or peritonitis
- Temperature greater than 40°C
- Inability to eat or drink
- No response to outpatient therapy
- Decreased resistance to infection because of her condition
- Inability to confirm diagnosis
- Lack of available follow-up
- Noncompliance with outpatient treatment plan.

Sexual assault

Sexual assault, commonly called *rape*, refers to sexual contact without the person's consent. It includes physical and psychological coercion and force – that result in varying degrees of physical and psychological trauma.

Most information related to sexual assault is derived from statistics involving women who have been sexually assaulted. However, men and children can also be victims.

What's in a name?

Persons who have experienced sexual assault may be referred to as survivors or victims. Some health care practitioners use the term *survivor* because it's empowering and positive. Others use the term *victim* because it underscores the event's overwhelming severity and devastation. However, other health care practitioners feel that the term *victim* denotes hopelessness and helplessness.

Rape-trauma syndrome

Persons who have been sexually assaulted or have experienced an attempted sexual assault may develop rape-trauma syndrome. This syndrome involves the victim's short- and long-term reactions to the trauma and the methods used to cope with it. With support and counselling to help the patient deal with her/his feelings, the prognosis is good.

What causes it

Sexual assault is the result of a crime involving power, anger and control. It isn't the result of wearing suggestive clothing, a secret desire to be raped or a specific sexual orientation. The person committing the assault uses sex as a means to control and humiliate the victim. In this situation, all options for choice are removed from the victim. Subsequently, the attacker uses sexual contact forcibly and degradingly.

What to look for

Sexual assault is commonly characterised by:
• Signs of physical trauma, including bruising, lacerations, abrasions and avulsions
• Clothing that's ripped, stained or cut
• Tearfulness, crying and shaking
• Withdrawal
• Anxiety.

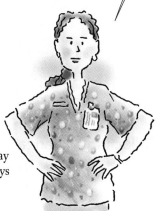

Sexual assault victims commonly display signs of withdrawal.

What tests tell you

Typically, several tests rule out possible STIs and pregnancy. Other tests may be done depending on the extent of the patient's injuries; for example, X-rays may be done to rule out fractures.

How it's treated

Treatment focuses on proper evidence collection, immediate care of apparent or life-threatening wounds or injuries and medication therapy to prevent STIs and pregnancy.

Each department has a specific protocol for specimen collection in cases involving sexual assault. Specimens can be collected from many sources. Typically, they include blood, hair, nails, tissues and body fluids, such as urine, semen, saliva and vaginal secretions. In addition, evidence can be obtained via the results of diagnostic tests, such as CT scan and radiography.

Regardless of the protocol or specimen source, accurate and precise specimen collection is essential in conjunction with thorough, objective documentation because, in many cases, this information will be used as evidence in legal proceedings.

In good hands

Many authorities have Sexual Assault Referral Centres (SARCS) to care for sexual assaulted victims. These are skilled rape-crisis professionals who can support the victim with medical treatment, counselling, provide legal advice and collect specimens. They may also be called upon at a later date to testify in legal proceedings. http://www.rapecrisis.org.uk/Referralcentres2.php.

What to do

When caring for the victim of a sexual assault, follow these steps:
• Stay with the patient at all times; offer comfort and support. Ask about calling a person for the patient who can also provide support, such as a friend, family member or counsellor
• Develop a therapeutic relationship with the patient; make sure that they have given informed consent for testing that may be performed
• Inform the patient of the department's responsibility in reporting the assault; make sure that the patient understands this responsibility. Arrange for an advocate to talk with the patient about her choices and decision-making
• Assist with history taking and physical examination; obtain the following key information: date and time of the assault; where it occurred and the surroundings; body areas penetrated, including the use of foreign objects; and other sexual acts
• Also ask about injuries occurring during the assault; actions after the assault, such as showering, urinating, changing clothing; recent gynaecologic treatment or surgery; and history of sexual intercourse within the past 72 hours.

Collecting evidence

• Make sure that the chain of custody for all evidence collected is maintained and logged according to the department protocol. Document all information completely; including the date and time that evidence was given to the police. Include the names of the individuals in the patient's medical record.

Medication and follow-up

• Administer medications as ordered to prevent STIs and pregnancy
• Review instructions with the patient about medications and follow-up and what to expect physically and psychologically

• Encourage the patient to have the support person accompany him/her home or to a safe place and stay with him/her
• Ensure that the patient has a follow-up appointment in 10 to 14 days with her health care practitioner or clinic and has the name and contact number of the rape crisis counsellor.

Quick quiz

1. When checking for costovertebral angle tenderness, where is the ball of nondominant hand placed?
    A. At the symphysis pubis.
    B. On the back at the level of the 12th rib.
    C. On the abdomen just below the rib cage.
    D. Just above the iliac crest.

Answer: B. When checking costovertebral angle tenderness, place the ball of your nondominant hand on the back at the costovertebral angle of the 12th rib.

2. When assessing a patient for PID, which would you **least** expect to find?
    A. Profuse vaginal discharge.
    B. Pain on palpation of the adnexa (fallopian tubes and ovaries).
    C. Fever greater than 40°C.
    D. Lower abdominal pain.

Answer: C. A patient with PID typically has a low-grade fever with malaise, profuse purulent vaginal discharge, pain on palpation of the adnexa and lower abdominal pain.

3. Which condition would you identify as a factor contributing to the development of renal calculi?
    A. Hypocalcaemia.
    B. Heart failure.
    C. Hypothyroidism.
    D. Changes in urine pH.

Answer: D. Urine that's consistently acidic or alkaline provides a favorable medium for calculus formation.

4. Which of the following electrolytes have an inverse relationship?
    A. Chloride and potassium.
    B. Sodium and magnesium.
    C. Calcium and phosphorus.
    D. Chloride and sodium.

Answer: C. Calcium and phosphorus have an inverse relationship – when one increases the other decreases.

Scoring

✰✰✰   If you answered all four questions correctly, get up and cheer! You're a GU and gynaecological genius!

✰✰   If you answered three questions correctly, pat yourself on the back! You're gearing up for GU success.

✰   If you answered fewer than three questions correctly, don't worry. Just review the chapter and give it another go.

11 Maxillofacial and ophthalmic emergencies

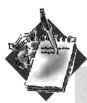

Just the facts

In this chapter, you'll learn:

♦ Emergency assessment of the face and associated structures of the eyes, ears, nose, mouth and throat

♦ Diagnostic tests and procedures for maxillofacial and ophthalmic emergencies

♦ Common maxillofacial and ophthalmic disorders in the emergency department and their treatments.

Understanding maxillofacial and ophthalmic emergencies

The face consists of various structures that are closely related and, as such, an injury in one area can affect surrounding areas as well. Numerous bones and the organs of sight, hearing, taste and smell are located on and in the face. In addition, the facial nerve (cranial nerve VII), its branches and several other cranial nerves provide motor and sensory function for the face.

Maxillofacial and ophthalmic emergencies typically involve some discomfort and pain. In addition, they may affect the patient's functional ability and physical appearance. Moreover, because of the proximity of the patient's airway to the structures of the face, there's always potential for the patient's airway to be compromised in some way, such as from oedema or extension of the injury.

Quickness counts

When faced with a maxillofacial or an ophthalmic emergency, you must assess the patient thoroughly and quickly, always staying alert for subtle changes that might indicate a potential deterioration in the patient's condition. A thorough assessment forms the basis for your interventions, which must be instituted quickly to minimise risks to the patient that can be life threatening. The following assessment of facial injuries should be carried out:

- Airway
- Breathing
- Cervical spine
- Bleeding
- Level of consciousness
- Pain
- Scalp injuries
- Facial structures
- Difficulty in swallowing or talking
- Missing or broken teeth
- Leakage from eyes, ears, mouth and/or nose. For example bleeding or cerebrospinal fluid
- Visual acuity.

As with any emergency, the primary survey is the priority (ABCDE).

Assessment

Assessment of a patient's face and associated structures includes a health history and physical examination. If you can't interview the patient because of his condition, you may gather information from the patient's medical record. In some cases, you may need to ask his family or the paramedic/ambulance crew that transported the patient to the emergency department (ED) for information.

Health history

To obtain a health history, begin by introducing yourself and explaining what happens during the health history and physical examination. Use a systematic approach, focusing on one area of the face and then proceeding to another to gather information on the patient's chief complaint, past health status, family history and cultural factors that may influence your assessment.

Chief complaint

When obtaining the patient's history, adapt the questions to the patient's specific complaints. Focus your questions on the onset, location, duration and characteristics of the symptom as well as what aggravates or relieves it.

Be sure to question the patient about complaints of pain or changes or loss of function in the area as well as the use of medications such as eyedrops.

Physical examination

Maxillofacial and ophthalmic emergencies affect people of all ages and can take many forms. To best identify abnormalities, use a consistent, methodological approach to the physical examination. Because of the emergency nature of the patient's condition, remember that you may need to limit your examination to specific problem areas or stop it entirely to intervene should the patient exhibit signs and symptoms of a deteriorating condition.

Examination of extraophthalmic structures

Start by observing the patient's face. With the scalp line as the starting point, check that his eyes are in a normal position – about one-third of the way down the face and about one eye's width apart from each other.

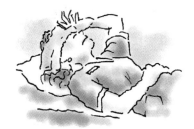

Frequent headaches can be symptoms of larger problems, so be sure to ask about them.

Eye spy

Key questions related to the eye should address:
* Routine problems with the eyes
* Use of glasses or contact lenses and why
* Problems with blurred vision or changes in the visual field
* History of eye surgery or injury, glaucoma or cataracts
* Medications to treat eye problems.

Earmark past problems

Key questions related to the ears, nose and throat should address:
* Changes in hearing, smell or the ability to taste or swallow
* Complaints of frequent headaches, nasal discharge or postnasal drainage
* History of ear infections, sinus infections or nosebleeds.

Personal and family health and lifestyle

Next, question the patient about possible familial disorders related to the eyes, ears, nose and throat. Also explore the patient's daily habits that might affect these structures. Appropriate questions may include:
* Does your occupation require intensive use of your eyes or require you to be exposed to loud noises or chemicals?
* Does the air where you work or live contain anything that causes you problems?
* Do you wear safety equipment, such as goggles and ear protection?

Visual acuity testing

Visual acuity testing is performed on the patient with an ophthalmic emergency or who complains of eye or vision problems. In most cases, it's the first test performed; however, if the patient has experienced chemical exposure to the eyes, it follows eye irrigation.

A very telling Snellen

To test your patient's distant and near vision, use a Snellen chart and a near-vision chart. (See *Visual acuity charts*.) To test his peripheral vision, use confrontation. Before each test, ask the patient to remove corrective lenses if he wears them.

Have the patient sit or stand 6 metres (20 ft) from the chart, and then cover his left eye with an opaque object. Ask him to read the letters on one line of the chart and then to move downward to increasingly smaller lines until he can no longer discern all of the letters. Have him repeat the test covering his right eye. Lastly, ask him to read the smallest line he can read with both eyes uncovered to test his binophthalmic vision.

If the patient wears corrective lenses, have him repeat the test wearing them. Record the vision with and without correction.

With these methods, be sure to document the distance at which the patient identified or perceived it.

E for everyone else

Use the Snellen E chart to test visual acuity in a young child and a patient who can't read. Cover the patient's left eye to check the right eye; point to an E on the chart and ask him to indicate which way the letter faces. Repeat the test on the other side.

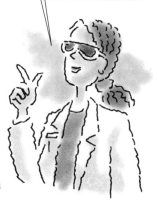

If your patient wears corrective lenses, have him repeat the Snellen test without them and record the difference.

Visual acuity charts

The most commonly used charts for testing vision are the Snellen alphabet chart (left) and the Snellen E chart (right), which is used for young children and adults who can't read. Both charts are used to test distance vision and measure visual acuity. The patient reads each chart at a distance of 6 m (20 ft).

Recording results

Visual acuity is recorded as a fraction. The top number (6) is the distance between the patient and the chart. The bottom number is the distance from which a person with normal vision could read the line. The larger the bottom number, the poorer the patient's vision.

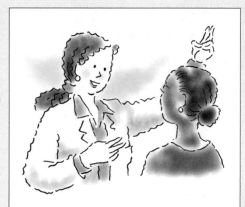

Using confrontation

Follow these steps to assess peripheral vision with confrontation:
- Sit directly across from the patient and ask her to focus her gaze on your eyes
- Place your hands on either side of the patient's head at ear level so that they're about 61 cm (2') apart (as shown)
- Tell the patient to focus her gaze on you as you gradually bring your wiggling fingers into her visual field
- Instruct the patient to tell you as soon as he can see your wiggling fingers; he should see them at the same time you do
- Repeat the procedure while holding your hands at the superior and inferior positions.

If the test values between the two eyes differ by two lines – for example, 6/24 in one eye and 6/12 in the other – suspect an abnormality, such as amblyopia, especially in children.

To test near vision, cover one of the patient's eyes with an opaque object and hold a Rosenbaum near-vision card 14 inches from his eyes. Have him read the line with the smallest letters he can distinguish. Repeat the test with the other eye. If the patient wears corrective lenses, have him repeat the test while wearing them. Record the visual accommodation with and without lenses.

To assess peripheral vision, use a method known as *confrontation*. (See *Using confrontation*.)

Then assess the eyelid, conjunctiva, cornea, anterior chamber, iris and pupil.

Looking at lids

To examine the eyelid, follow these steps:
- Inspect the eyelids; each upper eyelid should cover the top quarter of the iris so the eyes look alike
- Check for an excessive amount of visible sclera above the limbus (corneoscleral junction)
- Ask the patient to open and close his eyes to see if they close completely
- If the downward movement of the upper eyelid in down gaze is delayed, the patient has a condition known as *lid lag*, which is a common sign of hyperthyroidism
- Assess the lids for redness, oedema, inflammation or lesions
- Check for a stye, or hordeolum, a common eyelid lesion. Also check for excessive tearing or dryness
- The eyelid margins should be pink and the eyelashes should turn outward

- Observe whether the lower eyelids turn inward toward the eyeball (called *entropion*) or outward (called *ectropion*)
- Examine the eyelids for lumps
- Put on examination gloves and gently palpate the *nasolacrimal sac*, the area below the inner canthus. Note any tenderness, swelling or discharge through the lacrimal point, which could indicate blockage of the nasolacrimal duct.

Nice to meet ya, conjunctiva

Next, inspect the conjunctiva. To inspect the *bulbar conjunctiva* (the delicate mucous membrane that covers the exposed surface of the sclera), ask the patient to look up and gently pull his lower eyelid down. The bulbar conjunctiva should be clear and shiny; note excessive redness or exudate.

With the lid still secured, inspect the bulbar conjunctiva for colour changes, foreign bodies and oedema. Also observe the sclera's colour, which should be white. In a black patient, you may see flecks of tan. A bluish discolouration may indicate scleral thinning.

To examine the *palpebral conjunctiva* (the membrane that lines the eyelids), ask the patient to look down. Then lift the upper lid, holding the upper lashes against the eyebrow with your finger. The palpebral conjunctiva should be uniformly pink. In the patient with a history of allergies, the palpebral conjunctiva may have a cobblestone appearance.

Corneal matters

Examine the cornea by shining a penlight from both sides and then from straight ahead. The cornea should be clear without lesions. Test corneal sensitivity by lightly touching the cornea with a wisp of cotton. (See *Tips for assessing corneal sensitivity*.)

Tips for assessing corneal sensitivity

To test corneal sensitivity, touch a wisp of cotton from a cotton ball to the cornea, as shown below.

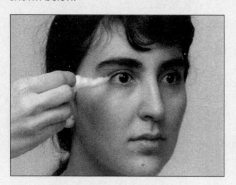

The patient should blink. If she doesn't, she may have suffered damage to the sensory fibres of cranial nerve V or to the motor fibers controlled by cranial nerve VI.

Keep in mind that people who wear contact lenses may have reduced sensitivity because they're accustomed to having foreign objects in their eyes.

Just a wisp

Remember that a wisp of cotton is the only safe object to use for this test. Even though a 4" × 4" gauze pad or tissue is soft, it can cause corneal abrasions and irritation.

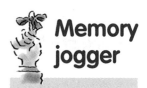

Memory jogger

To make sure that your pupil assessment is complete, think of the acronym PERRLA.
Pupils
Equal
Round
Reactive
Light-reacting
Accommodation.

Observe the iris, which should appear flat, and the cornea, which should appear convex. The irises should be the same size, colour and shape.

Pupil examination

Each pupil should be round, equal in size and about one-fourth the size of the iris in average room lighting. About one person in four has asymmetrical pupils without disease. Unequal pupils generally indicate neurologic damage, iritis, glaucoma or therapy with certain drugs. A fixed pupil that doesn't react to light can be an ominous neurologic sign.

Testing

Test the pupils for direct and consensual response. In a slightly darkened room, hold a penlight about 51 cm (20 in) from the patient's eyes and direct the light at the eye from the side. Note the reaction of the pupil you're testing (direct response) and the opposite pupil (consensual response). They should both react the same way. Also, note sluggishness or inequality in the response. Repeat the test with the other pupil. *Note*: If you shine the light in a blind eye, neither pupil will respond. If you shine the light in a seeing eye, the pupils will respond consensually.

To test the pupils for accommodation, place your finger approximately 10 cm (4 in) from the bridge of the patient's nose. Ask the patient to look at a fixed object in the distance and then at your finger. His pupils should constrict and his eyes converge as he focuses on your finger.

Assessment of ophthalmic muscle function

Evaluation of ophthalmic muscle function involves assessing the corneal light reflex and the cardinal positions of gaze.

To assess the corneal light reflex, ask the patient to look straight ahead; then shine a penlight on the bridge of his nose from about 30.5 cm to 38 cm (12 in to 15 in) away. The light should fall at the same spot on each cornea. If it doesn't, the eyes aren't being held in the same plane by the extraophthalmic muscles. This inequality commonly occurs in a patient who lacks muscle coordination, a condition called *strabismus* (cross-eye).

Cardinal concerns

Cardinal positions of gaze evaluate the oculomotor, trigeminal and abducent nerves as well as the extraophthalmic muscles. To perform this test, ask the patient to remain still while you hold a pencil or other small object directly in front of his nose at a distance of about 46 cm (18 in). Ask him to follow the object with his eyes without moving his head. Then move the object to each of the six cardinal positions, returning to the midpoint after each movement. The patient's eyes should remain parallel as they move. Note abnormal findings, such as nystagmus and amblyopia (the failure of one eye to follow an object; also called *lazy eye*). (See *Cardinal positions of gaze*, page 398.)

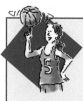

Stay on the ball

Cardinal positions of gaze

This illustration identifies the six cardinal positions of gaze.

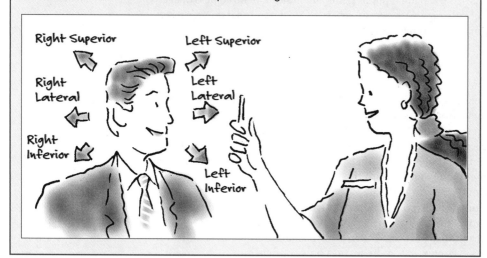

Right Superior

Left Superior

Right Lateral

Left Lateral

Right Inferior

Left Inferior

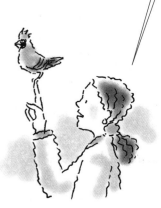

When testing with 'cardinal' positions of gaze, make sure that the patient's head stays still.

Peek-a-boo!

If time and the patient's condition allow, you may perform the cover-uncover test. This test usually isn't done unless you detect an abnormality when assessing the corneal light reflex and cardinal positions of gaze.

Ask the patient to stare at a wall on the other side of the room. Cover one eye and watch for movement in the uncovered eye. Remove the eye cover and watch for movement again. Repeat the test with the other eye.

Eye movement while covering or uncovering the eye is considered abnormal. It may result from weak or paralysed extraophthalmic muscles, which may be caused by cranial nerve impairment.

Diagnostic tests

Fluorescein staining

Fluorescein staining is used to evaluate ophthalmic structures, specifically the cornea. It uses a stain that, when applied to the conjunctival sac, is distributed

Stay on the ball

Technique for fluorescein staining

When performing fluorescein staining, depending on which application you have, be sure to touch the dampened edge of the fluorescein strip to the conjunctiva at the inner canthus of the lower eyelid. Or, other applicators may require you to just drop the fluorescein into the conjunctiva at the inner canthus of the lower eyelid. Ensure you follow individual instructions.

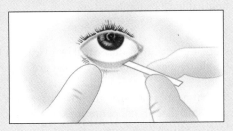

over the cornea. The cornea is then examined using a cobalt blue light; colours denote corneal irregularities. For example, corneal abrasions appear bright yellow like a highlighter and loss of the protective conjunctiva appears as orange-yellow. Foreign bodies can vary in colour depending on their material.

Practice pointers

• Explain the procedure and the reason for its use to the patient; and gain consent
• Make sure that he has removed his contact lenses if he wears them
• Put on gloves and remove the strip from the package, being sure to keep the strip sterile
• Moisten the strip with normal saline solution
• Using your nondominant hand, gently pull down the eye's lower lid
• Touch the tip of the fluorescein strip to the inner canthus of the lower lid. (See *Technique for fluorescein staining*.)
• Have the patient blink several times so that his tears can help transport the stain throughout the eye
• Examine the patient's eye under cobalt blue light, looking for coloured areas or spots
• After completion, flush the patient's eye with normal saline solution to remove the stain
• Instruct the patient to wait at least 1 hour before inserting his contact lenses.

Ultrasonography

Ultrasonography involves the transmission of high-frequency sound waves. For ophthalmic emergencies, the transmission of high-frequency sound waves through the eye are measured based on their reflection from ophthalmic structures.

Illustrating the eyes' structures through ultrasound especially helps to evaluate a fundus clouded by an opaque medium, such as a cataract, or changes in density due to fractures. This test can identify pathologies that are normally undetectable through ophthalmoscopy. Ophthalmic ultrasonography may also be performed before such surgeries as cataract removal or intraophthalmic lens implantation.

Practice pointers

- Tell the patient that a small transducer will be placed on his closed eyelid and will transmit high-frequency sound waves that are reflected by the structures in the eye
- Tell the patient that he may be asked to move his eyes or change his gaze during the procedure and that his cooperation is required to ensure accurate determination of test results
- After the test, remove the water-soluble gel that was placed on the patient's eyelids.

Treatments

Treatments vary depending on the specific ophthalmic emergency. Common treatment measures include drug therapy, ophthalmic agents and surgery.

Drug therapy

Various drugs may be used in ophthalmic emergencies. Topical and systemic medications, including analgesic, antibiotic and anti-inflammatory agents, are commonly employed.

Ophthalmic agents

Ophthalmic agents are usually administered in drop form but may also come in ointment form. Generally, ophthalmic agents fall into one of two groups:

 Miotics

 Mydriatics.

Miotics constrict the pupil; mydriatics dilate the pupil. In most cases, mydriatics are anticholinergic agents that also paralyse the muscle of accommodation (termed *cycloplegics*). (See *Examples of miotics and mydriatics*.)

Nursing considerations

- Administer the agent as ordered; making sure that the proper form is used
- Instill topical agents appropriately, making sure you keep the tip of the applicator (eyedrop bottle or ointment tip) sterile

Examples of miotics and mydriatics

Commonly used miotics include:
- Carbachol
- Pilocarpine
- Betaxolol
- Levobunolol
- Timolol.

Commonly used mydriatics include:
- Atropine
- Cyclopentolate
- Homatropine
- Tropicamide.

- Provide patient teaching about the proper method for instilling eye ointment and eyedrops, especially if the patient is to continue the medication at home. (See *Instilling eye ointment and eyedrops*.)

Common ophthalmic disorders

Common ophthalmic emergencies you're likely to 'face' include:
- Chemical burns to the eye
- Corneal abrasion
- Retinal detachment.

Regardless of the disorder, the priorities are always to ensure vital functioning (the ABCDEs).

Chemical burns to the eye

Chemical burns to the eye can cause serious eye injury. These injuries may be work-related or may occur while using common household products.

Education edge
Instilling eye ointment and eyedrops

To teach about instilling eye ointment, instruct the patient to:
- Hold the tube for several minutes to warm the ointment
- Squeeze a small amount of ointment – 0.5 to 1.5 cm – (¼" to ½") inside the lower lid
- Gently close the eye and roll the eyeball in all directions with the eye closed
- Wait 10 minutes before instilling other ointments.

To teach about instilling eyedrops, instruct the patient to:
- Tilt his head back and pull down on his lower lid
- Drop the medication into the conjunctival sac
- Apply pressure to the inner canthus for 1 minute after administration
- Wait 5 minutes before instilling a second drop or other eye solutions.

What causes it

Chemical injury to the eye involves splashing or spraying hazardous materials into the eyes. It may also result from exposure to fumes or aerosols. Chemical burns may be caused by an acidic or alkaline substance or an irritant:

• Alkaline substances have a high pH and tend to cause the most severe ophthalmic damage. Examples include lye, cement, lime and ammonia

• Acidic substances have a low pH and tend to cause less severe damage. (Even so, hydrofluoric acid, found in rust removers, aluminum brighteners and heavy-duty cleaners, is an exception and causes severe burns.) An automobile battery explosion, causing a sulphuric acid burn, is the most common injury to the eye involving an acidic substance. Other common acids that can cause chemical burns include sulphurous acid, hydrochloric acid, nitric acid, acetic acid and chromic acid

• Irritant substances have a neutral pH and tend to cause discomfort, rather than ophthalmic damage. Examples of irritants include pepper spray and many household detergents.

How it happens

The severity of chemical injury to the eye depends on the chemical's pH, the duration of contact with the chemical, the amount of chemical and the chemical's ability to penetrate the eye.

Alkaline substances can penetrate the surface of the eye into the anterior chamber within 5 to 15 minutes, causing damage to such internal structures as the iris, ciliary body, lens and trabecular network.

Acidic substances can't penetrate the corneal epithelial layer of the eye, which limits injury to superficial, nonprogressive damage. However, because hydrofluoric acid has properties similar to alkaline substances, it can cause more progressive and severe damage.

What to look for

• Obtain the patient's history; ask about a chemical spraying or splashing in the face or exposure to fumes or aerosols. Also ask about the use of cleaning solutions, solvents or lawn and garden chemicals

• Ask the patient about pain, irritation, inability to keep his eyes open, blurred vision and a sensation of having something in the eye

• Note patient complaints of severe pain and burning; observe for extreme redness, irritation and excessive tearing.

What tests tell you

Chemical burns to the eye are an immediate threat to the patient's vision and are considered the most urgent of all ophthalmic emergencies. Typically, no diagnostic tests are initially performed because eye irrigation takes priority.

Household cleaning solutions carry with them a risk of eye irritation. As if you needed another excuse not to clean!

How it's treated

The patient's eye is irrigated continuously with copious amounts of normal saline solution. Irrigation continues for at least 30 minutes and until the ophthalmic pH reaches the desired level. Topical antibiotics, cycloplegic agents and corticosteroids are ordered; opioid analgesia may also be ordered. Referral or follow-up care with an ophthalmologist is essential.

What to do

• If the patient has face burns from an alkaline substance, assess him for tracheal or oesophageal burns; these burns can be life-threatening injuries
• Assess the patient's eye pH before irrigating the eye with sterile normal saline solution. Assessing the patient's visual acuity can be delayed until after irrigation
• Flush the patient's eyes with large amounts of sterile isotonic saline solution for at least 30 minutes. Intermittently check the pH of the eye (because ophthalmic pH may be increased if the offending chemical is alkaline, decreased if it's acidic or neutral if it's an irritant). Continue to irrigate until the pH returns to a normal level (6.5 to 7.6). (See *Eye irrigation for chemical burns*.)

Eye irrigation for chemical burns

The patient's eye may be irrigated using a Morgan lens or an intravenous (I.V.) tube.

Morgan lens

Connected to irrigation tubing, a Morgan lens permits continuous lavage and also delivers medication to the eye. Use an adapter to connect the lens to the I.V. tubing and the solution container. Begin the irrigation at the prescribed flow rate. To insert the device, ask the patient to look down as you insert the lens under the upper eyelid (as shown). Then have him look up as you retract and release the lower eyelid over the lens.

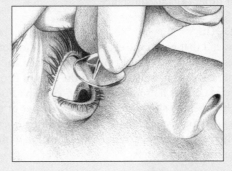

I.V. tube

If a Morgan lens isn't available, set up an I.V. bag and tubing without a needle. Direct a constant, gentle stream at the inner canthus so that the solution flows across the cornea to the outer canthus (as shown). Flush the eye for at least 15 minutes.

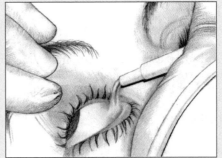

- After irrigation, inspect for conjunctival and scleral redness and tearing and corneal opacification
- Prepare the patient for an ophthalmic examination
- Provide analgesics as needed for pain
- Administer other medications – topical or oral antibiotics, cycloplegics to prevent ciliary spasms and reduce inflammation and topical lubricants – as ordered
- Because burns resulting from hydrofluoric acid may cause severe hypocalcaemia, monitor serum calcium levels as ordered
- Apply eye dressings or patches as needed to reduce eye movement
- Teach the patient how to apply ophthalmic medications as necessary
- Strongly advise patients to wear protective goggles or eyewear when working with toxic substances and to keep all toxic home products out of children's reach.

Corneal abrasion

A corneal abrasion is a scratch on the surface epithelium of the cornea. With treatment, prognosis is usually good.

What causes it

A corneal abrasion usually results from a foreign body – such as a cinder or a piece of dust, dirt or grit – becoming embedded under the eyelid. Additional causes include small pieces of metal, improperly fitted contact lenses or falling asleep wearing hard contact lenses or other items, such as a fingernail, piece of paper or other organic substance.

How it happens

Small pieces of metal that get in the eyes of workers who don't wear protective glasses quickly form a rust ring on the cornea and cause corneal abrasion. Such abrasions are also common in the eyes of people who fall asleep wearing hard contact lenses or whose lenses aren't fitted properly. A corneal scratch caused by a fingernail, a piece of paper or other organic substance may cause a persistent lesion. The epithelium doesn't always heal properly, possibly resulting in recurrent corneal erosion with delayed effects more severe than the original injury.

What to look for

- Reports of eye trauma or wearing contact lenses for a prolonged period
- Complaints of a sensation of something in the eye, sensitivity to light, decreased visual acuity (if the abrasion occurs in the pupillary region) and pain
- Redness, increased tearing
- Evidence of a foreign body on the cornea or eyelid.

What tests tell you

Fluorescein staining confirms the diagnosis. The practitioner uses a cobalt-blue light and slit-lamp examination. The injured area appears yellow like a highlighter when examined.

How it's treated

If a foreign body is identified, the eye is irrigated and a topical anaesthetic eyedrop is used. A foreign body spud is used to remove a superficial foreign body. If the foreign body is a rust ring, it must be removed by the physician using an ophthalmic burr. When only partial removal is possible, a referral to an ophthalmologist maybe required, for re-epithelialisation lifts what remains of the ring to the surface so that removal can be completed the next day.

What to do

• Assist with the eye examination. Check visual acuity before beginning treatment
• If a foreign body is visible, carefully irrigate the eye with normal saline solution
• Instill topical anaesthetic eyedrops in the affected eye before assisting the practitioner with removal
• Instill broad-spectrum antibiotic eyedrops in the affected eye every 3 to 4 hours
• Reassure the patient that the corneal epithelium usually heals in 24 to 48 hours
• Provide tetanus prophylaxis. Many places will refer patients back to their GP for tetanus prophylaxis to ensure continuity of immunisation records.

Practice pointers

• Check the patient's name
• Check doctor's instructions
• Wash hands prior to instilling medication
• Cleanse the eyelids and lashes with cotton buds moistened with normal saline
• Use each cotton bud for only one stroke, moving from the inner to the outer aspect of the eye
• Tilt the patient's head back slightly if he is sitting or place the head over a pillow if he is lying down
• Hold the applicator in one hand, then:
  • Using the forefinger of your other hand, pull the lower lid down gently to expose inner the surface of eye-lid
  • Instruct patient to look upward
  • Hold the applicator close to the eye but avoid touching the eyelids and eyeball
  • Allow the prescribed number of drops to fall in the lower conjunctival sac but do not allow to fall onto the cornea
  • Release the lower lid after the drops are instilled. Instruct the patient to close eyes slowly, move the eye and not to squeeze or rub
  • Wipe off excess solution with gauze or cotton balls.

To patch or not to patch

• If a patch is ordered, tell the patient to leave it in place for 6 to 12 hours. Warn him that a patch alters depth perception and advise caution in performing

Corneal ulceration

A major cause of blindness worldwide, corneal ulcers result in corneal scarring or perforation. They occur in the central or marginal areas of the cornea, vary in shape and size and may be singular or multiple. Prompt treatment (within hours of onset) can prevent vision impairment.

Corneal ulcers generally result from bacterial, protozoan, viral or fungal infections, but other causes may include ophthalmic trauma, exposure, toxins and allergens.

Signs and symptoms

Typically, corneal ulceration begins with pain (aggravated by blinking) and photophobia, followed by increased tearing. Eventually, central corneal ulceration produces pronounced visual blurring. The eye may appear red. Purulent discharge is possible if a bacterial ulcer is present.

Treatment

Prompt treatment is essential for all forms of corneal ulcer to prevent complications and permanent vision impairment. Treatment aims to eliminate the underlying cause of the ulcer and relieve pain.

A corneal ulcer should never be patched because patching creates the dark, warm, moist environment ideal for bacterial growth. However, it should be protected with a perforated shield. Antibiotics, antivirals or antifungals are prescribed based on culture and sensitivity findings. Artificial tears and lubricating ointments may be prescribed as needed.

Nursing considerations

- Because corneal ulcers are quite painful, give analgesics as needed
- Watch for signs of secondary glaucoma (transient vision loss and halos around lights)
- The patient may be more comfortable in a darkened room or when wearing dark glasses.

daily activities, such as climbing stairs or stepping off a curb. (Patching is no longer routinely recommended in the treatment of corneal abrasions)
- Stress the importance of instilling antibiotic eyedrops as ordered because an untreated corneal abrasion, if infected, can lead to a corneal ulcer and permanent vision loss. Teach the patient the proper way to instill eye medications. (See *Corneal ulceration*.)
- Advise the patient who wears contact lenses to abstain from wearing them until the corneal abrasion heals
- Urge the patient to wear safety glasses to protect his eyes from flying fragments
- Review instructions for wearing and caring for contact lenses to prevent further trauma.

Retinal detachment

Retinal detachment occurs when the outer retinal pigment epithelium splits from the neural retina, creating a subretinal space. This space then fills with fluid, called *subretinal fluid*.

Retinal detachment usually involves only one eye, but may later involve the other eye. Surgical reattachment is typically successful. However, the prognosis for good vision depends on which area of the retina has been affected.

What causes it

Predisposing factors include high myopia and cataract surgery. The most common causes are degenerative changes in the retina or vitreous humour. Other causes include:
- Trauma or inflammation
- Systemic diseases such as diabetes mellitus.

Retinal detachment is rare in children. However, it occasionally develops as a result of retinopathy of prematurity, tumours (retinoblastomas), trauma or myopia, which tends to run in families.

How it happens

A retinal tear or hole allows the vitreous humour to seep between the retinal layers, separating the retina from its choroidal blood supply. Retinal detachment may also result from seepage of fluid into the subretinal space or from traction placed on the retina by vitreous bands or membranes. (See *Understanding retinal detachment*.)

Understanding retinal detachment

Traumatic injury or degenerative changes cause retinal detachment by allowing the retina's sensory tissue layers to separate from the retinal pigment epithelium. This permits fluid – for example, from the vitreous humour – to seep into the space between the retinal pigment epithelium and the rods and cones of the tissue layers.

The pressure that results from the fluid entering the space balloons the retina into the vitreous cavity away from choroidal circulation. Separated from its blood supply, the retina can't function. Without prompt repair, the detached retina can cause permanent vision loss.

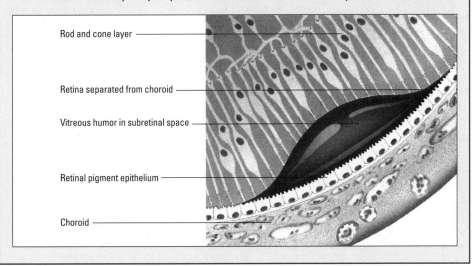

Rod and cone layer

Retina separated from choroid

Vitreous humor in subretinal space

Retinal pigment epithelium

Choroid

What to look for

Signs and symptoms of retinal detachment include:
- Floaters
- Light flashes
- Sudden, painless vision loss that may be described as a curtain that eliminates a portion of the visual field
- Wavy or watery vision.

What tests tell you

Ophthalmoscopic examination through a well-dilated pupil confirms the diagnosis. It shows the usually transparent retina as gray and opaque; in severe detachment, it reveals folds in the retina and ballooning out of the area. Indirect ophthalmoscopy is also used to search the retina for tears and holes. Ophthalmic ultrasonography may be necessary if the lens is opaque or if the vitreous humour is cloudy.

How it's treated

Treatment depends on the location and severity of the detachment:
- Admission to an ophthalmic ward is necessary
- Eye movements are restricted through bed rest and sedation. If the patient's macula is threatened, his head may be positioned so the tear or hole is below the rest of the eye before surgical intervention
- Bed rest is typically ordered with bilateral eye patching
- A hole in the peripheral retina can be treated with cryotherapy; a hole in the posterior portion, with laser therapy
- Retinal detachment rarely heals spontaneously. Surgery – including scleral buckling, pneumatic retinopexy or vitrectomy (or a combination of these procedures) – can reattach the retina.

What to do

- Provide emotional support because the patient may be distraught about his vision loss
- Maintain complete bed rest and instruct the patient to restrict eye movements until surgical reattachment is performed
- To avoid pressure to the globe of the eye, which could cause further extrusion of intraophthalmic contents into the subretinal space, apply goggles or a metallic eye shield
- Urge the patient to avoid activities in bed that could increase intraophthalmic pressure (IOP), such as straining at stool, bending down, forceful coughing, sneezing or vomiting
- Prepare the patient for surgery; if indicated, wash the patient's face with no-tears shampoo. Give antibiotics and cycloplegic-mydriatic eyedrops
- Provide preoperative and postoperative teaching, including care measures to avoid increased IOP. (See *Teaching tips for the patient with retinal detachment*.)

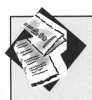

Teaching tips for the patient with retinal detachment

- Explain to the patient undergoing laser surgery that he may have blurred vision for several days afterward
- Show the patient having scleral buckling how to instill eyedrops properly. Remind him to lie in the position recommended by the practitioner after surgery
- Reinforce the need to rest and avoid driving, bending, heavy lifting and other activities that affect intraophthalmic pressure (IOP) for several days after eye surgery. Discourage activities that could cause the patient to bump the eye
- Review early symptoms of retinal detachment and emphasise the need for immediate treatment.

Maxillofacial emergencies

Examination of the nose and sinuses

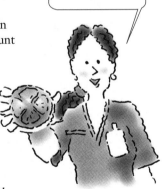

When life gives you lemons, use them to test cranial nerve I!

Begin by observing the patient's nose for position, symmetry and colour. Note such variations as discolouration, swelling and deformity. Variations in size and shape are largely caused by differences in cartilage and in the amount of fibroadipose tissue.

Observe for nasal discharge or flaring. If discharge is present, note the colour, quantity and consistency; if you notice flaring, observe for other signs of respiratory distress.

Test nasal patency and olfactory nerve (cranial nerve I) function. Ask the patient to block one nostril and inhale a familiar aromatic substance through the other nostril. Possible substances include soap, coffee, citrus, tobacco or nutmeg. Ask him to identify the aroma and then repeat the process with the other nostril using a different aroma.

Now, inspect the nasal cavity. Ask the patient to tilt his head back slightly and then push the tip of his nose up. Use the light from the otoscope to illuminate his nasal cavities. Check for severe deviation or perforation of the nasal septum. Examine the vestibule and turbinates for redness, softness, swelling and discharge.

Upon closer inspection

Examine the nostrils by direct inspection, using a nasal speculum, a penlight or small flashlight or an otoscope with a short, wide-tip attachment. Have the patient sit in front of you with his head tilted back. Put on gloves and insert

Inspecting the nostrils

This illustration shows the proper placement of the nasal speculum during direct inspection and the structures you should be able to see during this examination.

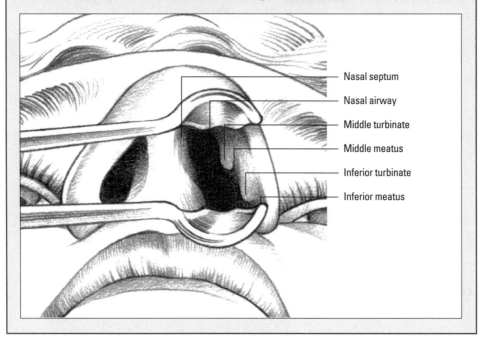

- Nasal septum
- Nasal airway
- Middle turbinate
- Middle meatus
- Inferior turbinate
- Inferior meatus

the tip of the closed nasal speculum into one nostril to the point where the blade widens. Slowly open the speculum as wide as possible without causing discomfort. Shine the flashlight in the nostril to illuminate the area.

Observe the colour and patency of the nostril and check for exudate. The mucosa should be moist, pink to light red and free from lesions and polyps. After inspecting one nostril, close the speculum, remove it and inspect the other nostril. (See *Inspecting the nostrils*.)

Lastly, palpate the patient's nose and surrounding soft tissue with your thumb and forefinger, assessing for pain, tenderness, swelling and deformity.

Face and sinuses

Next, examine the facial structures, using both hands and simultaneously palpating for irregularities and crepitus. Palpate in an upward fashion and then laterally. Observe the patient's face using a downward approach from the eyebrows to the chin. Then observe in the opposite manner to identify deformities.

Examine the sinuses. Remember, only the frontal and maxillary sinuses are accessible; you won't be able to palpate the ethmoidal and sphenoidal sinuses. Begin by checking for swelling around the eyes, especially over the sinus area. Then palpate the sinuses, checking for tenderness. To palpate

Stay on the ball

Transilluminating the sinuses

Transillumination of the sinuses helps detect sinus tumours and obstruction and requires only a penlight. However, only an appropriately qualified and experienced nurse should attempt this procedure, especially in patients who may also have a nasal (cribriform)/facial fracture.

Before you start, darken the room and have the patient close her eyes.

Frontal sinuses

Place the penlight on the supraorbital ring and direct the light upward to illuminate the frontal sinuses just above the eyebrow, as shown here.

Maxillary sinuses

Place the penlight on the patient's cheekbone just below her eye and ask her to open her mouth, as shown here. The light should transilluminate easily and equally.

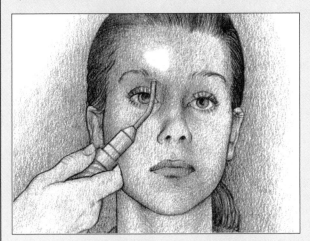

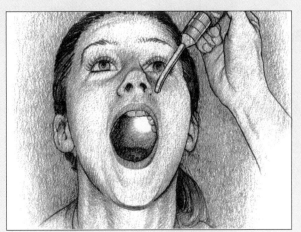

the frontal sinuses, place your thumbs above the patient's eyes just under the bony ridges of the upper orbits and place your fingertips on his forehead. Apply gentle pressure. Next, palpate the maxillary sinuses.

If the patient complains of tenderness during palpation, use transillumination to see if the sinuses are filled with fluid or pus. Transillumination can also help reveal tumours and obstructions. (See *Transilluminating the sinuses*.)

Examination of the mouth and throat

First, inspect the patient's lips. They should be pink, moist, symmetrical and without lesions. A bluish hue or flecked pigmentation is common in dark-skinned patients.

Use a tongue blade and a bright light to inspect the oral mucosa. Have the patient open his mouth and then place the tongue blade on top of his tongue. The oral mucosa should be pink, smooth, moist and free from lesions and unusual odours. Increased pigmentation is seen in dark-skinned patients.

Gag order

Inspect the patient's oropharynx by asking him to open his mouth while you shine the penlight on the uvula and palate. You may need to insert a tongue blade into the mouth and depress the tongue. Place the tongue blade slightly off centre to avoid eliciting the gag reflex. The uvula and oropharynx should be pink and moist, without inflammation or exudate. The tonsils should be pink and shouldn't be hypertrophied. Ask the patient to say 'Ahhh' Observe for movement of the soft palate and uvula.

Lastly, palpate the lips, tongue and oropharynx. Note lumps, lesions, ulcers or oedema of the lips or tongue. Assess the patient's gag reflex by gently touching the back of the pharynx with a cotton-tipped applicator or the tongue blade. This should produce a bilateral response.

Gums...

Next, observe the gingivae or gums; they should be pink, moist and have clearly defined margins at each tooth. They shouldn't be retracted. Inspect the teeth, noting their number, condition and whether any are missing or crowded. If the patient is wearing dentures, ask him to remove them so that you can inspect the gums underneath. Ask the patient to open his jaw and palpate the interior of the mouth while wearing gloves.

...and tongues

Lastly, inspect the tongue. It should be midline, moist, pink and free from lesions. The posterior surface should be smooth and the anterior surface should be slightly rough with small fissures. The tongue should move easily in all directions and it should lie straight to the front at rest.

Ask the patient to raise the tip of his tongue and touch his palate directly behind his front teeth. Inspect the ventral surface of the tongue and the floor of the mouth. Next, wrap a piece of gauze around the tip of the tongue and move the tongue first to one side then the other to inspect the lateral borders. They should be smooth and even textured.

Diagnostic tests

Diagnostic tests include computed tomography (CT) scan and facial X-rays.

CT scan

A CT scan aids in diagnosing complex facial fractures. It's considered the standard for assessing soft tissue and bony injury and provides useful information in identifying soft tissue injury involving the optic nerve. It also confirms the diagnosis of cervical spine injury, which may be present in a maxillofacial or ophthalmic emergency patient.

It's orbital

Performed specifically for an ophthalmic emergency, an orbital CT scan allows visualisation of abnormalities not readily seen on standard X-rays, such as size and position delineation and relationship to adjoining structures. Contrast media may be used in orbital CT scanning to define ophthalmic tissues and help confirm a suspected circulatory disorder or haemangioma.

The application of CT scanning to ophthalmology extends beyond the evaluation of the orbital and adjoining structures; it also permits precise diagnosis of many intracranial lesions that affect vision.

Practice pointers

• Check the patient's history for hypersensitivity reactions to iodine, shellfish or radiographic contrast agents
• Tell the patient that he'll be positioned on a CT scan table and that the table's head will be moved into the scanner, which will rotate around his head
• If a contrast medium will be used, tell the patient that he may feel that he has 'wet' himself, nausea or vomiting, flushed and warm and may experience a metallic taste in his mouth. Reassure him that these reactions are typical.

Facial X-rays

Various types of X-rays may be used to determine maxillofacial injury. These include:
• *Posteroanterior*, considered the most useful X-ray in helping to identify problems in the orbital rim and floor
• *Anterior, posterior and lateral views*, which provide information about the skull, sinuses and roof of the orbit
• *Occipito mental views* 15 and 30 degrees, which detect facial fractures
• *Submental vertex*, which provides information about the zygomatic arch and base of the skull
• *Anteroposterior and lateral oblique views* to detect injuries to the condylar and coronoid processes and the symphysis (of the mandible)
• *Orthopantomogram (OPT)*, which detects problems in the mandible and teeth.

Practice pointers

• Prepare the patient for the X-ray to be performed; inform him of the reason for the X-ray and gain consent
• Verify that the X-ray order includes a pertinent history, such as trauma, and identifies the site of tenderness or pain
• Make sure that the patient removes all jewellery from the head and neck area.

Common disorders

Common emergencies you're likely to 'face' include:
* Soft tissue facial injuries
* Epistaxis
* Facial fractures
* Foreign body in the ear
* Foreign body in the nose
* Nasal fracture
* Orbital fracture
* Tonsillitis
* Quinsy (Peritonsillar abcess)
* Dental abscess.

Regardless of the disorder, the priorities are always to ensure vital functioning (the ABCDEs).

Soft tissue facial injuries

Soft tissue facial injuries include contusions, lacerations, abrasions and friction injuries. These injuries are problematic because they can cause considerable upset or changes in physical appearance. Therefore, facial lacerations are typically repaired as soon as possible.

What causes it

Soft tissue facial injuries can be the result of numerous causes; playing sport and road traffic collisions are a common one. Air bag deployment commonly causes minor abrasions of the face, neck and upper chest.

Lacerations and contusions may result from blunt or penetrating trauma. Friction injuries and animal or human bites are a common cause of lacerations.

How it happens

During the trauma, the skin of the face comes in contact with the offending cause. For example, in the case of a bite, the animal's teeth penetrate the outer layer of the skin, causing damage to the underlying tissue. Contact of skin leads to shearing of the outer surface and abrasion.

What to look for

Signs and symptoms associated with soft tissue facial injuries may include:
* Superficial to deep lacerations on any area of the face, including the ears
* Evidence of skin opening or revealing teeth marks
* Epidermal staining (friction injuries)
* Intraoral deformities, including lacerations and bleeding.

If the patient sustains deep lacerations of the cheek, you may note:
* Forehead asymmetry due to damage of the temporal branch of the facial nerve

- Inability to close the eye on the affected side due to damage of the temporal or zygomatic branch of the facial nerve
- Inability to purse lips due to damage to the buccal branch of the facial nerve
- Elevation of the lower lip at rest with an inability to lower the lower lip from damage to the mandibular branch.

What tests tell you
Facial X-rays, CT scan and magnetic resonance imaging (MRI) aid in diagnosing the extent of injury and ruling out fractures.

How it's treated
Treatment of soft tissue facial injuries varies, depending on the type of injury and its severity. Regardless, bleeding is controlled and the wound area is cleaned and irrigated if necessary. In addition:
- Superficial lacerations are sutured as soon as possible to minimise cosmetic disfigurement
- Lacerations due to bites are thoroughly cleaned and irrigated; consultation with a plastic surgeon or a maxillofacial surgeon is recommended for the decision to close the wounds to minimise possible disfigurement. Animal bites require rabies evaluation and tetanus prophylaxis
- Friction injuries are vigorously scrubbed with mild soap; dermabrasion may be needed
- Ear cartilage lacerations should be sutured by the skin alone – not the cartilage
- Perichondrial haematomas (cauliflower ears) should be aspirated
- Surgical exploration and repair is conducted for large or deep lacerations
- Debridement is conducted for wounds that are extensively contaminated
- Antibiotic therapy is instituted to prevent and treat infection.

What to do
- Assess the patient's ABCDEs and intervene as necessary to stabilise him
- Apply direct pressure to any openly bleeding wounds. Pressure bandages made need to be used, e.g. bleeding perichondrial haematoma
- Clean all wounds and irrigate as ordered; apply sterile dressings as appropriate.

Epistaxis

Epistaxis refers to a nosebleed. Such bleeding in children generally originates in the anterior nasal septum and tends to be mild. In adults, such bleeding most likely originates in the posterior septum and can be severe.

What causes it
Epistaxis may be a primary disorder or may occur secondary to another condition. It usually follows trauma from external or internal causes, such as a blow to the nose, nose picking or insertion of a foreign body. Less commonly,

it results from polyps, inhalation of chemicals that irritate the nasal mucosa, vascular abnormalities or acute or chronic infections, such as sinusitis or rhinitis, that cause congestion and eventual bleeding from capillary blood vessels. Epistaxis may also follow sudden mechanical decompression and strenuous exercise.

How it happens
A rich supply of fragile blood vessels makes the nose particularly vulnerable to bleeding. Air moving through the nose can dry and irritate the mucous membranes, forming crusts that bleed when they're removed. Dry mucous membranes are also more susceptible to infections, which can lead to epistaxis as well. In addition, trauma to the mucous membranes leads to bleeding.

What to look for
The patient with epistaxis commonly comes to the ED holding bloody tissues, towels or cloths. Bleeding from one or both nostrils is visible and may range from a slow trickle to a profuse continuous flow. Unilateral bleeding is typical; bilateral bleeding suggests a blood dyscrasia or severe trauma.

Bright red blood oozing from the nostrils suggests anterior bleeding. Blood visible in the back of the throat originates in the posterior area and may be dark or bright red. It's commonly mistaken for haemoptysis because of expectoration.

The patient's history may reveal trauma to the nose or evidence of a predisposing factor, such as anticoagulant therapy, hypertension, chronic aspirin use, high altitudes and dry climate, sclerotic vessel disease, Hodgkin's disease, vitamin K deficiency or blood dyscrasias.

Life at a high altitude can predispose you to two things. One is yodeling. The other is epistaxis.

What tests tell you
Diagnosis is determined by assessment findings. Facial X-rays may be done to determine if a fracture is present. If the patient's bleeding is severe, full blood count and coagulation studies may be done to evaluate the patient's status. In addition, blood typing and crossmatching is done if the patient requires a transfusion because of blood loss.

How it's treated
Ensure protective equipment is worn, including, gown, gloves and eye protection. The nose is cleared of blood clots by having the patient blow his nose or with suctioning. If the bleeding is anterior, treatment typically includes stopping the bleeding with topical vasoconstrictors, direct pressure for 5 to 10 minutes, cautery (chemical or electrical) and packing (tampons) if needed. Nasal packing (tampons), which is coated with an antibiotic ointment before insertion, can be in the form of petroleum iodoform gauze, which requires removal in 24 to 72 hours, or commercial packing (tampons) products that dissolve and don't require removal.

Posterior bleeding is treated with nasal packing (tampons) in the form of nasal sponges, special epistaxis balloon devices or a urinary catheter (with the distal tip removed). This type of packing (tampons) is usually removed in 2 to 3 days. Drug therapy to treat an underlying condition, such as hypertension, is ordered. If bleeding doesn't respond to treatment, surgery involving ligation or embolisation may be necessary.

What to do
• Assess the patient's ABCDEs including signs of hypovolaemic shock. If bleeding is severe or if there's associated trauma, institute emergency interventions as necessary, such as suctioning, oxygen saturation monitoring and oxygen therapy, insertion of large bore cannula, obtain blood samples, I.V. therapy and cardiac monitoring
• Determine the location of the bleeding (anterior or posterior) and whether epistaxis is unilateral or bilateral. Inspect for blood seeping behind the nasal septum, in the middle ear and in the corners of the eyes
• Apply direct pressure to the soft portion of the nostrils against the septum continuously for 5 to 10 minutes. Maintain the patient in an upright position with his head tilted slightly downward as you compress the nostrils
• Apply an ice collar or cold compresses to the nose. Bleeding should stop after 10 minutes
• Assist with treatment for anterior bleeding, including the application of external pressure and a topical vasoconstrictor (such as a cotton ball saturated with topical cocaine solution or a solution of lignocaine and topical adrenaline) to the bleeding site, followed by cauterisation with electrocautery or a silver nitrate stick. If these measures don't control bleeding, petroleum gauze nasal packing (tampons) may be needed. (See *Types of nasal packing (tampons)*, page 418.)

Pack it up

• Assist with treatment for posterior bleeding, including the use of a nasal balloon catheter to control bleeding effectively, gauze packing (tampons) inserted through the nose or postnasal packing (tampons) inserted through the mouth, depending on the bleeding site
• If local measures fail to control bleeding, assist with additional treatment, which may include supplemental vitamin K and, for severe bleeding, blood transfusions and surgical ligation or embolisation of a bleeding artery
• Monitor the patient's vital signs and skin colour; record blood loss
• Assess oxygen saturation levels via pulse oximetry and administer oxygen as needed
• Tell the patient to breathe through his mouth and not to swallow blood, talk or blow his nose
• Keep vasoconstrictors, such as phenylephrine (Neo-Synephrine) nasal spray, on hand
• Reassure the patient and his family that epistaxis usually looks worse than it is
• Administer antibiotics as ordered if packing (tampons) must remain in place for longer than 24 hours

Types of nasal packing (tampons)

Nosebleeds may be controlled with anterior or posterior nasal packing (tampons).

Anterior nasal packing (tampons)

The practitioner may treat an anterior nosebleed by packing the anterior nasal cavity with an antibiotic-impregnated petroleum gauze strip (shown at right) or with a nasal tampon.

A nasal tampon is made of tightly compressed absorbent material with or without a central breathing tube. The practitioner inserts a lubricated tampon along the floor of the nose and, with the patient's head tilted backward, instills 5 to 10 ml of antibiotic or normal saline solution. This solution causes the tampon to expand, stopping the bleeding. The tampon should be moistened periodically and the central breathing tube should be suctioned regularly.

In a patient with blood dyscrasias, the practitioner may fashion an absorbable pack by moistening a gauzelike, regenerated cellulose material with a vasoconstrictor. Applied to a visible bleeding point, this substance will swell to form a clot. The packing (tampons) is absorbable and doesn't need removal.

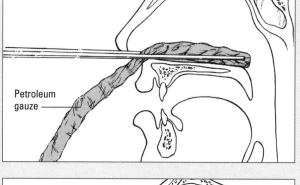

Petroleum gauze

Posterior nasal packing (tampons)

Posterior packing consists of a gauze roll shaped and secured by three sutures (one suture at each end and one in the middle) or a balloon-type catheter. To insert the packing, the practitioner advances one or two soft catheters into the patient's nostrils (shown at right). When the catheter tips appear in the nasopharynx, the practitioner grasps them with a clamp or forceps and pulls them forward through the mouth. He secures the two end sutures to the catheter tip and draws the catheter back through the nostrils.

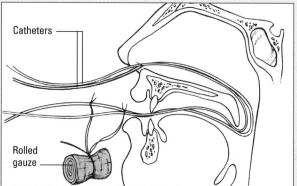

Catheters

Rolled gauze

This step brings the packing (tampons) into place with the end sutures hanging from the patient's nostril. (The middle suture emerges from the patient's mouth to free the packing, when needed.)

The practitioner may weight the nose sutures with a clamp. Then he'll pull the packing (tampons) securely into place behind the soft palate and against the posterior end of the septum (nasal choana).

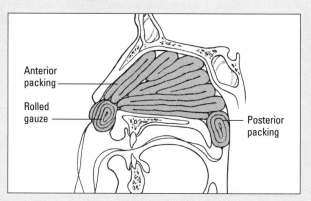

Anterior packing

Rolled gauze

Posterior packing

After the practitioner examines the patient's throat (to ensure that the uvula hasn't been forced under the packing, he inserts anterior packing (tampons) and secures the whole apparatus by tying the posterior pack strings around rolled gauze or a dental roll at the nostrils (shown at right).

Education edge

Teaching tips to prevent epistaxis

Epistaxis can be a frightening experience for a patient, especially if he requires interventions other than just applying pressure to the nostril area. Therefore, educating the patient in measures to prevent epistaxis can help to alleviate his anxiety and decrease the risk of a recurrent episode. Be sure to include the following information in your discharge teaching:

• If the patient required anterior packing, instruct him to return to the emergency department (ED) or make an appointment with the practitioner for packing removal
• Tell the patient to return to the ED if bleeding recurs or if packing (tampons) becomes dislodged
• Instruct the patient not to insert foreign objects into his nose and to avoid bending and lifting
• Instruct the patient to sneeze with his mouth open
• Emphasise the need for follow-up examinations and periodic blood studies after an episode of epistaxis. Advise the patient to seek prompt treatment for nasal infection or irritation
• Suggest a humidifier if the patient lives in a dry climate or at a high elevation or if his home is heated with circulating hot air
• Caution the patient against inserting cotton or tissues into his nose because these objects are difficult to remove and may further irritate nasal mucosa.

• If the bleeding is controlled effectively, prepare the patient for discharge; if the patient required posterior nasal packing (tampons), prepare him for admission. (See *Teaching tips to prevent epistaxis*.)

Facial fractures

A facial fracture refers to an injury that results in a broken bone or bones of the face. Facial fractures may involve damage to almost any of the bone structures of the face, including the nose, zygoma (cheekbone), mandible, frontal region, maxilla and supraorbital rim. Nasal bone fractures are the most common type of facial fracture.

What causes it
Many facial fractures result from sports-related injuries. Other mechanisms of injury may include road traffic accidents, manual blows to the face and falls.

How it happens
The amount of force necessary to fracture bones of the face varies depending on the bone. Nasal fractures require the least amount of force, whereas fractures of the supraorbital rim require the greatest amount of force.

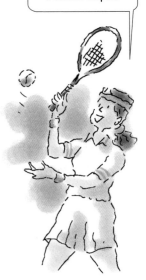

Watch that return! Sports-related injuries are a main facial-fracture culprit.

Assessing facial fractures

When a patient experiences a facial fracture, signs and symptoms vary based on the area of injury. This chart highlights some of the common assessment and diagnostic test findings associated with various facial fracture areas.

Fracture area	Assessment findings	Diagnostic test findings
Nasal	• Pain • Changes in vision • Oedema of the periorbital area and upper face • Bruising • Epistaxis • Crepitus • Possible intracranial injuries	Facial computed tomography (CT) scan or nasal bone X-ray revealing disruption of the bone
Zygomatic arch	• Pain in the lateral cheek • Difficulty closing the jaw • Swelling and crepitus • Visible asymmetry	Facial X-ray or facial CT scan showing depressed arch
Mandibular	• Point tenderness • Crepitus • Trismus (tonic contracture of chewing muscles) • Asymmetrical facial appearance • Swelling • Bruising • Malocclusion • Possible lower lip and chin paresthesia • Inability to grasp a tongue blade between his teeth	Facial X-ray or CT scan revealing displacement at the site of fracture (most commonly mandibular angle, condyle, molar and mental areas)
Maxillary	• Severe facial pain • Lack of sensation or paraesthesia of the upper lip • Vision changes • Severe facial oedema and bruising • Elongated facial appearance • Periorbital or orbital oedema • Subconjunctival haemorrhage • Facial asymmetry • Malocclusion • Rhinorrhoea • Moveable maxilla	Facial X-ray revealing displacement and site of fracture; CT scan identifying the extent and severity of the fracture

What to look for

General findings related to facial fractures include:

* Swelling
* Displacement
* Bruising
* Pain
* Possible loss of function.

Specific signs and symptoms vary depending on the areas and structures involved. (See *Assessing facial fractures*.)

What tests tell you

Typically, facial X-rays reveal the type of fracture and its location. CT scan may be used to determine the injury's extent.

How it's treated

Treatment of facial fractures involves stabilising the patient's airway, including frequent suctioning if bleeding and secretions are profuse, and ruling out cervical spine injury. Endotracheal intubation is preferred for airway maintenance, if required. Oxygen therapy and assisted ventilation are used as necessary. Haemorrhage is treated with direct pressure, ice packs or an external compression dressing. Nasal fractures require splinting and setting of the bone. Surgery with open reduction and internal fixation or wiring is used to treat mandibular fractures.

What to do

• Because facial fractures typically involve structures located near the airway, immediately assess ABCDEs. If the patient has sustained severe facial trauma, oral airway insertion or endotracheal intubation and mechanical ventilation may be necessary
• Immobilise the cervical spine until spinal injury is ruled out. Because of the force needed to cause a facial fracture, cervical spine injury may be present in 1% to 4% of those with facial fractures
• Obtain facial X-rays and/or a CT scan of the face as ordered to locate the fracture and determine the level of severity
• Initiate measures to reduce swelling and control bleeding (which may include elevating the patient's head if cervical spine injury has been ruled out); apply ice to the area
• Administer analgesics and other medications as ordered, including tetanus prophylaxis
• Prepare the patient for surgery as indicated.

Foreign body in the ear

Foreign body in the ear, as the name suggests, refers to any object in the ear canal that causes some obstruction. This problem is most commonly associated with children ages 9 months to 4 years.

What causes it

The most common cause of a foreign body in the ear is cerumen (earwax), commonly as a result of inserting cotton swabs into the ear and pushing cerumen further into the ear canal. Cerumen impaction is another cause, most commonly seen in the older adult. Other causes include insects and such objects as beads, small stones, beans, corn and dry cereal.

How it happens

The object becomes lodged in the ear canal. Cerumen blocks the transmission of sound to the eardrum. Other objects, such as beans or insects, become lodged in the canal, leading to inflammation, pain and possible infection.

What to look for

Typically, the patient reports a change in hearing. He may complain of ear pain or feelings of fullness. Signs and symptoms of ear infection or purulent foul-smelling drainage may be seen. If an insect is the cause, the patient commonly reports a feeling of buzzing or something moving in the ear.

Hearing acuity testing

Test your patient's gross hearing acuity. Ask him to occlude one ear or occlude it for him. Then stand at a distance of 30.5 to 61 cm (1′ to 2′) away, exhale fully and whisper softly toward the unoccluded ear. Choose numbers or words that have two syllables that are equally accented such as 'nine-four' or 'baseball'. If you note diminished hearing, you should seek further senior professional advice, such as an ear, nose and throat specialist or audiologist.

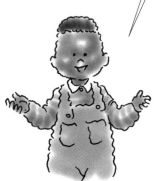

Little hands, big trouble! Children ages 9 months to 4 years are the usual suspects when it comes to foreign bodies in the ear.

What tests tell you

Gross hearing screening may be done to estimate the degree of hearing loss. Otoscopic examination reveals evidence of an obstruction.

How it's treated

Removal of the foreign body is key. This removal may be achieved with suctioning, irrigation or special tools while directly visualising the ear canal. These tools may include an ear curette, right-angle hook, suction catheter or forceps. Eardrops may be used to help soften impacted cerumen. If a patient has a live insect in his ear, mineral oil or 2% lignocaine may be used to kill the insect before its removal.

What to do

• Assess the patient's gross hearing acuity and determine evidence of obstruction
• Prepare the patient for ear irrigation; provide comfort to the patient and his family
• Explain procedures and treatments to the patient and family to help alleviate anxiety and gain consent
• If ordered, administer eardrops to soften cerumen or insert mineral oil or 2% lignocaine to kill a live insect
• Irrigate the ear as ordered using warm tap water or a solution of warm water; make sure that the solution is warmed to body temperature to prevent stimulating the inner ear, which could lead to dizziness, nausea and vomiting. (See *Contraindications for irrigation*.)
• Assist with the instrument removal of a foreign object.

Foreign body in the nose

A foreign body in the nose refers to any object in the nasal cavity that causes some obstruction. This problem is most commonly associated with children

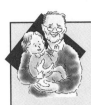

Ages and stages

Contraindications for irrigation

Remember that ear irrigation is contraindicated in patients:
- Younger than 5 years old
- With a ruptured tympanic membrane
- With an ear infection
- With a vegetable or soft foreign body that would absorb water.

but can also be associated with adults who have a psychiatric illness. They are often accompanied by their distressed parents or carer who will need comforting and reassurance.

What causes it
Normally, the object is from an item or a toy that the child has been playing with, such as, beads, small stones, beans, corn and dry cereal.

What to look for
In most cases, information is provided from the person who has witnessed the insertion of the foreign body. It is important to gain a thorough history from the patient (if possible) and his or her primary carer. If help is delayed, the patient may present a nasal discharge, nasal irritation, epistaxis, sneezing, snoring, sinusitis, stridor, wheezing or fever.

What to do
Examining the nasal cavity is essential for diagnoses. Positioning the patient in a relaxed position is of utmost importance as the inspection of the nasal cavity can be uncomfortable. Using a bright lamp/torch, the nostrils should be inspected, possibly assisted with a nasal speculum, although good visualisation can be obtained by using your thumb to pull the nose upward. (See *Inspecting the nostrils*, page 410.)

Visualise the tympanic membranes for signs of acute otitis media, assess for sinusitis, check for nuchal rigidity in the toxic child and auscultate the chest and neck for wheezing or stridor, which may be a sign of an aspirated foreign body.

Be aware that there could be more foreign bodies in other cavities that need exploration and removal.

How it's treated
Be aware that when you try and remove the foreign body you may push the object further down the nasal cavity. All the necessary equipment should

therefore be at hand, including airway adjuncts. Depending on the nature and material of the foreign body, different techniques can be used:

- Direct instrumentation, e.g. forceps
- Balloon catheters, e.g. insert the catheter beyond the object, inflate the balloon and pull out the foreign body
- Positive pressure, e.g. blocking one nostril and asking the patient to blow out of the other nostril
- Suction, e.g. using a catheter and suction
- Magnet, e.g. if the foreign body is made from metal.

If the foreign body cannot be removed with any of these techniques the patient should be referred to an ENT surgeon for further examination.

Nasal fracture

This is a common facial fracture, normally caused by blunt trauma and assaults.

What to look for

The injury is sometimes obvious, with a presentation of:

- Unconventional nasal shape
- Swelling
- Pain
- Epistaxis.

What tests tell you

Tests are not normally ordered as they don't change the management of the injury. However, X-rays maybe requested and performed for medicolegal reasons.

How it's treated

The nose should be inspected for any confirmation of:

- Cerebrospinal fluid (CSF)
- Rhinorrhoea
- Fractures to the cribriform plate.

Due to the swelling there is not much treatment that can be carried out initially for 5 to 10 days. The patient should therefore be referred and followed up by an ENT surgeon. The nasal bones will start to reset after approximately 3 weeks. If reduction is required, the patient should be admitted for this procedure within 1 to 2 weeks following the injury.

What to do

- Evaluate the patient's ABCDEs and intervene as necessary
- Determine the type of injury, including the mechanism, time, force and object causing the trauma
- The patient may require his visual acuity tested
- Apply ice and elevate the patient's head, unless a spinal injury is suspected
- Provide reassurance to help alleviate anxiety
- Refer the patient to an ENT consultant/specialist as indicated
- Administer analgesia as prescribed.

Tonsillitis

This is a common throat infection caused by a variety of viruses or bacteria.

What to look for

The patient may present with all or some of the following presentation:
- Sore throat
- Fever
- Headache
- Dysphagia
- Bad breath
- Swollen neck
- Cough.

What tests tell you

Inspection of the throat may reveal inflamed tonsils and a bacterial infection will be diagnosed if pus is present. General lymphadenopathy may suggest glandular fever. Throat swabs maybe necessary to test for the source of infection.

How it's treated

Treatment to reduce the discomfort and pain may include paracetamol or/and an anti-inflammatory such as ibuprofen. Lozenges and warm liquids may also help relieve the soreness.

Oral antibiotics rarely treat the symptoms; however, if the tonsillitis is caused by considerable exudate or group A streptococcus, then antibiotics are useful with penicillin or amoxicillin being the preferred choice. Erythromycin is used for patients allergic to penicillin. Normally tonsillitis starts to clear within a week but if symptoms persist the patient should visit their GP.

What to do

- Evaluate the patient's ABCDEs and intervene as necessary
- Provide reassurance to help alleviate anxiety
- Refer the patient to their GP or an ENT specialist as indicated
- Administer analgesia and antibiotics as prescribed.

Quinsy (Peritonsillar abscess)

This is a condition when the infection from tonsillitis spreads to the surrounding areas.

What to look for

The patient may present with a history of tonsillitis:
- Sore throat (usually on one side)
- Swollen neck
- High temperature of 38 C or above

- Headache
- Dysphagia
- Bad breath
- Cough
- Trismus (difficulty opening the mouth)
- Change in voice.

How it's treated

Analgesia is prescribed and normally the patient is admitted for intravenous antibiotics and steroids. A needle aspiration may be used to drain the abscess. The fluid that is removed from the abscess will be sent for analysis so that the bacteria that caused the infection can be identified.

In severe cases or when the patient has reoccurring problems the patient will require a tonsillectomy.

Dental abscess

A dental abscess is a bacterial infection which causes pus in the teeth or gums.

What to look for

The patient may present with all or some of the following presentation:
- Airway/breathing problems
- Pain
- Swelling of the face/tooth/gum
- Swelling of lymph glands
- Dysphagia
- Bad breath
- Fever
- Disturbed sleep.

How it's treated

The only way to cure a dental abscess is to anaesthetise the area, cut out the abscess and drain away the pus that contains the infectious bacteria. A rapid referral to a specialist such as a dentist or oral surgeon should be made. However, the patient may not be able to see a specialist straight away and will attend an ED; the primary goal is to reduce the pain, swelling and discomfort by administering prescribed:
- Painkillers, such as ibuprofen and paracetamol or codeine phosphate, depending on contraindications and the severity of pain
- Antibiotics, such as amoxicillin or metronidazole.

What to do

- Evaluate the patient's ABCDEs and intervene as necessary
- Provide reassurance to help alleviate anxiety
- Refer the patient to their dentist
- Administer analgesia and antibiotics as prescribed
- Apply an ice pack which may help alleviate the swelling.

Quick quiz

1. When preparing to assess a patient's corneal sensitivity, you should use:
   A. A wisp of cotton.
   B. A tissue.
   C. A gauze pad.
   D. Ophthalmoscopy.

Answer: A. A wisp of cotton is the only safe object to use for assessing corneal sensitivity. Even though a gauze pad or tissue is soft, it can cause corneal abrasions and irritation.

2. Which cranial nerve would you expect to be possibly affected with a soft tissue injury of the face?
   A. IX.
   B. VII.
   C. II.
   D. I.

Answer: B. With a soft tissue facial injury, the most commonly affected cranial nerve would be cranial nerve VII, the facial nerve, because its branches are responsible for sensory and motor function of various facial structures.

3. Which drug should you identify as a mydriatic?
   A. Pilocarpine.
   B. Epinephrine.
   C. Betaxolol.
   D. Timolol.

Answer: B. Epinephrine is a mydriatic agent. Pilocarpine, betaxolol and timolol are miotic agents.

Scoring

☆☆☆ If you answered all three questions correctly, give a big grin! You're tops when it comes to maxillofacial and ophthalmic emergencies.

☆☆ If you answered two questions correctly, say 'Eye caramba!' You're ahead of the competition in this emergency category.

☆ If you answered fewer than two questions correctly, don't frown. Keep your eyes on the prize as you look through the chapter again.

Environmental emergencies

Just the facts

In this chapter, you'll learn:

♦ Assessment methods for environmental emergencies

♦ Some types of environmental emergencies

♦ Treatment and management of the emergencies.

Understanding environmental emergencies

Environmental emergencies are emergencies that occur because of exposure to, or contact with, the environment. Environmental emergencies include injuries from fire, electricity, lightning, water, animals, insects, cold and heat.

Your environmental emergency assessment will depend on the type of injury and its location. Like all emergencies, first and foremost, assess the patient's airway, breathing, circulation, disability and exposure (ABCDE). (See *Priorities first*.)

Common disorders

There are so many disorders that can present to the emergency department (ED) that it would be impossible to cover them all. However, there are some common environmental emergencies which include burns, wounds, bites and stings, caustic substance ingestion (poisoning), hyperthermia and hypothermia.

Insects and lightning and fire – oh my! Environmental emergencies give new meaning to 'the great outdoors!'

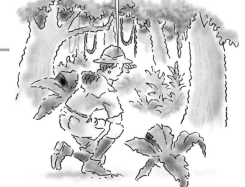

Priorities first

The primary survey is described in more detail in Chapter 3, *Initial assessment in emergency departments*, but the priority consists of airway, breathing, circulation, disability and exposure.

A is for airway

Remember as you assess the airway of an environmental emergency patient to ensure cervical spine immobilisation; any patient who has sustained a major trauma must be assumed to have a cervical spine injury until proven otherwise.

B is for breathing

A patient who has sustained major trauma requires high-flow oxygen to maintain blood oxygenation. If the patient doesn't have spontaneous respirations or has ineffective respirations, ventilate him using a bag-valve mask device until you can achieve endotracheal tube intubation.

C is for circulation

All patients who have sustained major trauma need two large-bore I.V. lines. Because these patients may require large amounts of fluids and blood, use a fluid warmer if possible. If external bleeding is present, apply direct pressure over the site.

If the patient has no pulse, cardiopulmonary resuscitation must be started. If there is a suspected injury to the heart (such as a knife wound or gunshot), the doctor may elect to perform an emergency thoracotomy in the emergency department in an effort to repair the wound.

D is for disability

Assess the patient using the mnemonic AVPU:
- A stands for alert and oriented
- V stands for responds to voice
- P stands for responds to pain
- U stands for unresponsive.
  If the patient isn't alert and oriented, conduct further assessments during the secondary survey.

E is for exposure

Expose the patient, whilst maintaining their dignity and warmth, to perform a thorough assessment.

Remember that ABCDE is a rapid assessment designed to identify life-threatening emergencies. Treat any life-threatening emergencies before continuing your assessment.

Burns

A burn is a tissue injury resulting from contact with fire, a thermal chemical, or an electrical source. It can cause cellular skin damage and a systemic response that leads to altered body function.

What causes it

Thermal burns, the most common type of burn, typically result from residential fires, road traffic collisions, playing with matches, improper handling of fireworks or bonfires, scalding and kitchen accidents (such as a child climbing on top of a stove or grabbing a hot iron), abuse (in children and older adults).

It's electric

Electrical burns usually result from contact with faulty electrical wiring or high-voltage power lines. Tissue damage is normally evident along the

---

Electrical burn care

Keep these tips in mind when caring for a patient with an electrical burn:
- Stay alert for ventricular fibrillation as well as cardiac and respiratory arrest caused by the electrical shock; begin cardiopulmonary resuscitation immediately
- Get an estimate of the voltage that caused the injury
- Tissue damage from an electrical burn is difficult to assess because internal destruction along the conduction pathway is usually greater than the surface burn would indicate
- An electrical burn that ignites the patient's clothes may also cause thermal burns.

---

path of a high - voltage source. There maybe no tissue damage visible but, the nurse should be aware of potential internal injuries, such as, cardiac arrythmias leading to a cardiac arrest and muscle damage. (See *Electrical burn care.*) Be vigilant to entry signs, which is normally the point of contact with the electrical source. The current can follow different pathways but usually follows the vessels. Also check for an exit point, which could include a wound or sweaty area around the distal areas of the feet, hands or potentially, any part of the body. This can depend upon the size of the current and tissue resistance. Remember, it doesn't matter how small the exit wound is, the damage can cause deep internal injury.

Scorching brews

Chemical burns result from contact, ingestion, inhalation, or injection of acids, alkalis, or vesicants.

How it happens
Specific pathophysiologic events depend on the cause and classification of the burn. (See *Visualising burn depth.*) The injuring agent modifies the molecular structure of cellular proteins. Some cells die because of traumatic or ischaemic necrosis. Loss of collagen cross-linking also occurs that moves intravascular fluid into interstitial spaces. Cellular injury triggers the release of mediators of inflammation, contributing to local and – in the case of major burns – systemic increases in capillary permeability.

Not just a matter of degrees anymore

Traditionally, burns were gauged only by degree. Today, however, most assessment findings use depth of tissue damage to describe a burn.

For your epidermis only

Superficial partial-thickness or first-degree burns are limited to the epidermis; these burns cause localised injury or destruction to the skin by direct or indirect contact. The barrier function of the skin remains intact.

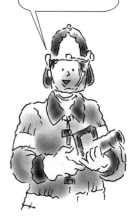

Thermal burn causes range from residential fires to kitchen accidents.

Visualising burn depth

The most widely used system of classifying burn depth and severity categorises burns by depth. However, it's important to remember that most burns involve tissue damage of multiple depths. This illustration may help you visualise burn damage at the various depth.

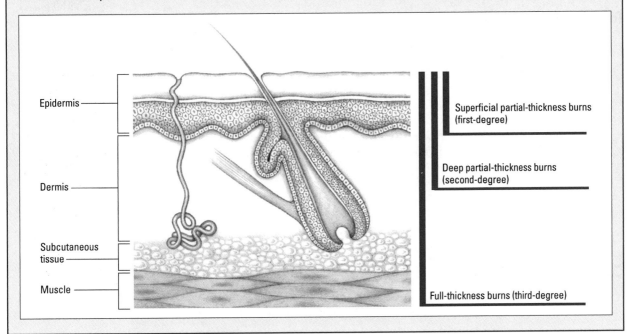

Epidermis

Dermis

Subcutaneous tissue

Muscle

Superficial partial-thickness burns (first-degree)

Deep partial-thickness burns (second-degree)

Full-thickness burns (third-degree)

Two differing degrees

Deep partial-thickness or second-degree burns involve destruction to the epidermis and some dermis. Pain and tactile responses remain intact, causing treatments to be very painful. The barrier function of the skin is lost.

In deep partial-thickness burns, destruction of the epidermis and dermis occur, producing blisters and mild to moderate oedema and pain. The hair follicles remain intact. These burns are less painful than second-degree, superficial partial-thickness burns because the sensory neurons have undergone extensive destruction. The areas around the burn are sensitive to pain because the barrier function of the skin is lost.

Third layer, third degree

Full-thickness or third-degree burns extend through the epidermis and dermis and into the subcutaneous tissue layer. These burns may also involve muscle, bone and interstitial tissues. Within hours, fluids and protein shift from capillary to interstitial spaces, causing oedema.

What to look for

Assessment provides a general idea of burn severity. First, determine the depth of tissue damage; a partial-thickness burn damages the epidermis and part of the dermis, while a full-thickness burn also affects subcutaneous tissue.

Tracking burn traits

People can have varying burn depths and the signs and symptoms depend on the type of burn:
- *Superficial burn* – localised pain and erythaema, usually without blisters in the first 24 hours
- *More severe superficial burn* – chills, headache, localised oedema and nausea and vomiting
- *Superficial partial-thickness burn* – thin-walled, fluid-filled blisters appear within minutes of the injury, with mild to moderate oedema and pain
- *Deep partial-thickness burn* – white, waxy appearance to damaged area
- *Full-thickness burn* – white, brown or black leathery tissue and visible thrombosed vessels due to destruction of skin elasticity, but without blisters (most commonly on the dorsum of the hand)
- *Electrical burn* – silver-coloured, raised or charred area, usually at the site of electrical contact.

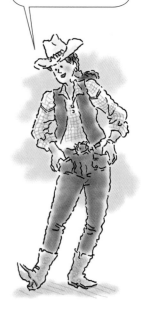

Whether white, brown, or black, full-thickness burn tissue tends to look as leathery as my boots here.

Configure this

Inspection reveals the burn's location and the extent. Note its configuration:
- If the patient has a circumferential burn on an extremity, he runs the risk of oedema occluding its circulation
- If the patient has burns on his neck, he may suffer airway obstruction
- Burns on the patient's chest can lead to restricted respiratory movement.

More than just skin deep

Inspect the patient for other injuries that may complicate recovery, such as signs of pulmonary damage from smoke inhalation – singed nasal hairs, mucosal burns, voice changes, coughing, wheezing, soot in the mouth or nose and darkened sputum.

What tests tell you

An assessment method that can be used to determine the size of a burn is the Rule of Nines chart, which determines the percentage of body surface area (BSA) covered by the burn. (See *Estimating burn size*.)

Burns may be classified into three categories:

 Major

 Moderate

 Minor.

BSA coverage is the main factor used to determine burn category.

Estimating burn size

Because body surface area (BSA) varies with age, two different methods are used to estimate burn size in adult and paediatric patients.

Rule of nines

You can quickly estimate the extent of an adult patient's burn by using the Rule of Nines. This method quantifies BSA in multiples of 9 (thus, the name). To use this method, mentally transfer the burns on your patient to the body charts below. Add the corresponding percentages for each body section burned. Use the total – a rough estimate of burn extent – to calculate initial fluid replacement needs.

Lund and browder classification

The Rule of Nines isn't accurate for infants or children because their body shapes, and therefore BSA, differ from those of adults. For example, an infant's head accounts for about 17% of his total BSA, compared with 7% for an adult. Instead, use the Lund and Browder classification to determine burn size for infants and children.

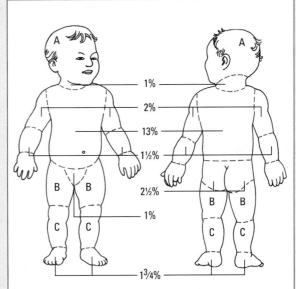

Percentage of burned body surface by age

At birth	0 to 1 year	1 to 4 years	5 to 9 years	10 to 15 years	Adult
9½%	8½%	6½%	5½%	4½%	3½%
2¾%	3¼%	4%	4¼%	4½%	4¾%
2½%	2½%	2¾%	3%	3¼%	3½%

Area
A = ½ of head
B = ½ of one thigh
C = ½ of one leg

Paging major burns

Major burns include:
- Full-thickness burns on more than 10% of BSA
- Deep partial-thickness burns on more than 15% of BSA in adults and more than 10% in children
- Burns on the hands, face, feet or genitalia
- Burns complicated by fractures or respiratory damage
- Electrical burns
- Any burn in a poor-risk patient.

Everything in moderation

Moderate burns include:
- Full-thickness burns on 2% to 10% of BSA
- Deep partial-thickness burns on 15% to 25% of BSA in adults and 10% to 20% of BSA in children.

Minor yours?

Minor burns include:
- Full-thickness burns on less than 2% of BSA
- Deep partial-thickness burns on less than 15% of BSA in adults and less than 10% of BSA in children.

Meanwhile, back in the lab

Here are some additional diagnostic test results related to the patient with burns:
- Arterial blood gas (ABG) levels may be normal in the early stages but reveal hypoxaemia and metabolic acidosis later
- Carboxyhaemoglobin level may reveal the extent of smoke inhalation due to carbon monoxide presence
- Full blood count (FBC) may reveal a decreased haemoglobin level due to haemolysis, increased haematocrit (HCT) secondary to haemoconcentration and leukocytosis resulting from a systemic inflammatory response or the possible development of sepsis
- Electrolyte levels may show hyponatraemia from massive fluid shifting and hyperkalaemia from fluid shifting and cell lysis
- Creatine kinase (CK) and myoglobin levels may be elevated. Keep in mind that CK and myoglobin are helpful indicators of muscle damage; the higher the CK or myoglobin level, the more extensive the muscle damage. The presence of myoglobin in urine may lead to acute tubular necrosis.

How it's treated

The initial assessment, resuscitation and stabilisation of the patient should be performed and then transportation should be arranged to a tertiary burns centre for on-going specialist care.

Rnitial burn treatments are based on the type of burn and may include:
- Removing the source of the burn and items that retain heat, such as clothing and jewellery
- Maintaining an open airway; assessing ABCDEs
- Preparing for endotracheal tube (ET) intubation if the airway is compromised
- Administering supplemental humidified oxygen
- Controlling active bleeding
- Preventing further contamination of the burns by using sterile gloves
- Covering deep partial-thickness burns that are more than 30% of BSA or full-thickness burns that are more than 5% of BSA with clean, dry, sterile sheets (because of the drastic reduction in body temperature, don't cover large burns with saline-soaked dressings). Burns can also be covered with cling film; this allows the area to be seen but protects without leaving fibres behind
- Fluid replacement. (See *A closer look at fluid replacement*, page 436.)

After stabilisation

- Antimicrobial therapy (for all patients with major burns)
- Pain medication as needed
- Laboratory tests such as FBC; electrolyte, glucose and serum creatinine levels; ABG analysis; typing and crossmatching and urinalysis for myoglobinuria and haemoglobinuria
- Close monitoring of fluid intake, output and vital signs
- Surgical intervention, including skin grafts and thorough surgical debridement for major burns
- Tetanus prophylaxis as ordered
- Nutritional therapy.

What to do
- Immediately assess the patient's ABCDEs, including the cervical spine. Carry out emergency resuscitative measures as necessary. Monitor arterial oxygen saturation and serial ABG values and anticipate the need for ET intubation and mechanical ventilation if the patient's respiratory status deteriorates, especially with facial or neck burns.

Listen to the lungs

- Auscultate lung sounds for crackles or stridor. Observe for signs of laryngeal oedema or tracheal obstruction, including laboured breathing, severe hoarseness, and dyspnoea
- Administer supplemental humidified oxygen as ordered
- Perform oropharyngeal or tracheal suctioning as indicated by the patient's inability to clear his airway or evidence of abnormal breath sounds
- Initiate continuous cardiac monitoring and monitor the patient's cardiac and respiratory status closely – at least every 15 minutes, or more frequently depending on his condition. Also, monitor the patient for cardiac arrhythmias. Assess his level of consciousness (LOC) for changes, such as increasing confusion, restlessness or decreased responsiveness.

A closer look at fluid replacement

Fluid replacement is essential for the patient with burns because of the massive fluid shifts that occur. However, you must be extreme cautious because of the risk of over replacement.

How much?

Various formulas may be used to determine the amount of fluid replacement to be administered during the first 24 hours after a burn injury. Typically, these formulas use body weight and the percentage of BSA burned. One of the most common formulas used is the Parkland formula shown here:

Total fluid requirement in 24 hours =
- 4 ml × (total burn surface area (%) × (body weight (kg)
- 50% given in first 8 hours
- 50% given in next 16 hours.

Children receive maintenance fluid in addition, at hourly rate of:
- 4 ml/kg for first 10 kg of body weight plus
- 2 ml/kg for second 10 kg of body weight plus
- 1 ml/kg for >20 kg of body weight.

End point
Urine adults 0.5 to 5 1.0 ml/kg/hour
Urine Children 1.0 to 1.5 ml/kg/hour
NB: Subtract any fluid already received from the amount required for first 8 hours to ensure accurate calculations.

OR

The Muir and Barclay formula:

$$\frac{\text{Percentage area of burn} \times \text{weight in kg}}{2}$$

This gives you the amount of fluid needed for each time period over 36 hours. For example:

$$\frac{20\% \times 80}{2} = 800 \text{ mls}$$

- Period 1 – will require 800 ml/4 hour for the first 12 hours
- Period 2 – will require 800 ml/6 hour for the second 12 hours
- Period 3 – will require 800 ml for the last 12 hours.

Totaling: 800 × 3 = 2,400 (Period 1)
800 × 2 = 1,600 (Period 2)
800 × 1 = 800 (Period 3)
= 4,800 ml over the first 36 hours post injury.

Which fluids?

There is no gold standard as to which type of fluids, whether it'll be crystalloid or colloid, used in resuscitating a burn – injured patient.

Crystalloid fluids include:
- Normal saline
- Hartmann's solution.

These are predominantly used as resuscitation fluids with the Parklands formula.

Colloid fluids include:
- Albumin
- Blood.

These are predominantly used as resuscitation fluids with the Muir and Barclay formula.

Too much or too little?

During fluid replacement, always stay alert for indications of over replacement and under replacement. Signs and symptoms of heart failure and pulmonary oedema suggest over replacement. Assessment findings of hypovolaemic shock suggest under replacement. Inhalation injuries accompanying thermal trauma increases the magnitude of total body injury and requires increased volumes of fluid and sodium to achieve resuscitation from early burn shock.

High voltage electrical injury can require more fluid due to the release of myoglobin and haemoglobin from damaged cells which collect in the renal tubules causing acute renal tubular necrosis. These patients usually require double the urine output to flush the kidneys of large myoglobin cells.

Minor burns
- Cool the burn with cold running water between 8° C (46° F) and 15° C (59° F) for approximately twenty minutes. Iced water should not be used as the severe cold will result in vasoconstriction and may cause further tissue damage.
- Cover the area with an antimicrobial agent and a nonstick bulky dressing after debridement
- Provide a prophylactic tetanus injection as needed.

Moderate or major burns
- Provide 100% oxygen, and prepare for ET intubation and mechanical ventilation if necessary
- If the patient has facial or neck burns, anticipate the need for early ET intubation to reduce the risk of airway obstruction.

Breathing

- Place the patient in an appropriate position to maximise chest expansion. Beware of positioning patients correctly with potential cervical spine injuries
- Control active bleeding
- Remove smoldering clothing (first soaking in saline solution if clothing is stuck to the patient's skin), rings and other constricting items
- Cover partial-thickness burns over 30% of BSA or full-thickness burns over 5% of BSA with a clean, dry, sterile sheet
- Because of the drastic reduction in body temperature, don't cover large burns with saline-soaked dressings
- You may need to prepare the patient for emergency escharotomy (a surgical incision used to release pressure from swollen tissues) of the chest and neck for deep burns or circumferential injuries to promote lung expansion
- Assist with central venous or pulmonary artery catheter placement as needed.

Consider in and out

- Insert an indwelling urinary catheter (if requested); monitor fluid intake and output
- Insert a nasogastric (NG) tube to decompress the stomach and prevent aspiration of stomach contents
- Maintain nil-by-mouth status
- Watch for signs and symptoms of infection
- For chemical burns, provide frequent wound irrigation with copious amounts of normal saline solution
- Prepare the patient for surgical intervention, including skin grafts and more thorough surgical debridement for major burns.

Administration station

Expect to administer:
- Pain medication as needed
- Analgesics I.V., rather than I.M., because tissue damage associated with the burn injury may impair absorption of the drug when given I.M.
- A fluid replacement formula to prevent hypovolaemic shock and maintain cardiac output
- Antimicrobial therapy
- Bronchodilators and mucolytics to aid in the removal of secretions.

Be vigilant

Although injuries from environmental factors are seen in EDs, they can occur from nonaccidental injuries with the child or adult being subjected to abuse. Chapter 3 (*Initial assessment in emergency departments*) provides more detail on this topic but some observations when treating patients should be noted:
- Injuries inconsistent with the information given
- Changing the history of the injury
- Injuries inappropriate to development stage, e.g. a 3-month-old baby rolling off the bed
- Cigarette burns
- Vague history
- Delay seeking medical attention
- Lack of concern from carer or guardian.

Managing difficult situations such as these should be taken extremely seriously but treated with caution. For example, a person with generalised bruising may have an underlying bleeding disorder which would explain such presentations. However, such presentations must be investigated further with the assistance of other multidisciplinary teams, if necessary, before a clinical diagnosis and judgment is made to implement the local safeguarding adult and children policies.

Wounds

Wounds can vary in nature and can be caused by different mechanisms of injury, some traumatic wounds include:
- Penetration (penetration of the skin and tissues): can be caused by an object, such as metal fragments
- Puncture (penetration of the skin and tissues): can be caused by an object, such as a screwdriver
- Laceration (tissues torn apart): can be caused by a pulling action, such as machinery
- Abrasion (scrape): can be caused by a fall
- Contusion (blow from a blunt instrument): can be caused by an object, such as a hammer
- Incision (a cut to the body tissue): can be caused by a knife.

Assessment

With all traumas, an assessment of life-threatening injuries (primary survey) should be carried out and the necessary interventions should be performed before an assessment of any wound which is not life threatening. Any bleeding should be controlled by applying a firm, direct pressure and elevate the patient's extremities. If bleeding continues, you may need to compress a pressure point above the wound.

Ask questions

It's very important to gain a history about the mechanism of the injury. For example, a presentation of a small 1-inch wound to a chest wall may appear nonconcerning; however, when questioning the patient, they tell you that it was caused by a 5-inch knife. You should start to think about the potential of a life-threatening problem, such as a tension pneumothorax or haemothorax. Some of the questions that you may want to include are:

- Mechanism of injury
- Time of injury
- Where did the injury happen (increase risk of infection)
- How much blood loss
- How much pain.

On examination

- Inspect the wound for any foreign bodies, bleeding, size, depth and damage to underlying anatomy, such as tendons and arteries
- Check for colour, movement and sensation of the limb
- Check capillary refill time and pulses of the distal aspect to the wound
- Palpate the injury and check for any other possible underlaying injuries, such as fractures.

What next

The patient may require an X-ray to check for any potential foreign bodies in the wound or for any potential fractures.

Closing up

Sutures or tissue adhesive can be used on wounds that have minimal tissue loss and if the edges of the wound can be brought together. Tissue adhesives, sometimes known as tissue glue, can be used alone to close superficial wounds or in conjunction with subcutaneous sutures to close dermal wounds where deeper wound stability is necessary. They may also minimise some of the problems associated with sutures such as premature absorption or reactivity as well as improve the final cosmetic outcome. Wound closure strips are useful for paediatric wounds or where the person may be very anxious about having the sutures applied. A local anaesthetic should be used prior to suturing.

Special considerations

When caring for a patient with a traumatic wound, pay particular attention to these aspects of care:

• Irrigate the wound to remove all visible contaminants from the wound bed prior to closure or dressing; this will help to decrease the risk of infection and tattooing (blue/purple scarring caused by debris remnants)

• Consider possibility of foreign bodies in the wound bed, seek specialist advice on identification (X-ray or ultrasound scan) and removal

• Avoid using high-pressure irrigation on wounds. High-pressure irrigation can seriously interfere with healing by destroying cells and forcing bacteria into the tissue

• Use sterile 0.9% normal saline to remove debris when cleaning the wound. Alternatively, hold the injury under a running tap of (drinkable) water

• Avoid using alcohol to clean a traumatic wound. It's painful for the patient and dehydrates tissue

• Never use a cotton ball or a cotton-filled gauze pad to clean a wound because cotton fibres left in the wound may cause contamination or a foreign body reaction

• If there are plans to debride the wound to remove dead tissue and reduce the risk of infection and scarring, loosely pack the wound with gauze pads soaked in 0.9% normal saline until it's time for the procedure

• Monitor closely for signs of developing infection, such as warm red skin or purulent discharge from the wound. Infection in a traumatic wound can delay healing, increase scarring and trigger systemic infections such as septicaemiae

• Inspect the dressing regularly. If oedema develops, adjust the dressing to ensure adequate circulation to the affected area of the wound

• Provide analgesia as necessary and ensure your patient understands the treatment he has received and when and where to return for follow-up care.

Bites

Special consideration for infection should be paid to all bite wounds, as the amount of pathogens found in human and animal mouths can cause painful and swollen limbs.

When assessing a bite wound, it's important to quickly discover the bite's source – cat, dog, spider, human? This will help determine which bacteria or toxins may be present and the likely type of tissue trauma.

Fancy a bite?

For example, a human bite can cause a puncture wound and introduce any one of the innumerable organisms present in the human mouth into the wound. *Staphylococcus aureus* and streptococci are two such organisms that can be transmitted to the wound or into the victim's bloodstream. Other serious diseases that can be transmitted in this way include human immunodeficiency virus infection, hepatitis B, hepatitis C, syphilis and tuberculosis.

Animal house

A bite from a dog, cat or rodent can introduce deadly infectious diseases, such as rabies, into a wound. Cats and other smaller mammals cause relatively little tissue damage. However, a dog can generate up to 200 psi of pressure when biting and if he shakes his head at the same time (which is usually the case), strong torsional force is brought to bear. Together, these forces can cause a massive amount of tissue damage.

Consider tendon damage with cat and rodent bites and consider the possibility of fractures with large dog bites.

What to do

Remove dead or damaged skin and cleanse the wound to reduce the likelihood of infection. Wounds to the face and hands may need to be closed sooner rather than later. However, wounds to other body parts may require closure after a few days to make sure there is no infection, especially if the wound is more than 6 hours old. Wide open wounds may need to be closed by using steri-strips, sutures or skin glue.

Antibiotics maybe prescribed for wounds:
- That are deep or large
- On the face, hand or foot
- Low immune system.

Check the patient's tetanus immunisation status and administer as prescribed.

Stings

Insects, including bees, ants and wasps, have a venom sac on their tail that they use to inject venom into humans and animals. In their venom are proteins and other substances which they use to kill or paralyse other insects. It is the proteins that cause allergic reactions in people.

Most people only experience redness, itching and mild pain and swelling at the site of the bite. Cleaning the area and applying ice are enough to relieve the symptoms. However, if the victim is allergic to the venom, then they may have an anaphylactic reaction, although an anaphylactic reaction does not usually occur on the first sting.

Most local reactions are not serious, although, if there are signs such as:
- Hives (swollen bumps on the skin)
- Significant swelling over major body parts – face, head, neck, arms/hands, legs/feet
- Difficulty breathing, wheezing or the feeling that the throat is closing
- Dizziness or fainting
- Chest pain or tachycardia
- Nausea, vomiting or diarrhoea.

Quick reactive attention needs to be carried out to secure the airway. Treatment such as adrenaline (also known as epinephrine) may need to be administered to constrict blood vessels, relax smooth muscles in the lungs which will improve breathing, stimulate the heartbeat and help to stop swelling around the face and lips.

The itching, pain and redness may last for several days but should improve gradually. Increasing redness, pain, swelling and warmth may signal an infection at the site. If this occurs, antibiotics may need to be commenced.

For more in-depth information on wound care, please see Vuolo J, Anderson I, & Fletcher J (2009): *Wound Care Made Incredibly Easy!* (1st UK Edition) Lippincott Williams & Wilkins.

Caustic substance ingestion

Caustic substances can be strong acids or strong bases. The most damaging substances are industrial products because they are highly concentrated. However, some common household products, including toilet and drain cleaners as well as some dishwasher detergents, contain damaging caustic substances, such as sodium hydroxide and sulphuric acid.

Caustic substances are available as solids and liquids. The fact that solids stick to a moist surface (such as the lips) may prevent a person from consuming a large amount of a solid product. Because liquids don't stick, it's easier to consume more of the product and possibly damage the entire oesophagus.

Regular offenders

Common acid-containing sources include:
- Toilet-cleaning products
- Automotive battery liquid
- Rust-removal products
- Metal-cleaning products
- Cement-cleaning products
- Drain-cleaning products
- Soldering flux containing zinc chloride.
  Common alkaline-containing sources include:
- Drain-cleaning products
- Ammonia-containing products
- Oven-cleaning products
- Swimming pool cleaning products
- Automatic dishwasher detergent
- Hair relaxers
- Bleaches
- Cement.

What causes it

Ingestion of a caustic substance can be accidental, such as ingestion by a young child, or deliberate, as in an attempted suicide.

How it happens

The extent of the injury is determined by the amount of the ingested material, its concentration and form and whether the patient has vomited or aspirated.

- After ingestion, an extreme inflammatory reaction occurs that results in erythema and oedema of the superficial layers
- Ingestion of caustic substances can cause oesophageal stricture and laryngeal stenosis and can increase the risk of oesophageal cancer
- Alkaline cleaners, such as drain cleaner, are generally tasteless and odourless, allowing larger amounts to be ingested. These substances tend to cause injury to the mucosa and submucosa of the oesophagus. Alkaline substances cause liquefication necrosis, a process in which necrosis continues from the superficial layers into the deeper tissues
- Acidic cleaners, such as chlorinated household cleaners, undergo oxygenation reactions and form hydrochloric acid, which causes gastric injury if ingested. These agents cause coagulation necrosis, a process in which a protective layer forms at the site of the injury and limits its depth.

What to look for

- Airway, breathing and circulation
- Abdominal pain or guarding
- Altered mental status
- Burns around the mouth
- Diarrhoea
- Drooling
- History of ingesting poisons
- Nausea and vomiting
- Odd breath odours. (See *Identifying breath odour*, page 444.)
- Saliva or foaming at the mouth
- Unresponsiveness.

What tests tell you

- pH testing of saliva determines whether the substance is an acid or base; however, a neutral pH can't rule out ingestion of a caustic substance. A pH of less than 2.0 (acidic substance) or greater than 12.5 (alkaline substance) indicates the potential for severe tissue damage
- FBC, urea and electrolytes, creatinine and ABG levels evaluate the patient's renal status and acid-base balance as well as his blood oxygen ventilation status
- Urinalysis can evaluate the patient's renal status because many toxic and caustic substances can be excreted through the kidneys
- Alcohol and toxicologic screens rule out or confirm cases of suspected intentional ingestion by evaluating the levels of these substances in the blood
- Chest X-ray may reveal mediastinitis, pleural effusions, pneumoperitoneum and aspiration pneumonitis
- Abdominal X-ray may reveal pneumoperitoneum or ascites.

Identifying breath odour

The patient's breath odour may help determine what he/she ingested, especially if he/she arrives at the emergency department unconscious.

Breath odour	Possible substance
Alcohol	• Chloral hydrate • Alcohol • Phenols
Acetone	• Acetone • Isopropyl alcohol • Salicylates
Bitter almond	• Cyanide
Coal gas	• Carbon monoxide
Garlic	• Arsenic • Organophosphates • Phosphorus
Nonspecific	• Possible inhalant use
Wintergreen	• Methylsalicylates

What to do

• Initiate universal precautions, such as, goggles (face mask), gown and gloves.
• If necessary provide supplemental oxygen and prepare the patient for emergency ET intubation, cricothyroidotomy or tracheostomy and mechanical ventilation if necessary
• Initiate suicide precautions if necessary
• Initiate resuscitation status
• Obtain the patient's history, including the substance and the amount ingested
• Assess the patient's LOC, airway and rate, depth and pattern of respirations
• Auscultate the lung and heart sounds
• Obtain the patient's vital signs, noting hypotension and fever; also observe the electrocardiogram tracing for arrhythmias
• Don't induce vomiting or perform gastric intubation and lavage, which may induce vomiting; inducing vomiting will reintroduce the caustic substances to the upper GI tract.

Call the pros

• Contact a poison control centre, e.g. Toxbase (http://www.toxbase.org/) and get a quick, accurate information, suggestions and recommendations if necessary

- Wash the mouth and face to remove any particles of the ingested substance
- You may need to administer broad-spectrum antibiotics and antireflux medication.

A stiff, boardlike abdomen is a sign of peritonitis.

Look, listen and ask

- Ask about chest pain
- Inspect the oropharyngeal cavity for burns and injury
- Observe for drooling and dysphagia
- Ask about vomiting
- Listen to the patient's voice to detect laryngitis, hoarseness, and dysphagia
- Observe for stridor
- Auscultate bowel sounds
- Assess for abdominal pain; a boardlike, rigid abdomen and other signs of peritonitis
- Signs and symptoms of peritonitis, fever, chest pain and hypotension suggest a full-thickness gastric injury or perforation, which requires immediate surgical intervention
- Monitor serum electrolyte levels
- Contact the safeguarding children team if abuse or neglect is suspected.

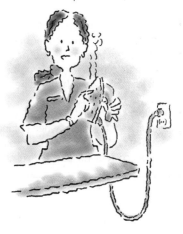

Prep for

Prepare the patient for:
- Chest X-ray to check the mediastinal width and detect free air in the mediastinum or abdomen
- Surgical intervention, such as exploratory laparotomy or thoracotomy with possible oesophagectomy, oesophagogastrectomy or gastrectomy for a full-thickness injury.

Investigations

The patient may need to be admitted for:
- Flexible nasopharyngoscopy, laryngoscopy or endoscopy to visualise the injuries
- Periodic oesophagography with water-soluble contrast and possible oesophageal stenting or dilatation with contrast to detect and correct dysphagia.

Hyperthermia

Hyperthermia refers to an elevation in body temperature to more than 37.2°C (99°F). It may result from environmental or internal conditions that increase heat production or impair heat dissipation.

Ages and stages

Heatstroke in older adults

With ageing, an individual's thirst mechanism and ability to sweat decreases. These factors put the older adult at risk for heatstroke, especially during hot summer days. Heatstroke must be treated rapidly to prevent serious complications or death. To help prevent heatstroke, teach your older patient to follow these instructions:

- Reduce activity in hot weather, especially outdoor activity
- Wear lightweight, loose-fitting clothing during hot weather; when outdoors, wear a hat and sunglasses, and avoid wearing dark colours that absorb sunlight
- Drink plenty of fluids, especially water, and avoid tea, coffee and alcohol because they can cause dehydration
- Use air conditioning or open windows and use a fan to help circulate air. If the patient doesn't have air conditioning at home, suggest that, during periods of excessive heat, he go to community resources that have air conditioning, community centres, libraries, and churches. Some community centres may even provide transportation for the patient.

What Causes it

Hyperthermia may result from excessive exercise, infection and drug use such as amphetamines. It may also result from an impaired ability to dissipate heat. (See *Heatstroke in older adults*.) Factors that impair heat dissipation include:

- High temperatures or humidity
- Lack of acclimatisation
- Excess clothing
- Cardiovascular disease
- Obesity
- Dehydration
- Sweat gland dysfunction
- Drugs, such as phenothiazines and anticholinergics.

How it happens

Humans normally adjust to excessive temperatures with complex cardiovascular and neurologic changes that are coordinated by the hypothalamus. Heat loss offsets heat production to regulate body temperature. The body loses heat by the process of evaporation or vasodilation, which cools the body's surface by radiation, conduction and convection. However, when heat loss mechanisms fail to offset heat production, the body retains heat.

Metabolism and increased body temperature

Central nervous system, cellular and cardiac function are greatly affected by increased body temperature. For every 1°C (1.8°F) rise in body temperature, the body's metabolic rate increases by 13%. The body can't tolerate this level of increased metabolic rate for long, and death can quickly occur if the temperature isn't lowered.

Body temperature	Percentage of metabolic increase
38°C (100.4°F)	13
39°C (102.2°F)	26
40°C (104°F)	39
41°C (105.8°F)	52
42°C (107.6°F)	Cellular needs can't be met because of insufficient oxygen

From ENA: *Sheehy's Manual of Emergency Care*, 6th ed. Newberry, L. and Criddle, L. (eds), Body Temperature and Metabolism, p. 505. © 2005, Reprinted with permission from Elsevier.

Good-bye fluid, hello hypovolaemic shock

If body temperature remains elevated, fluid loss becomes excessive and may lead to hypovolaemic shock. If untreated, the patient's thermoregulatory mechanisms can fail.

Feeling hot, hot, hot

Hyperthermia occurs in varying degrees:
• Mild hyperthermia (heat cramps) occurs with excessive perspiration and loss of salt from the body
• Moderate hyperthermia (heat exhaustion) occurs when the body is subjected to high temperatures and blood accumulates in the skin in an attempt to decrease the body's temperature. This accumulation causes a decrease in circulating blood volume, which decreases cerebral blood flow. Syncope then occurs
• Critical hyperthermia (heatstroke) occurs when the body's temperature continues to rise and internal organs become damaged, eventually resulting in death. (See *Metabolism and increased body temperature*.)

What to look for

Assessment findings vary with the degree of hyperthermia. (See *Hyperthermia signs and symptoms*, page 448.)

Hyperthermia signs and symptoms

Hyperthermia may be classified as mild (heat cramps), moderate (heat exhaustion) or critical (heatstroke). This table highlights the major assessment findings associated with each classification.

Classification	Assessment findings
Mild hyperthermia (heat cramps)	• Mild agitation (central nervous system findings otherwise normal) • Mild hypertension • Moist, cool skin and muscle tenderness; involved muscle groups possibly hard and lumpy • Muscle twitching and spasms • Nausea, abdominal cramps • Report of prolonged activity in a very warm or hot environment without adequate salt intake • Tachycardia • Temperature ranging from 37.2° to 38.9°C (99° to 102°F)
Moderate hyperthermia (heat exhaustion)	• Dizziness • Headache • Hypotension • Muscle cramping • Nausea and vomiting • Oliguria • Pale, moist skin • Rapid, thready pulse • Syncope or confusion • Thirst • Weakness • Temperature elevated up to 40°C (104°F)
Critical hyperthermia (heatstroke)	• Atrial or ventricular tachycardia • Confusion, delirium • Fixed, dilated pupils • Hot, dry, reddened skin • Loss of consciousness • Seizures • Tachypnoea • Temperature greater than 41.1°C (106°F)

What tests tell you

No single diagnostic test confirms hyperthermia, but these test results may help support the diagnosis:
• ABG results may reveal respiratory alkalosis and hypoxaemia
• FBC may reveal leukocytosis and increased HCT secondary to haemoconcentration
• Electrolyte levels may show hypokalaemia. Other blood studies may reveal elevated U&E level, increased bleeding and clotting times and fibrinolysis

- Urinalysis may show concentrated urine with elevated protein levels, tubular casts, and myoglobinuria.

How it's treated
Mild or moderate hyperthermia is treated by allowing the patient to rest in a cool environment. Oral or I.V. fluid and electrolyte replacement is administered as ordered.

Critical measures

Measures for treating critical hyperthermia include:
- Removing the patient's clothing and applying cool water to the skin, and then fanning the patient with cool air
- Controlling shivering by giving diazepam or chlorpromazine
- Applying hypothermia blankets and ice packs to the groin and axillae if necessary
- Continuing treatment until the patient's body temperature drops to 39°C (102.2°F).

In addition to the cool-down

Supportive measures for hyperthermia include:
- Oxygen therapy
- Central venous pressure
- ET intubation, if necessary.

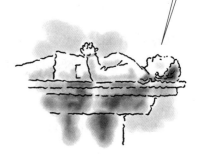

We could probably all use some rest in a cool environment, but for hyperthermia patients it's of the utmost importance.

What to do
- Assess the patient's ABCDEs and initiate emergency resuscitative measures as indicated. Remove as much of the patient's clothing as possible
- Assess oxygen saturation and administer supplemental oxygen as indicated and ordered. Monitor the patient's pulmonary status closely, including respiratory rate and depth and lung sounds; anticipate the need for ET intubation and mechanical ventilation if respiratory status deteriorates
- Monitor the patient's vital signs continuously, especially core body temperature. Although the goal is to reduce the patient's temperature rapidly, too rapid a reduction can lead to vasoconstriction, which can cause shivering. Shivering increases metabolic demand and oxygen consumption and should be prevented if possible
- Employ external cooling measures, such as cool sheets, tepid baths and cooling blankets
- Assess the patient's neurologic and cardiac status closely, including heart rate and rhythm. Institute continuous cardiac monitoring to evaluate for arrhythmias secondary to electrolyte imbalances. Monitor haemodynamic parameters; assess peripheral circulation, including skin colour, peripheral pulses and capillary refill
- Monitor fluid and electrolyte balance and laboratory test results. Assess renal function studies to evaluate for rhabdomyolysis.

Hypothermia

Hypothermia is defined as a core body temperature below 35°C (95°F); it may be classified as:
- *Mild* – 32° to 35°C (89.6° to 95°F)
- *Moderate* – 30° to 32°C (86° to 89.6°F)
- *Severe* – 25° to 30°C (77° to 86°F) which can be fatal.

What causes it

Hypothermia commonly results from near in cold water, prolonged exposure to cold temperatures, disease or debility that alters homeostasis or administration of large amounts of cold blood or blood products.

Likely candidates

The risk of serious cold injury, especially hypothermia, is higher in patients who are:
- Young
- Elderly
- Lacking in insulating body fat
- Wearing wet or inadequate clothing
- Abusing drugs or alcohol or smoking
- Suffering from cardiac disease
- Fatigued
- Malnourished with a depletion of calorie reserves.

How it happens

In hypothermia, metabolic changes slow down the functions of most major organ systems, resulting in decreased renal blood flow and decreased glomerular filtration. Vital organs are physiologically affected. Severe hypothermia results in depression of cerebral blood flow, diminished oxygen requirements, reduced cardiac output, and decreased arterial pressure.

What to look for

Obtaining the history of a patient with a cold injury may reveal:
- Cause of hypothermia
- Temperature to which the patient was exposed
- Length of exposure.

Temperature dependent

Assessment findings in a patient with hypothermia vary with the patient's body temperature:
- Mild hypothermia includes severe shivering, slurred speech and amnesia
- Moderate hypothermia includes unresponsiveness, peripheral cyanosis and muscle rigidity. If the patient was improperly rewarmed, he may show signs of shock

Clinical findings and body temperature

A patient's signs and symptoms can change, depending on his core body temperature. This chart lists body temperature ranges and their associated signs and symptoms.

Body temperature	Signs and symptoms
35.6° to 37.2°C (96° to 99°F)	• Loss of manual coordination • Shivering
32.8° to 35°C (91° to 95°F)	• Amnesia • Violent shivering • Slurred speech
30° to 32.2°C (86° to 90°F)	• Decreased shivering • Cyanosis • Muscular rigidity
<30°C (<86°)	• Atrial fibrillation • Rewarming shock
27.2° to 29.4°C (81° to 85°F)	• Patient is irrational • Stupor • Decreased pulse and respirations
25.6° to 26.7°C (78° to 80°F)	• Erratic heartbeat • Coma
<27.2°C (<81°F)	• Ventricular fibrillation
<25.6°C (<78°F)	• Cardiopulmonary arrest

From ENA: Sheehy's Manual of Emergency Care, 6th ed. Newberry, L., and Criddle, L. (eds), Clinical Manifestations of Hypothermia, p. 503. © 2005, Reprinted with permission from Elsevier.

• Severe hypothermia includes absence of palpable pulses, no audible heart sounds, dilated pupils and a rigor mortis-like state. In addition, ventricular fibrillation and a loss of deep tendon reflexes are common. (See *Clinical findings and body temperature*.)

How it's treated

Treatment for hypothermia consists of supportive measures and specific rewarming techniques, including:
• Passive rewarming (when the patient rewarms on his own)
• Active external rewarming with heating blankets, warm water immersion, heated objects such as water bottles, and radiant heat
• Active core rewarming with heated I.V. fluids, genitourinary tract irrigation, extracorporeal rewarming, haemodialysis and peritoneal, gastric and mediastinal lavage.

Cardiac concerns

Arrhythmias that develop usually convert to normal sinus rhythm with rewarming. If the patient has no pulse or respirations, cardiopulmonary resuscitation (CPR) is needed until rewarming raises the core temperature to at least 32°C (89.6°F).

Monitoring dependent

The administration of oxygen, ET intubation, controlled ventilation, I.V. fluids and treatment for metabolic acidosis depend on test results and careful patient monitoring.

What to do

• Assess the patient's ABCDEs and initiate CPR as appropriate. Keep in mind that hypothermia helps protect the brain from anoxia, which normally accompanies prolonged cardiopulmonary arrest. Therefore, even if the patient has been unresponsive for a long time, CPR may resuscitate him
• Administer supplemental oxygen, and prepare for ET intubation and mechanical ventilation if necessary
• Initiate continuous cardiac monitoring
• Initiate CPR if necessary
• Assist with rewarming techniques as necessary. (In moderate to severe hypothermia, only experienced personnel should attempt aggressive rewarming)
• During rewarming, provide supportive measures as ordered, including mechanical ventilation and heated, humidified therapy to maintain tissue oxygenation, and warmed I.V. fluids to correct hypotension and maintain urine output
• Continuously monitor the patient's core body temperature and other vital signs during and after initial rewarming. Continuously monitor his cardiac status, including continuous cardiac monitoring, for evidence of arrhythmias
• If using a hyperthermia blanket, discontinue the warming when core body temperature is within 0.6° to 1.1°C (1° to 2°F) of the desired temperature. The patient's temperature will continue to rise even when the device is turned off.

As time goes by

• If the patient has been hypothermic for longer than 45 to 60 minutes, administer additional fluids as ordered to compensate for the expansion of the vascular space that occurs during vasodilation in rewarming. Monitor the patient's heart rate and haemodynamic parameters closely to evaluate fluid needs and response to treatment

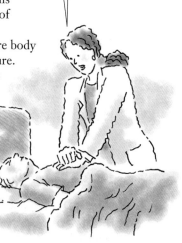

CPR is a-OK for hypothermia victims. Even when they've been unresponsive for a while, their lack of brain anoxia provides a chance for survival.

• Monitor the patient's hourly output, fluid balance and serum electrolyte levels, especially potassium. Stay alert for signs and symptoms of hyperkalaemia. If hyperkalaemia occurs, administer calcium chloride, sodium bicarbonate, glucose and insulin as ordered. If his potassium level is extremely elevated, he may require dialysis.

Poisoning

Poisoning refers to inhalation, ingestion and injection of, or skin contamination from, any harmful substance. It's a common environmental emergency. The prognosis depends on the amount of poison absorbed, its toxicity and the time interval between poisoning and treatment.

What causes it

Because of their curiosity and ignorance, children are common poison victims, usually from the ingestion of salicylates (aspirin), cleaning agents, insecticides, paints, cosmetics and plants.

In adults, poisoning is most common among chemical company employees – particularly those in companies that use chlorine, carbon dioxide, hydrogen sulphide, nitrogen dioxide and ammonia – and in companies that ignore safety standards. Other causes of poisoning in adults include improper cooking, canning, and storage of food; ingestion of or skin contamination from plants (e.g., Dieffenbachia, mistletoe, azalea, and philodendron) and accidental or intentional drug overdose (usually barbiturates) or chemical ingestion. (See *Poisoning facts.*)

How it happens

The pathophysiology of poisons depends on the substance that's inhaled or ingested. The extent of damage depends on the pH of the substance, the amount ingested, its form (solid or liquid) and the length of exposure to it.

Substances with an alkaline pH cause tissue damage by liquefaction necrosis, which softens the tissue. Acids produce coagulation necrosis. Coagulation necrosis denatures (changes the molecular composition of) proteins when the substance contacts tissue. This limits the extent of the injury by preventing penetration of the acid into the tissue.

The mechanism of action for inhalants is unknown, but they're believed to act on the CNS similarly to a very potent anaesthetic. Hydrocarbons sensitise the myocardial tissue and allow it to be sensitive to catecholamines, resulting in arrhythmias.

What to look for

The patient's history should reveal the poison's source and form of exposure (ingestion, inhalation, injection or skin contact). Assessment findings vary with the poison. (See *Pinpointing poison's effects*, page 454.)

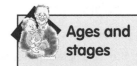

Ages and stages

Poisoning facts

Adolescents tend to overdose on over-the-counter drugs instead of prescription drugs. Older adults who overdose do so usually because of polypharmacy, improper use of their prescribed medication, improper storage of the medication (not in its original container) or mistaking the identity of the medication.

Pinpointing poison's effects

Review the assessment findings and possible toxins listed below to help determine what type of poison is causing your patient's signs and symptoms.

Agitation, delirium

Alcohol, amphetamines, atropine, barbiturates, neostigmine

Coma

Atropine, barbiturates, bromide, carbon monoxide, chloral hydrate, alcohol, salicylates.

Constricted pupils

Barbiturates, chloral hydrate, morphine.

Sweating

Alcohol, fluoride, insulin.

Diarrhoea, nausea, vomiting

Alcohol (ethanol, methanol, ethylene glycol), heavy metals (lead, arsenic), morphine and its analogues, salicylates.

Dilated pupils

Alcohol, amphetamines, belladonna alkaloids (such as atropine), cocaine, cyanide, ephedrine.

Dry mouth

Antihistamines, belladonna alkaloids, morphine, phenothiazines, tricyclic antidepressants.

Extrapyramidal tremor

Phenothiazines.

Haematemesis

Fluoride, mercuric chloride, phosphorus, salicylates.

Kussmaul's respirations

Ethanol, ethylene glycol, methanol, salicylates.

Partial or total blindness

Methanol.

Pink skin

Atropine (flushed, dry skin), carbon monoxide, cyanide, phenothiazines.

Seizures

Alcohol (ethanol, methanol, ethylene glycol), amphetamines, carbon monoxide, salicylates.

What tests tell you

- Toxicology studies (including drug screens) of poison levels in the mouth, vomitus, urine, stool or blood, or on the victim's hands or clothing, confirm the diagnosis. If possible, have the family or patient bring the container holding the poison to the ED for comparable study
- In inhalation poisoning, chest X-rays may show aspiration pneumonia. In petroleum distillate inhalation, they may show pulmonary infiltrates or oedema. Abdominal X-rays may reveal iron pills or other radiopaque substances
- ABG analysis, serum electrolyte levels and FBC are used to evaluate oxygenation, ventilation and the metabolic status of seriously poisoned patients.

What to do
- Initial treatment includes emergency resuscitation, support of the patient's ABCDEs and prevention of further poison absorption. Secondary treatment consists of continuing supportive or symptomatic care and, when possible, administration of a specific antidote
- A poisoning victim who exhibits altered LOC routinely receives oxygen, glucose and naloxone. Activated charcoal is effective in eliminating many toxic substances. Specific treatment depends on the poison
- Carefully monitor the patient's vital signs and LOC. If necessary, begin CPR
- Depending on the poison, prevent further absorption by administering activated charcoal. For specific treatment, contact the poison centre (local or national), e.g. National Poisons Information Services (NPIS). The treatment's effectiveness depends on the speed of absorption and the time elapsed between ingestion and removal.

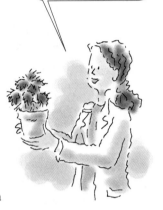

It doesn't look tasty to me, but household plant ingestion is one of the most common poisoning sources in children.

Vomiting
- Never induce vomiting if you suspect corrosive acid poisoning, if the patient is unconscious or has seizures or if the gag reflex is impaired, even in a conscious patient. Instead, neutralise the poison by instilling the appropriate antidote by an NG tube. Common antidotes include milk and activated charcoal
- When possible, add the antidote to water or juice.

Enter the I.V.
- If several hours have passed since the patient ingested the poison, use large quantities of I.V. fluids to force the poison through the kidneys to be excreted. The kind of fluid you use depends on the patient's acid-base balance and cardiovascular status and on the flow rate necessary for effective diuresis of poison.

Give him some air
- To prevent further absorption of inhaled poison, remove the patient to fresh or uncontaminated air. Provide supplemental oxygen and, if needed, ET intubation. To prevent further absorption from skin contamination, remove the clothing covering the contaminated skin and immediately flush the area with large amounts of water
- If the patient is in severe pain, give analgesics as ordered; frequently monitor fluid intake and output, vital signs and LOC
- Keep the patient warm and provide support in a quiet environment
- If the poison was ingested intentionally, refer the patient for counselling/crises resolution team to help prevent future attempts at suicide.

Quick quiz

1. Your patient has partial- and full-thickness burn injuries to his anterior chest, anterior abdomen and entire right arm. Using the Rule of Nines, the percent of total body surface area involved can be estimated at:

    A.   18%.
    B.   27%.
    C.   45%.
    D.   50%.

Answer: *B.* The anterior chest and abdomen constitute 18% of the BSA, and the entire right arm is 9%, for a total of 27%.

2. A patient admitted to the ED is suspected of taking an overdose of atropine. Which clinical finding would you look for?

    A.   Kussmaul's respirations.
    B.   Diarrhoea and nausea and vomiting.
    C.   Flushed, dry skin.
    D.   Extrapyramidal tremors.

Answer: *C.* A patient who has overdosed on atropine will have flushed, dry skin and dilated pupils.

3. Your patient has a core body temperature of 26.7°C (80°F). Which classification of hypothermia is this?

    A.   Low.
    B.   Mild.
    C.   Moderate.
    D.   Severe.

Answer: *D.* Severe hypothermia is a core body temperature of 25° to 30°C (77° to 86°F).

4. An unconscious patient is admitted to the ED with a very strong wintergreen odour on his breath. What might he have ingested?

    A.   Ethanol.
    B.   Acetone.
    C.   Methylsalicylates.
    D.   Cyanide.

Answer: *C.* If a patient has ingested methylsalicylates, his breath will have a wintergreen odour.

Scoring

✩✩✩   If you answered all four questions correctly, stop and smell the roses! You're quite erudite when it comes to environmental emergencies.

✩✩   If you answered three questions correctly, breathe a sigh of relief, you're burning for success!

✩   If you answered fewer than three questions correctly, don't let it rain on your parade. Review the chapter again and give it another try.

Glossary

abduct: move away from the midline of the body; opposite of *adduct*

adduct: move towards the midline of the body; opposite of *abduct*

advance directive: written legal document that identifies a patient's advance wishes regarding the types of health care he desires if he becomes unable to decide for himself

agonist: drug that binds to a receptor to elicit a physiologic response

alveolus: in the lung, a small saclike dilation of the terminal bronchioles

anaerobic: oxygen not required for growth

angina: pain felt in the chest region; typically associated with a heart attack

anion: ion with a negative electrical charge

anorexia: loss of appetite

antagonist: drug that binds to a receptor but doesn't produce a response or blocks the response at the receptor

anterior: front or *ventral;* the opposite of *posterior* or *dorsal*

antibody: immunoglobulin produced by the body in response to exposure to a specific foreign substance (antigen)

antigen: foreign substance that causes antibody formation when introduced into the body

anuria: urine output of less than 100 ml in 24 hours

aphasia: language disorder characterized by difficulty expressing or comprehending speech

apnoea: cessation of breathing

apraxia: inability to perform coordinated movements, even though no motor deficit is present

arthrosis: joint or articulation

ascites: accumulation of fluid in the abdominal cavity

assessment: first step in the nursing process that involves data gathering

ataxia: uncoordinated actions when voluntary muscle movements are attempted

atrophy: wasting away

automaticity: ability of the heart to generate its own electrical impulse

avulsion fracture: fracture that occurs when a joint capsule, ligament, tendon or muscle is pulled from a bone

axonal injury: diffuse brain injury that usually results from tension and shearing forces

Battle's sign: bruising immediately behind the ear that usually indicates a fracture of the posterior portion of the skull

Biot's respirations: respirations that are rapid, deep and alternate with abrupt periods of apnoea

blepharitis: inflammation of the eyelids

body mechanics: use of body positioning or movement to prevent or correct problems related to activity or immobility

borborygmi: loud sounds produced by the normal movement of air through the intestines

bradycardia: abnormally slow heart rate; usually less than 60 beats per minute

bradypnoea: abnormally slow respiratory rate; usually less than 10 breaths per minute

bruit: abnormal sound heard over peripheral vessels that indicates turbulent blood flow

buccal: pertaining to the cheek

bursa: fluid-filled sac lined with synovial membrane

capillary: microscopic blood vessel that links arterioles with venules

cardiac cycle: period from the beginning of one heartbeat to the beginning of the next; includes two phases: systole and diastole

carpal: pertaining to the wrist

cartilage: connective supporting tissue occurring mainly in the joints, thorax, larynx, trachea, nose and ear

coeliac: pertaining to the abdomen

central nervous system: one of the two main divisions of the nervous system; consists of brain and spinal cord

cognition: thinking and awareness

colloid: fluid containing starches or proteins

consciousness: state involving full awareness and ability to respond to stimuli

contralateral: on the opposite side; opposite of *ipsilateral*

coronary: pertaining to the heart or its arteries

cortex: outer part of an internal organ; the opposite of *medulla*

costal: pertaining to the ribs

crackles: intermittent, nonmusical, crackling breath sounds that are caused by collapsed or fluid-filled alveoli popping open

crepitus: noise or vibration produced by rubbing together irregular cartilage surfaces or broken ends of a bone; also the sound heard when air in subcutaneous tissue is palpated

cutaneous: pertaining to the skin

cyanosis: bluish discoloration of the skin or mucous membranes

debridement: removal of dead tissue or foreign material from a wound

dehiscence: separation of a wound's edges

deltoid: shaped like a triangle (as in the deltoid muscle)

dermis: skin layer beneath the epidermis

diaphragm: membrane that separates one part from another; the muscular partition separating the thorax and abdomen

diastole: resting portion of the cardiac cycle where the coronary arteries are filling with blood and the ventricles are relaxed

distal: far from the point of origin or attachment; the opposite of *proximal*

diuresis: formation and excretion of large amounts of urine

dorsal: pertaining to the back or posterior; the opposite of *ventral* or *anterior*

dysarthria: speech defect commonly related to a motor deficit of the tongue or speech muscles

dysphagia: difficulty swallowing

dyspnoea: difficult or laboured breathing

empathy: process of putting oneself into the feelings of another

endocardium: interior lining of the heart

endocrine: pertaining to secretion into the blood or lymph rather than into a duct; the opposite of *exocrine*

endometrium: inner mucosal lining of the uterus

epidermis: outermost layer of the skin; lacking vessels

Erb's point: auscultatory point on the precordium at the third intercostal space to the left of the sternum

evisceration: internal organ protrusion through an opening in a wound

exocrine: pertaining to secretion; the opposite of *endocrine*

exophthalmos: abnormal protrusion of the eyeball

fistula: abnormal opening between organs or between an organ and body surface

flaccidity: decrease in muscle tone that causes muscle to become weak or flabby

fluid wave: rippling across the abdomen during percussion; indicative of the presence of ascites

fremitus: palpable vibration that results from air passing through the bronchopulmonary system and transmitting vibrations to the chest wall

gastric lavage: instillation of solution into the stomach and subsequent withdrawal to remove stomach contents

glomerulus: compact cluster; the capillaries of the kidney

haematuria: blood in the urine

haemoglobin: protein found in red blood cells that contains iron

haemoptysis: blood in the sputum

hordeolum: inflammation of the sebaceous gland of the eyelid; also called *stye*

hydrocele: accumulation of serous fluid in a saclike structure such as the testes

hyperopia: defect in vision that allows a person to see objects clearly at a distance but not at close range; also called *farsightedness*

hyperresonance: increased resonance produced by percussion

hypertonic: having a greater concentration than body fluid

hypotonic: having a lesser concentration than body fluid

hypoxaemia: state in which the blood contains a lower than normal amount of oxygen

hypoxia: state in which the tissues have a decreased amount of oxygen

infarction: death of tissue due to ischaemia

inferior: lower; the opposite of *superior*

infiltration: seepage or leakage of fluid into the tissues

informed consent: a patient (or legal guardian for children) giving permission for a procedure after the patient has demonstrated understanding of the procedure

ipsilateral: on the same side; opposite of *contralateral*

ischaemia: insufficient blood supply to a part

isotonic: having the same concentration as body fluid

Korotkoff sounds: sounds heard when auscultating blood pressure denoting systolic and diastolic pressures

laceration: wound caused by tearing of the tissues

lacrimal: pertaining to tears

lateral: pertaining to the side; the opposite of *medial*

lethargy: slowed responses, sluggish speech and slowed mental and motor processes in a person oriented to time, place and person

living will: advance directive that states the medical care that persons would want or refuse should the person be unable to give consent or refusal

lumbar: pertaining to the area of the back between the thorax and the pelvis

maceration: tissue softening as a result of excessive moisture

manubrium: upper part of the sternum

meatus: opening or passageway

medial: pertaining to the middle; opposite of *lateral*

myocardium: thick, contractile layer of muscle cells that forms the heart wall

nephron: structural and functional unit of the kidney

neutropenia: decreased number of neutrophils

neutrophil: white blood cell that removes and destroys bacteria, cellular debris and solid particles

Nitrazine paper: treated paper used to detect pH and determine the presence of amniotic fluid

nociceptors: nerve endings that respond to noxious stimuli

oedema: accumulation of fluid in the interstitial space

olfactory: pertaining to the sense of smell

oliguria: urine output of less than 500 ml in 24 hours

ophthalmic: pertaining to the eye

pectoral: pertaining to the chest or breast

percussion: use of tapping on a body surface with fingers

pericardium: fibroserous sac that surrounds the heart and the origin of the great vessels

peristalsis: movement through the intestines

phrenic: pertaining to the diaphragm

plantar: pertaining to the sole

pleura: thin serous membrane that encloses the lung

plexus: network of nerves, lymphatic vessels or veins

popliteal: pertaining to the back of the knee

posterior: back or dorsal; the opposite of *anterior* or *ventral*

pronate: to turn the hand or forearm so that the palm faces down or back, or to rotate the foot so that the inner edge of the sole bears the weight of the body; opposite of *supinate*

proximal: situated nearest the centre of the body; opposite of *distal*

pruritus: itching

pulse deficit: difference between the apical and radial pulse rates

pulse pressure: difference between the systolic blood pressure and diastolic blood pressure readings

purulent: pus-producing or pus-containing

range of movement: extent to which a person can move his joints or muscles

sanguinous: referring to or containing blood

serosanguineous: containing blood and serum

spasticity: sudden, involuntary increase in muscle tone or contractions

sprain: complete or incomplete tear in the supporting ligaments surrounding a joint

station: relationship of the presenting part to the ischial spines

strain: injury to the muscle or tendinous attachment

striated: marked with parallel lines, such as striated (skeletal) muscle

subcutaneous: related to the tissue layer under the dermis

sublingual: under the tongue

superior: higher; opposite of *inferior*

supinate: to turn the palm or forearm upwards; the opposite of *pronate*

systole: period of ventricular contraction

tachycardia: rapid heart rate; usually more than 100 beats per minute

tachypnoea: rapid respiratory rate, usually more than 20 breaths per minute

tendon: band of fibrous connective tissue that attaches a muscle to a bone

toco transducer: external mechanical device that translates one physical quantity to another, most commonly seen in capturing foetal heart rates and transmitting and recording the value onto a foetal monitor

Valsalva manoeuvre: forceful exhalation with a closed glottis; bearing down

ventral: pertaining to the front or *anterior;* the opposite of *dorsal* or *posterior*

ventricle: small cavity, such as one of several in the brain or one of the two lower chambers of the heart

viscera: internal organs

xiphoid: sword-shaped; the lower portion of the sternum

Selected references and internet resources

Selected references

Alfaro R. *Applying Nursing Diagnosis and Nursing Process: A Step by Step Guide*, 2nd ed. London. J.B: Lippincott Company, 1990:90.

Nor AM, Davis J, Sen B, et al. The Recognition of Stroke in the Emergency Room (ROSIER) Scale. Development and validation of a stroke recognition instrument. *Lancet Neurology* 2005;4:727–734.

Devitt P, Thain J. *Children's & Young People's Nursing Made Incredibly Easy*. UK. Lippincott Williams & Wilkins, 2011.

Dolan B, Holt L. *Accident and emergency theory into practice,* 2nd ed. Edinburgh: Bailliere Tindall, 2007.

Evans D, Allen H. *Mental Health Nursing Made Incredibly Easy*, 1st ed. UK. Lippincott Williams & Wilkins, 2009.

Griffith R, Tengnah C. *Law and Professional Issues in Nursing*, 2nd ed. Exeter. Learning matters, 2010.

Stiell IG, Greenberg GH, McKnight RD, et al. A study to develop clinical decision rules for the use of radiography in acute ankle injuries. *Ann Emerg Med* 1992;21:384–390.

Le Duc Jimmerson C, Lomuas G. Facial, ophthalmic and otolaryngeal trauma. In: Driscoll PA, Gwinnutt CL, LeDuc Jimmerson C, Goodall O (eds.). *Trauma Resuscitation: The Team Approach*. Basingstoke: Macmillan, 2010.

Lewis SJ, Heaton KW. Stool form scale as a useful guide to intestinal transit time. *Scand J Gastroenterol* 1997;32(9):920–924. doi:10.3109/00365529709011203.

Mackway-Jones K, Marsden J, Windle J. *Manchester Triage Group. Emergency Triage* 2nd ed. Blackwell Publishing Ltd, 2006.

National Health Service. *Your Guide to the NHS: Getting the Most from Your Department of Health*. 2001.

National Health Service Modernisation Agency. *See and Treat*. London: NHS Modernisation Agency. 2002.

Patient at Risk Scoring: Reproduced with permission from, Abertawe Bro Morgannwg (ABM) University Health Board copyright 2010.

Paw RC. Emergency department staffing in England and Wales, April 2007. *Emerg Med J* 2008;25:420–423. doi: 10.1136/emj.2007.054197.

Ramrakha P, Moore K. *Oxford Handbook of Acute Medicine*. Oxford: Oxford University Press, 2004.

Royal College of Psychiatrists. *Psychiatric Services to Accident & Emergency Departments*, council report CR118. LONDON: British Association for Accident & Emergency Medicine, RCP, 2004.

Stiell IG, Wells GA, Hoag RH, Sivilotti ML, Cacciotti TF, Verbeek PR, Greenway KT, McDowell I, Cwinn AA, Greenberg GH, Nichol G, Michael JA. Implementation of the Ottawa knee rule for the use of radiography in acute knee injuries. *JAMA* 1997;278:2075–2079.

Vuolo J, Anderson I, Fletcher J. *Wound Care Made Incredibly Easy*, 1st ed. UK: Lippincot Williams & Wilkins, 2009.

Internet resources

British National Formulary (2010): *British National Formulary*, http://bnf.org/bnf/index.htm

Department of Health (2001): Reforming Emergency care, http://www.dh.gov.uk/en/Publicationsandstatistics/Publications/PublicationsPolicyAndGuidance/DH_4092955

Faculty of Emergency Nursing (FEN), www.fen.uk.com

National Institute for Clinical Excellence (2004): *Chronic obstructive pulmonary disease. Management of chronic obstructive pulmonary disease in adults in primary and secondary care*, http://www.nice.org.uk

National Institute for Clinical Excellence (2004): *The epilepsies: diagnosis and management of the epilepsies in adults in primary and secondary care*, http://www.nice.org.uk

National Institute for Clinical Excellence (2007): *Head injury. Triage, assessment, investigation and early management of head injury in infants, children and adults*, http://www.nice.org.uk

National Institute of Clinical Excellence (2008): *Stroke. Diagnosis and initial management of acute stroke and transient ischemic attack (TIA)*, http://www.nice.org.uk/

National Institute for Clinical Excellence (2010): *Chest pain of recent onset. Assessment and diagnosis of recent onset cardiac pain or discomfort of suspected cardiac origin*, http://www.nice.org.uk

National Institute for Clinical Excellence (2010): *Unstable angina and NSTEMI. The early management of unstable angina and non-S-T segment-elevation myocardial infarction*, http://www.nice.org.uk

National Institutes of Health Stroke Scale (NLHSS), http:///nihstrokescale.org (accessed 04/07/2010)

National Institute for mental health in England, Crisis resolution & home treatment, http://www.ccmh.uce.ac.uk/home_treatment_final.pdf

National services frameworks, department of health (DoH), *www.dh.gov.uk*

Revised National service guide: A Resource for developing sexual assault referral centres department of health, http://www.dh.gov.uk/prod_consum_dh/groups/dh_digitalassets/@dh/@en/@ps/@sta/@perf/documents/digitalasset/dh_108350.pdf

Scottish Intercollegiate Guidelines Network (2008): *Management of patients with stroke or TIA: Assessment, investigation, medical management and secondary prevention*, http://www.sign.ac.uk

The Resuscitation Council (UK) (2008): *Emergency treatment of anaphylactic reactions. Guidelines for healthcare providers*, http://www.resus.org.uk

The Resuscitation Council (UK) (2010), http://www.resus.org.uk

Index

Note: Page number followed by i and t indicates illustration and table respectively.

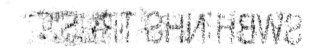